# Radiofrequency Ablation for Cancer

# Springer

*New York*
*Berlin*
*Heidelberg*
*Hong Kong*
*London*
*Milan*
*Paris*
*Tokyo*

# Radiofrequency Ablation for Cancer

## Current Indications, Techniques, and Outcomes

Lee M. Ellis, MD
Professor of Surgical Oncology and Cancer Biology
Department of Surgical Oncology
The University of Texas M.D. Anderson Cancer Center
Houston, Texas, USA

Steven A. Curley, MD
Professor, Department of Surgical Oncology
Chief of Gastrointestinal Tumor Surgery
The University of Texas M.D. Anderson Cancer Center
Houston, Texas, USA

Kenneth K. Tanabe, MD
Chief, Division of Surgical Oncology
Massachusetts General Hospital
Associate Professor of Surgery
Harvard Medical School
Boston, MA, USA

Editors

With 85 Illustrations

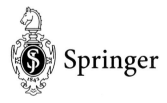

Springer

Lee M. Ellis, MD
Professor of Surgical Oncology
  and Cancer Biology
Department of Surgical Oncology
The University of Texas
  M.D. Anderson Cancer Center
Houston, TX 77030

Steven A. Curley, MD
Professor, Department of
  Surgical Oncology
Chief of Gastrointestinal
  Tumor Surgery
The University of Texas
  M.D. Anderson Cancer Center
Houston, TX 77030

Kenneth K. Tanabe, MD
Chief, Division of Surgical
  Oncology
Massachusetts General
  Hospital
Associate Professor of
  Surgery
Harvard Medical School
Boston, MA 02114-2167

Library of Congress Cataloging-in-Publication Data
Radiofrequency ablation for cancer : current indications, techniques, and outcomes
/ editors, Lee M. Ellis, Steven A. Curley, Kenneth K. Tanabe.
        p. ; cm.
      Includes bibliographical references and index.
      ISBN 0-387-95564-X (h/c : alk. paper)
      1. Cancer—Thermotherapy.   2. Catheter ablation.   I. Ellis, Lee M.   II. Curley,
    Steven A.   III. Tanabe, Kenneth K.
      [DNLM:   1. Cancer Ablation.   2. Neoplasms—therapy.   QZ 266 R129 2003]
    RC271.T5 R336 2003
    616.99'40632—dc21                                          2002042727

Printed on acid-free paper.

Printed in the United States of America.

9 8 7 6 5 4 3 2 1

ISBN 0-387-95564-X                    SPIN 10890910

Springer-Verlag   New York  Berlin  Heidelberg
*A member of BertelsmannSpringer Science+Business Media GmbH*

# Preface

Technologic advances have provided new methods for the surgical treatment of malignant tumors. This minor revolution in surgical therapy began with the widespread use of laparoscopy for the diagnosis and treatment of various abdominal malignancies. More recently, radiofrequency ablation (RFA) has been used to treat malignant disease in the liver. Although prior ablative therapies such as cryotherapy or ethanol injection have been used for malignant liver tumors, the complication rates have been moderately high and efficacy has been suboptimal. There has been a great deal of enthusiasm for the increased use of RFA not only for liver tumors but also for tumors in other locations. It is well established that the complication rate associated with RFA for tumors in various anatomic locations is relatively low. Specifically, when compared to cryoablation of liver tumors, RFA of liver tumors is associated with reduced morbidity. However, RFA is not yet in widespread use for malignant disease, and the long-term outcome of this treatment modality has yet to be determined.

This book on RFA for cancer addresses mainly hepatic tumors. The use of RFA for malignant liver neoplasms is approved by the Food and Drug Administration (FDA) and is now becoming more widespread throughout the world. It is important to point out that the indications for the use of RFA for liver tumors vary among treating physicians. The gold standard for the treatment of malignant liver tumors remains resection until such time as long-term follow-up of patients treated with RFA demonstrates equivalent or better results with respect to survival, morbidity, and quality of life. The use of RFA for malignant hepatic tumors has increased the number of patients who are now surgical candidates because RFA can be used in combination with hepatic resection for bilobar tumors that would otherwise be deemed unresectable. Experienced oncologists recognize that highly aggressive tumors are infrequently affected by surgical therapy. Therefore, the addition of chemotherapy to RFA of malignant hepatic tumors is a natural strategy to explore, and this topic is carefully considered in this book. With the relatively low complication rate associated with RFA, surgeons now have the option of "debulking" hepatic tumors. In the past this approach was not considered to be beneficial because of the relatively high complication rates of aggressive resections combined with the minimal benefits (if any) in survival for patients with biologically aggressive tumors. Despite the fact that some patients may have small-volume extrahepatic disease, it is the opinion of most oncologists that the tumor in the liver is the ultimate cause of patient demise. Currently, it is unknown if resection and ablation of the bulk of the tumor mass in the liver prolong survival or improve quality of life. Furthermore, it should be recognized that while the complications of RFA are uncommon, treatment-related complications and deaths do occur. Issues pertinent to complications of RFA are addressed. As with any technical procedure, there is a learning curve for RFA that affects the efficacy of the therapy and the risk for adverse events.

Recognizing that RFA can produce complete thermal tumor necrosis and is associated with relatively low complication rates, clinicians have investigated the use of RFA for benign and malignant tumors at other anatomic sites. Although one might anticipate that the complication rate for RFA of pulmonary and thyroid tumors would be high, initial experience suggests that RFA for lesions in these sites is feasible. The results reported in this book are in a highly selective group of patients studied on clinical protocols. Although the editors have selected such topics for discussion here, further studies published in peer-reviewed journals and evaluated by the FDA are critical before widespread use of these techniques for tumors at these extrahepatic sites can be recommended.

Lastly, it is critically important to understand the role of radiographic imaging in directing and monitoring the ablative process. It is also necessary for radiologists and oncologists to understand the radiographic changes associated with successful ablation versus recurrent disease. The use of radiographic imaging for RFA is covered in a separate section in this book.

Although RFA is rapidly being adopted as a treatment modality, universally accepted guidelines for its use have not been established. Even among the various authors in this book, there is little consensus as to the appropriate patient population that should be treated with this modality. Furthermore, some of the data may be difficult to interpret because RFA equipment continues to evolve; more powerful and larger arrays are continually being developed. Thus the early results of RFA where the arrays were relatively small with lower power generators may not be applicable to the results obtained at the present time with arrays that approach 7 cm and generators of 200 W. Therefore, clinicians are encouraged to stay abreast of the current literature in directing their practice.

LEE M. ELLIS, MD
STEVEN A. CURLEY, MD
KENNETH K. TANABE, MD

May 2003

# Contents

# Contributors

MUNEEB AHMED, MD
Beth Israel Deaconess Medical Center, Harvard Medical School
Department of Radiology
Boston, Massachusetts 02215
USA

EREN BERBER, MD
The Cleveland Clinic Foundation
Department of General Surgery / A 80
Cleveland, Ohio 44195
USA

ANTON BILCHIK, MD, PhD
John Wayne Cancer Institute
Department of Surgery
Santa Monica, California 90404
USA

RICHARD J. BLEICHER, MD
Attending Surgeon, Department of Surgery
The Palo Alto Medical Foundation and Clinic
795 El Camino Real
Palo Alto, California 94301
USA

CHUSILP CHARNSANGAVEJ, MD
The M.D. Anderson Cancer Center
Department of Radiology
Houston, Texas 77030
USA

HAESUN CHOI, MD
The M.D. Anderson Cancer Center
Department of Radiology
Houston, Texas 77030
USA

MICHAEL A. CHOTI, MD
The Sidney Kimmel Comprehensive Cancer Center at
    Johns Hopkins
Johns Hopkins Colon Cancer Center
Departments of Surgery and Oncology
The Johns Hopkins Hospital
Baltimore, Maryland 21287
USA

RAYMOND A. COSTABILE, MD
Uniformed Services University of Health Sciences
Madigan Army Medical Center
Department of Surgery Urology Service
Tacoma, Washington 98431
USA

STEVEN A. CURLEY, MD
The M.D. Anderson Cancer Center
Department of Surgical Oncology
Houston, Texas 77030
USA

DAMIAN E. DUPUY, MD
Brown University School of Medicine
Rhode Island Hospital
Department of Diagnostic Imaging
Providence, Rhode Island 02903
USA

LEE M. ELLIS, MD
The M.D. Anderson Cancer Center
Department of Surgical Oncology
Houston, Texas 77030
USA

HIRAN C. FERNANDO, MD
University of Pittsburgh School of Medicine
Department of Surgery, Division of Thoracic Surgery
Pittsburgh University Hospital
Pittsburgh, Pennsylvania 15213
USA

BRUNO D. FORNAGE, MD
The M.D. Anderson Cancer Center
Department of Diagnostic Radiology
Houston, Texas 77030
USA

DOUGLAS L. FRAKER, MD
University of Pennsylvania Medical Center
Department of Surgery
Philadelphia, Pennsylvania 19104
USA

S. NAHUM GOLDBERG, MD
Beth Israel Deaconess Medical Center
Harvard Medical School
Department of Radiology
Boston, Massachusetts 02215
USA

LUIS J. HERRARA, MD
University of Pittsburgh School of Medicine
Department of Surgery
Pittsburgh, Pennsylvania 15213
USA

FRANCESCO IZZO, MD
National Cancer Institute of Naples
Department of Surgical Oncology
Naples, Italy 80131

JONATHAN S. LEWIN, MD
University Hospitals of Cleveland
Department of Radiology
Cleveland, Ohio 44106
USA

EVELYNE M. LOYER, MD
The M.D. Anderson Cancer Center
Department of Radiology
Houston, Texas 77030
USA

JAMES D. LUKETICH, MD
University of Pittsburgh School of Medicine
Department of Surgery
Division of Thoracic Surgery
Pittsburgh University Hospital
Pittsburgh, Pennsylvania 15213
USA

JOHN M. MONCHIK, MD
Brown University School of Medical School
Rhode Island Hospital
Department of Surgery
Providence, Rhode Island 02903
USA


SHERIF GAMAL NOUR, MD
University Hospitals of Cleveland
Department of Radiology
Cleveland, Ohio 44106
USA


ALEXANDER A. PARIKH, MD
M.D. Anderson Cancer Center
Department of Surgical Oncology
Houston, Texas 77030
USA


MARK ROH, MD
Drexel University College of Medicine
Department of Surgery, Allegheny General Hospital
Pittsburgh, Pennsylvania 15212
USA


DANIEL I. ROSENTHAL, MD
Division of Musculoskeletal Radiology
Department of Radiology
Massachusetts General Hospital
Boston, Massachusetts 02114
USA


MERRICK I. ROSS, MD
M.D. Anderson Cancer Center
Department of Surgical Oncology
Houston, Texas 77030
USA


ALLAN SIPERSTEIN, MD
The Cleveland Clinic Foundation
Department of General Surgery / A 80
Cleveland, Ohio 44195
USA

Kenneth K. Tanabe, MD
Division of Surgical Oncology
Massachusetts General Hospital
Department of Surgery
Harvard Medical School
Boston, Massachusetts 02214
USA

Martin Torriani, MD
Division of Musculoskeletal Radiology
Massachusetts General Hospital
Department of Radiology
Boston, Massachusetts 02214
USA

Jack R. Walter, MD
Madigan Army Medical Center
Department of Surgery Urology Service
Tacoma, Washington 98431
USA

# Principles of
# Radiofrequency Ablation

# 1

# Radiofrequency Tissue Ablation: Principles and Techniques

Muneeb Ahmed and S. Nahum Goldberg

Percutaneous radiofrequency (RF) ablation has received much attention as an image-guided minimally invasive strategy for the treatment of focal malignant disease.[1] This chapter reviews the concept of thermal ablation and the principles of RF application. The early limitations in success and subsequent developments in RF technology are also discussed. Finally, recent advancements in RF ablation and current directions of research, including possible combination and adjuvant therapies are highlighted. A clear understanding of the underlying principles of RF ablation can facilitate its application to clinical practice with favorable results.

## Physics of RF

RF energy, a well-defined portion of the electromagnetic spectrum (10 kHz to 2.59 GHz), forms relatively long wavelengths when electrical charges are accelerated.[2] Body tissues are permeated by a saline solution and are relatively poor conductors. Hence, when RF current flows through the body, it results in lost energy in the form of moving ions and water molecules. This "ionic agitation" is manifest as tissue heating that is directly proportional to current density (Fig. 1.1). Direct heating by RF is localized to the active electrode, as current density, defined as current flow per unit area of the electrode, falls rapidly with distance from the electrode. Generated heat spreads into surrounding tissue by conduction until a steady state is achieved, described as

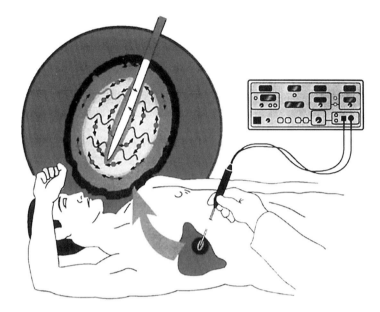

**Figure 1.1.** Schematic illustration of percutaneous radiofrequency (RF) ablation in the liver. This figure demonstrates the insertion of an RF electrode into a tumor within the liver. The electrode is connected to the RF generator. Resistive heating occurs as a result of ionic agitation surrounding the electrode as the RF energy oscillates during attempts to reach its ground (in this case, the grounding pad is not visualized on the patient's back).

thermal equilibrium. Higher energy amounts are required for ablating larger volumes of tissue. However, high current densities that have been applied too rapidly desiccates tissue immediately surrounding the probe, resulting in small, irregular ablation volumes. Desiccated cellular tissue functions as an electrical insulator, which reduces the electrode surface and further increases current density. Eventually, charring, tissue adherence, and associated thrombus formation results in dielectric breakdown if power is not terminated. However, large ablation volumes can be achieved by carefully regulating energy deposition to achieve maximum current density without overheating.

## Induction of Coagulation Necrosis

Thermal strategies for ablation attempt to destroy tumor tissue in a minimally invasive manner while limiting injury to nearby structures.[3–6] Treatment also includes a 5- to 10-mm surgical margin of normal tissue, based on the uncertainty concerning the exact tumor margin and the possibility of potential microscopic disease in the rim of tissue immediately surrounding visible tumor.[3,4] Cosman et al[7] have shown that the resistive heating produced by RF ablation techniques leads to heat-based cellular death via thermal coagulation necrosis.[7] Therefore, generated temperatures, and their pattern of distribution within treated tissues, determine the amount of tumor destruction.

Prior work has shown that cellular homeostatic mechanisms can accommodate slight increases in temperature (to 40°C). Though increased susceptibility to damage by other mechanisms (radiation, chemotherapy) is seen at hyperthermic temperatures between 42° and 45°C, cell function and tumor growth continue even after prolonged exposure.[8,9] Irreversible cellular injury occurs when cells are heated to 46°C for 60 minutes, and occurs more rapidly as temperature rises.[10] The basis for immediate cellular damage centers on protein coagulation of cytosolic and mitochondrial enzymes, and nucleic acid–histone protein complexes.[11–13] Damage triggers cellular death over the course of several days. "Coagulation necrosis" describes this thermal damage, even though ultimate manifestations of cell death may not fulfill strict histopathologic criteria of coagulative necrosis. This has significant implications with regard to clinical practice, as percutaneous biopsy and histopathologic interpretation may not be a reliable measure of adequate ablation. Optimal desired temperatures for ablation range from 50° to 100°C. Extremely high temperatures (>105°C) result in tissue vaporization, which in turn impedes the flow of current and restricts total energy deposition.[14]

## Bioheat Equation

Success of thermal ablative strategies, whether the source is RF, microwave, laser, or high-intensity focused ultrasound, is contingent on adequate heat delivery. The ability to heat large volumes of tissue in different environments is dependent on several factors encompassing both RF delivery and local physiologic tissue characteristics. Pennes[15] first described the relationship between this set of parameters as the bioheat equation:

$$\rho_t c_t \partial T(r,t)/\partial t = \nabla(k_t : \nabla T) - c_b \rho_b m \rho_t (T - T_b) + Q_p(r,t) + Q_m(r,t)$$

where $\rho_t$, $\rho_b$ = density of tissue, blood (kg/m$^3$)

$c_t$, $c_b$ = specific heat of tissue, blood (W s/kg C)

$k_t$ = thermal conductivity of tissue

$m$ = perfusion (blood flow rate/unit mass tissue) (m$^3$/kg s)

$Q_p$ = power absorbed/unit volume of tissue

$Q_m$ = metabolic heating/unit volume of tissue

This complex equation was further simplified to a first approximation by Goldberg et al[5] to describe the basic relationship guiding thermal ablation–induced coagulation necrosis as "coagulation necrosis = energy deposited × local tissue interactions − heat loss." Based on this equation, several strategies have been pursued to increase the amount of coagulation necrosis by improving tissue–energy interactions during thermal ablation. Discussed below, these strategies have centered on altering one of the three parameters of the simplified bioheat equation, either by increasing RF energy deposition or by modulating tissue interactions or blood flow.

## RF Energy Deposition

### Conventional Monopolar Electrodes

Initially, application of RF technology for thermal ablation occurred within the scope of cardiac and neurosurgical indications. Early studies documented its use in treating hyperactive neurologic foci[16,17] and aberrant intracardiac conductive pathways.[18–20] RF techniques were particularly well suited for these indications because of its ability to reproducibly induce small but well-defined areas of tissue destruction. Early studies of RF applied in a percutaneous manner used these conventional monopolar electrodes to generate up to 1.6 cm of coagulation.[21,22]

Goldberg et al[23] proceeded to study the effects of modifying electrode size, treatment duration, and tip temperature on the amount of coagulation necrosis. Using a 500-kHZ sinusoidal waveform generator, experiments were conducted demonstrating that RF duration to 6 minutes, diameter (12–24 gauge), and length to 3 cm increased amounts of necrosis to no more than 1.8 cm. A tip length increase from 0.5 to 8 cm was associated with a linear increase in the length of coagulation along the electrode shaft from 0.9 to 8.0 cm ($R^2 = 0.996$).

Characterization of electrode surface temperatures during RF heating was subsequently described.[14] Highest temperatures were observed at the ends of the exposed electrode. Nonuniform temperatures were seen in between these two points, with variability increasing with electrode length. The diameter of actual RF-induced necrosis was dependent on the overall local mean temperature during the application. No coagulation was identified when temperatures were below 50°C. Above 50°C, lesion size increased progressively with increasing temperature until 110°C. Beyond this threshold, tissue boiling took place, leading to a rise in local impedance and reduced RF output, resulting in variable and reduced amounts of coagulation necrosis.

## Techniques to Improve Potential RF Output

Complete and adequate destruction by RF ablation requires that an entire tumor be subjected to cytotoxic temperatures. The studies described in the previous section demonstrated that early use of RF as a strategy for percutaneous thermal ablation was inadequate for tumors larger than 1.8 cm. Of the strategies to improve results of RF ablation, enhancement of the electrode design has played an essential role in achieving acceptable tissue tumor coagulation.

## Modification of Probe Design

### Multiprobe Arrays
Though lengthening the RF probe tip increased the volume of coagulation necrosis, the cylindrical lesion shape does not correspond well with the spherical geometry of most tumors. In an attempt to address this inadequacy, several groups tried to repeatedly insert multiple RF electrodes into tissue to increase heating in a more uniform manner.[24,25] However, complete ablation requires multiple overlapping treatments in a contiguous fashion to adequately treat tumors. Hence, the time and effort required makes it impractical for use in a clinical setting.

Subsequent work centered on using several conventional monopolar RF electrodes employed simultaneously in an array to determine the effect of probe spacing, configuration, and RF application method on the size and shape of the induced necrosis.[26] Spacing no greater than 1.5 cm between individual probes produced uniform and reproducible tissue necrosis, with simultaneous application of RF energy producing more necrosis than sequential application. Lesion shape was further dependent on spacing and the number of probes and most often corresponded to the array shape. This improvement in RF application technique results in a significant increase in the volume of inducible tissue necrosis, increasing coagulation volume by up to 800% over RF application with a single conventional probe with similar tip exposure.

Working to overcome the technical challenges of multiprobe application, umbrella RF electrodes with multiple probes, or tines, have been developed. These systems, produced by two commercial vendors, involve the deployment of a varying number of multiple thin, curved tines in the shape of an umbrella from a central cannula.[27,28] This surmounts earlier difficulties by allowing easy placement of multiple probes to create large, reproducible volumes of necrosis. LeVeen,[29] using a 12-hook array, was able to produce lesions measuring up to 3.5 cm in diameter in in-vivo porcine liver by administering increasing amounts of RF energy from a 50-W RF generator for 10 minutes. More recently, high-power systems (up to 250 W) have been developed with complex multitine electrode geometries. With these systems, preliminary reports claim coagulation up to 3.5 cm in diameter[30,31] (Fig. 1.2A).

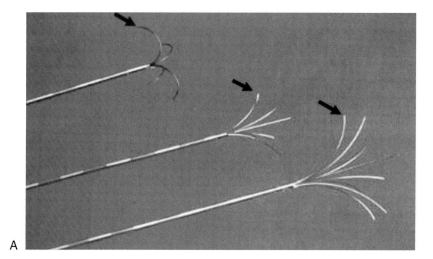

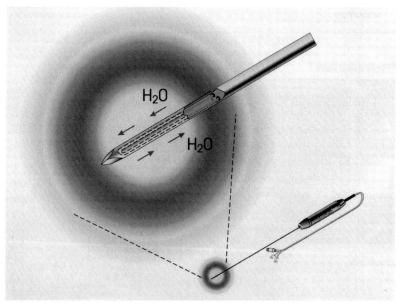

**Figure 1.2.** A: Hooked array radiofrequency needles. Multiple thin curved monopolar electrodes extend from the central cannula of these electrodes (arrows). RF emanates from each of these hooks, resulting in increased coagulation compared to a single conventional electrode. Successive generations of this electrode type have provided additional tines that permit the deposition of RF over larger tissue volumes. (Photograph courtesy of RITA Medical Systems, Mountain View, CA.) B: Internally cooled RF electrode. The shaft of these 18-gauge electrodes is electrically insulated with acrylic resin, with only 1 to 3 cm of exposed metallic tip from which RF emanates. Two central lumina extend to the electrode tip. One lumen is used to deliver chilled perfusate to the tip of the electrode, and the second returns the warmed saline effluent to a collection unit outside of the body. Arrows indicate the direction of flow. In this closed system no saline is deposited into the tissues being treated.

## Bipolar Arrays

Several groups have worked with bipolar arrays as compared to the conventional monopolar system to increase the volume of coagulation created by RF application. In these systems, applied RF current runs from an active electrode to a second grounding electrode in place of a grounding pad. Heat is generated around both electrodes, creating elliptical lesions. McGahan et al[32] used this method in ex-vivo liver to induce necrosis of up to 4.0 cm in the long axis diameter, but could only achieve 1.4 cm of necrosis in the short diameter. Though this results in an overall increase in coagulation volume, the shape of necrosis is unsuitable for actual tumors, making the gains in coagulation less clinically significant.

Desinger et al[33] have described another bipolar array that contains both the active and return electrodes on the same 2-mm-diameter probe.[33] This arrangement of probes eliminates the need for surface grounding pads and the risk of grounding pad burns (see below). Though there has been limited clinical experience with this device, studies report coagulation of up to 3 cm in ex-vivo liver.

## Internally Cooled Electrodes

One of the limitations to greater RF energy deposition has been overheating surrounding the active electrode leading to tissue charring, rising impedance, and RF circuit interruption. To address this limitation, internally cooled electrodes have been developed that are capable of greater coagulation compared to conventional monopolar RF electrodes. These electrodes contain two hollow lumina that permit continuous internal cooling of the tip with a chilled perfusate, and the removal of warmed effluent to a collection unit outside of the body (Fig. 1.2B). This reduces heating directly around the electrode, tissue charring, and rising impedance, allowing greater RF energy deposition. Goldberg et al[34] studied this method using an 18-gauge electrode. With internal electrode tip cooling (of $15 \pm 2°C$ using $0°C$ saline perfusate), RF energy deposited into tissue and resultant coagulation necrosis were significantly greater ($p < .001$) than that achieved without electrode cooling (Fig. 1.3). With this degree of cooling, significantly greater RF current could be applied without observing tissue charring. The maximum diameter of coagulation measured 2.5, 3.0, 4.5, and 4.4 cm for the 1, 2, 3, and 4 cm electrode tips, respectively. With tip temperatures of 25° to 35°C (less cooling), tissue charring occurred with reduced RF application with resulting necrosis decreasing from 4.5 to 3.0 cm in diameter. Similar results have been reported by Lorentzen,[35] who applied RF to ex-vivo calf liver using a 14-gauge internally cooled electrode and 20°C perfusate.

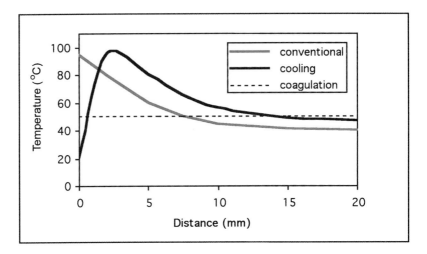

**Figure 1.3.** Thermal profile of tissues surrounding conventional and internally cooled electrodes. The figure depicts the maximum temperatures achieved when applying sufficient RF energy to generate 100°C temperatures in the tissue. Internal cooling (or pulsing of RF) permits greater energy deposition, and thus greater tissue heating.

Subsequent in-vivo studies were performed in normal porcine liver and muscle tissue. Within muscle tissue, lesion diameter increased from 1.8 to 5.4 cm for 12 minutes of RF. Nevertheless, in normal liver only 2.3 cm of coagulation was observed regardless of current applied or treatment duration (to 30 minutes). Thus, necrosis was significantly less than that observed for ex-vivo liver using identical RF parameters ($p < .01$). In clinical studies, Solbiati et al[36] demonstrated $2.8 \pm 0.4$ cm of coagulation for liver metastases.

*Cluster RF*
Based on success in inducing greater volumes of necrosis by using both multiprobe arrays and cooling, initial experiments were performed to study the use of internally cooled electrodes in an array.[37] Three 2-cm-tip exposure internally cooled electrodes were placed at varying distances in ex-vivo liver for simultaneous RF application (1100 mA for 10 minutes). At spacing distances of 0.5 to 1.0 cm apart, a uniform circular cross-sectional area of coagulation necrosis measuring 4.1 cm in diameter was achieved. In contrast, electrode spacing of 1.5 to 2.5 cm resulted in cloverleafed lesions with areas of viable tissue within the treatment zone.

Using an optimized 0.5-cm spacing distance between probes, Goldberg et al[37] proceeded to study variations in electrode tip length and duration of application on coagulation volume. Tip lengths of 1.5 to 3.0 cm were used in ex-vivo liver and in-vivo porcine liver and muscle systems for varied RF application (1400–2150 mA) and duration (5–60 minutes). In ex-vivo liver, simultaneous RF application to internally cooled electrode clusters for 15, 30, and 45 minutes produced 4.7, 6.2, and 7.0 cm of coagulation, respectively. In contrast, RF application for 45 minutes to a single internally cooled electrode resulted in only 2.7 cm of coagulation ($p < .01$).

RF applied for 12 minutes to electrode clusters produced 3.1 cm of coagulation in in-vivo liver and 7.3 cm in in-vivo muscle. This was significantly greater than the 1.8- and 4.3-cm sized lesions in in-vivo liver and muscle, respectively, that was seen with the use of single internally cooled electrode with similar technique ($p < .01$). When RF current (2000 mA) was applied for 30 minutes in in-vivo muscle, 9.5 cm of coagulation was observed, including extension into the retroperitoneum and overlying tissues.

In the initial clinical use of this clustered electrode device, 10 patients with large solitary intrahepatic colorectal metastases (4.2–7.0 cm) were treated with a single RF application (12–15 minutes, 1600–1950 mA).[37] Contrast-enhanced computed tomography (CT) postablation showed induced coagulation necrosis measuring $5.3 \pm 0.6$ cm with a minimum short axis diameter of 4.2 cm. The overall shape of coagulation was not spherical in several cases, and generally conformed to the tumor shape. In two cases, large blood vessels limited the size of induced coagulation.

The use of three internally cooled electrodes arranged in a cluster array for simultaneous RF application offers the potential of large-volume coagulation for clinical tumor ablation as compared to conventional monopolar RF electrodes or single internally cooled electrodes. Clearly, spacing distances of less than 1 cm between individual electrodes produce more spherical zones of necrosis with no intervening viable tissue as compared to greater spacing distances. While these results appear counterintuitive, postulating that these electrodes function as a single large electrode can explain this phenomenon of greater coagulation necrosis with relatively closely spaced electrodes.

*Pulsed RF Application*
Pulsing of energy is another strategy that has been used with RF and other energy sources such as laser to increase the mean intensity of energy deposition. When pulsing is used, periods of high-energy deposition are rapidly alternated with periods of low-energy deposition. If a proper balance between high- and low-energy deposition is achieved, preferential tissue cooling occurs adjacent to the electrode during periods of minimal energy deposition without significantly decreasing heating deeper in the tissue. Thus, even greater energy can be applied during periods

of high-energy deposition, thereby enabling deeper heat penetration and greater tissue coagulation.[37] Synergy between a combination of both internal cooling and pulsing has resulted in greater coagulation necrosis and tumor destruction than either method alone.[37]

Clearly, optimization is required for each system. Currently, at least one manufacturer has incorporated a pulsing algorithm into its generator design based on the work of Goldberg et al.[38] This group designed an optimal algorithm with a variable peak current for a specified minimum duration. Maximum coagulation, which measured 4.5 cm in diameter, was achieved using initial currents greater than 1500 mA, a minimum RF duration of 10 seconds of maximum deliverable current, with a 15-second reduction in current to 100 mA following impedance rises. This latter algorithm produced $3.7 \pm 0.6$ cm of necrosis in in-vivo liver, compared to 2.9 cm without pulsing ($p < .05$). Remote thermometry further demonstrated more rapid temperature increases and higher tissue temperatures when pulsed-RF techniques were used. Thus, an optimized algorithm for pulsed-RF deposition can increase coagulation over other pulsed and conventional RF ablation strategies.

## Protocols for Clinical RF Application

While modifications in electrode design have yielded significant increases in coagulation volume compared to conventional monopolar RF systems, work has also been done on optimizing clinical RF application protocols to further augment achievable tumor destruction. It is important to remember that tumor heating at a distance from the electrode surface requires application of energy for sufficient time to enable the heat to radiate from the high-temperature electrode source to deeper into the tissues. These properties of heat conduction are innate to the tissue, and cannot be readily overcome with increased energy deposition. If anything, increased energy usually leads to rapid tissue boiling and decreased coagulation. As a result, longer ablation times have been required when using the modified RF electrodes to increase coagulation volume. For example, while thermal equilibrium is achieved between 4 and 6 minutes for a monopolar electrode, a minimum of 12 minutes is required to achieve thermal equilibrium in ex-vivo liver using an internally cooled electrode.

Each probe modification requires individual optimization of its energy delivery paradigm to appropriately heat the volume tissue based on the specific characteristics of the electrode design. Thus, different algorithms have been constructed. Currently, the three major electrode manufacturers have used three alternative strategies for energy application. For the Radionics internally cooled electrodes, a pulsing algorithm as was previously described is used to apply energy for 12 to 15 minutes.[38] For multitined Radiotherapuetics devices, the applied RF energy is slowly increased in incremental steps so as to not induce tissue boiling early in the procedure.[39] As the applied energy increases, tissue boiling occurs surrounding some (i.e., the hottest), but not all, of the electrode tines. This increases energy application and heating at other tines, which is measured as a slowly increasing tissue impedance. The procedure concludes with the marked rise in impedance that denotes tissue boiling around all electrode tines. Because there are a large number of tines encompassing the entire tissue volume, this algorithm permits contiguous coagulation throughout a 3.5-cm tissue volume. The algorithm for the RITA configuration relies on a novel approach of initially heating a volume of 3 cm of tissue by extending the electrode tines only 3 cm.[30] This is followed by successive 10 minutes of heating of 4- and 5-cm tissue volumes, accomplished by further extension of the active electrode tines. Close temperature monitoring with automated feedback prevents tissue boiling. The principle is to create a hot core of ablated tissue that establishes a thermal gradient toward more peripheral tissue. This enables the creation of coagulation to 3 to 5 cm in diameter. With increased understanding of RF principles, the paradigms currently used by all manufacturers are continually changing, with improvements such as reduced RF application time undoubtedly to be achieved in the near future.

Presently, many RF ablation devices are being studied based on the principles outlined above. Multiple commercial devices are now available, with several companies committed to ongoing development of improved RF electrode and generator technology. Given the rapid pace of evolution in the state of the art for ablation technologies, it is too early to confidently predict which method, if any, will prove dominant for any given clinical application. Competitive technologies must be able to ablate the desired volume of tissue in a reproducible and predictable fashion. However, it is more than likely that other factors, including ease of clinical use, the duration of the procedure, and cost, will play a role in determining which of these technologies will receive the greatest attention.

### Factors Limiting Coagulation Volume In Vivo

Although modifications in electrode design and application protocols have yielded significant increases in coagulation volume compared to conventional monopolar RF systems, further gains through RF equipment modifications have not produced equivalent increases in clinical settings. This is largely due to multiple and often tissue-specific limitations that prevent heating of the entire tumor volume.[6,14] Most importantly, there is heterogeneity of heat deposition throughout a given lesion to be treated. Recent attention has centered on altering underlying tumor physiology as a means to advance RF thermal ablation. Based on the simplified bioheat equation described earlier, these efforts can be divided into two broad categories. One area examines altering local tissue interactions to permit greater RF energy input by altering tissue conductivity or increasing local heat conduction, while the other explores reducing heat loss by modulating blood flow within treatment zones. As will be shown, certain modifications can have several simultaneous effects. For example, saline and iron compounds have been useful for improving energy deposition, while continuous injection of saline during ablation has facilitated the spread of heat from the RF electrode into deeper tissues. Modulation of blood flow during RF application can improve ablation by limiting perfusion-mediated tissue cooling.

### Local Tissue Interactions

The effect of local tissue characteristics is defined by thermal and electrical conductivity of surrounding tissue. Altering both of these either separately or simultaneously can alter the pattern of thermal distribution with treated tissue.

### Improved Tissue Heat Conduction

Improved heat conduction within the tissues by injection of saline and other compounds has been proposed. The heated liquid spreads thermal energy farther and faster than heat conduction in normal "solid" tissue. An additional potential benefit of simultaneous saline injection is increased tissue ionicity, thereby enabling greater current flow. Similarly, amplification of current shifts using iron compounds, injected or deposited in the tissues prior to ablation, has been used for RF and microwave. For example, these authors have shown that increased ferric ions, in the form of high doses of supraparamagnetic iron oxide magnetic resonance (MR) contrast agent, can raise the temperature of polyacrylamide phantoms during RF ablation.[40]

### Altered Tissue Thermal and Electrical Conductivity

For a given RF current, the power deposition at each point in space is strongly dependent on the local electrical conductivity. Several investigators have demonstrated the ability to increase coagulation volume by altering electrical conductivity in tissues through saline injection prior to or during RF ablation. Curley and Hamilton[41] infused up to 10 mL/min of normal saline in ex-vivo liver for 4 minutes during RF application and achieved co-

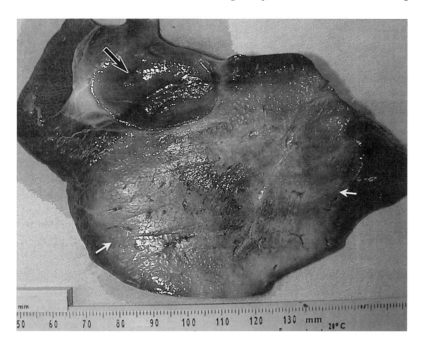

**Figure 1.4.** Large-volume coagulation with altered tissue electrical conductivity: 6.5 cm of coagulation was obtained in normal in vivo pig liver by applying RF for 12 minutes using a 3-cm tip internally cooled electrode (white arrows). Electrical conductivity was altered using pretreatment with 12 cc of 38.5% NaCl. However, coagulation extends to involve the entire thickness of the gallbladder wall (black arrow), an injury that potentially could lead to perforation or cholecystitis.

agulation measuring 2.6 cm in diameter. Similarly, Livraghi et al[42] have reported coagulation of up to 4.1 cm in diameter using continuous infusion of normal saline at 1 mL/min in experimental animal models and human liver tumors. Miao et al[43,44] used a novel "cooled-wet" technique to significantly increase RF-induced coagulation in both ex-vivo and in-vivo tissue using a continuous saline infusion combined with an expandable electrode system (Fig. 1.4).

However, saline can have multiple effects, and in these studies the mechanisms responsible for the increase in coagulation were not well characterized. This strategy seemed to confirm an initial hypothesis that high local ion concentration from NaCl injection could increase the extent of coagulation necrosis by effectively increasing the area of the active surface electrode. Other possible explanations for the increase in coagulation include reduced effects of tissue vaporization (i.e., allowing for probe to tissue contact despite the formation of electrically insulating gases), or improved thermal conduction caused by diffusion of boiling solution into the tissues.

More recent study has centered on exploring the effect of volume and concentration of NaCl on RF coagulation volume. In normal porcine liver and agar tissue phantom models, Goldberg et al[45] have demonstrated that both NaCl concentration and volume influenced RF coagulation. These experiments demonstrated that increased NaCl concentration increases electrical conductivity (which is inversely proportional to the measured impedance) and enables greater energy deposition in tissues without inducing deleterious high temperatures at the electrode surface. However, this effect is nonlinear with markedly increased tissue conductivity decreasing tissue heating. Under many circumstances (i.e., in the range of normal tissue conductivities) the increased conductivity can be beneficial for RF ablation in that it enables increased energy deposition that increases tissue heating. However, given less intrinsic electrical resistance, increased tissue conductivity also increases the energy required to heat a given volume of tissue. When this amount of energy cannot be delivered (i.e., it is beyond the maximum generator output), the slope is negative and less tissue heating (and coagulation) will result. Thus, to achieve clinical benefit (i.e., an increase in RF-induced coagulation), optimal parameters for NaCl injection need to be determined for each type of RF apparatus used and for the different tumor types and tissues to be treated.

In an attempt to optimize the effects of altered conductivity using injectable therapies, Goldberg et al[45] initially investigated the effect of injecting different volumes of high-concentration NaCl on the extent of RF-induced coagulation. Using an iterative, nonlinear simplex optimization strategy, parameters for NaCl injection were studied in in-vivo porcine liver over varying concentrations (0.9–38%) and injection volume (0–25 mL) using internally cooled electrodes following pulsed-RF algorithms for 12 minutes. Significant increases in generator output, tissue heating, and coagulation volume were seen when NaCl was injected ($p < .001$), with maximum heating and coagulation occurring with 6 mL of 36% NaCl solution. Regression analysis demonstrated that both volume and concentration of NaCl injected significantly influenced tissue heating and coagulation.

In a subsequent study, Lobo et al[46] explored the relationship between NaCl volume and concentration in a reproducible, static agar tissue phantom model. Using a protein gel with varying NaCl concentration (0–35%) in different sized wells (0–38 cc) surrounding the electrode to simulate tissue injection, various parameters of RF application (power, current, impedance, temperature) were recorded. Using mathematical modeling, they derived two equations, one describing the multivariate relationship to a peak point, representing maximum generator output. The other describes the relationship when temperature decreases as generator output is exceeded. Both equations predict the effect of volume and concentration of NaCl with an $R^2 = 0.96$. Based on this finding, the investigators reexamined the earlier reported trials in normal porcine liver to correlate results with these equations. Though the constants changed, the equations were able to account for 86% of the variance seen in those data. Clearly, this mathematical characterization is a significant step toward reliably predicting the effects of NaCl when combined with RF ablation.

### Reducing Blood Flow

Biophysical aspects of tumor–heat interaction must be taken into account when performing thermal ablation therapies. Based on the simplified form of the bioheat equation, the third component defining thermal-induced coagulation necrosis is heat loss. RF ablation outcomes in in-vivo models have been less successful and more variable as compared to reported reproducible ex-vivo results for identical RF protocols. RF-induced necrosis in vivo is also often shaped by the presence of hepatic vasculature in the vicinity of the ablation. This reduced RF coagulation necrosis in in-vivo settings is most likely a result of perfusion-mediated tissue cooling (vascular flow) that functions as a heat sink (Fig. 1.5). By drawing heat from the treatment zone, this effect reduces the volume of tissue that receives the required minimal thermal dose

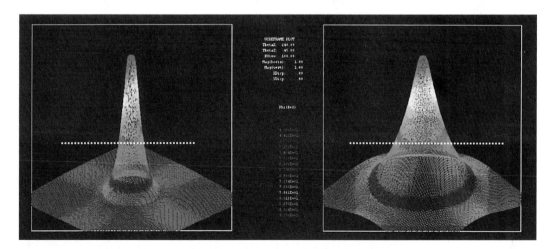

**Figure 1.5.** Modeling of the thermal gradient about a monopolar RF electrode. In these simulations, RF power was titrated to a maximum tissue temperature of 95°C for 6 minutes. Temperature is highest superiorly, and drops interiorly. In the absence of blood flow (left figure), the 50°C isotherm (the lower limit of the coagulation necrosis threshold[24]), shown as a dashed line, measures 1.8 cm in diameter. This compares favorably with the 0.7-cm diameter achieved in the presence of normal blood flow (10 mg/100 mL/min).

for coagulation. Several studies exploring altered tissue perfusion to increase the ablative zone through either mechanical occlusion or pharmacologic agents strongly support the contention that perfusion-mediated tissue cooling is responsible for this reduction in observed coagulation.

*Mechanical Occlusion*
Using internally cooled electrodes, Goldberg et al[47] applied RF to normal in-vivo porcine liver without and with balloon occlusion of the portal vein, celiac artery, or hepatic artery, and to ex-vivo calf liver. Increased coagulation was observed with RF ablation combined with portal venous occlusion as compared to RF without occlusion ($p < .01$). The differences seen in coagulation correlated to an approximate reduction in hepatic blood flow.

Several clinical studies provide additional data supporting the role of mechanical blood flow reduction in improving RF ablation efficacy. Goldberg et al[47] performed mechanical blood flow occlusion in three patients with hepatic colorectal metastases undergoing intraoperative RF ablation. Two similar-sized hepatic colorectal metastases (2.2–4.2 cm) were treated with identical RF parameters in each patient. In each case, one lesion was treated with normal blood flow, and the second was treated during portal flow occlusion (Pringle maneuver) by clamping the hepatic artery and portal vein to eliminate all intrahepatic blood flow. In each case, coagulation was increased with inflow occlusion (4.0 cm vs. 2.5 cm, $p < .05$). Hepatic inflow occlusion was performed in additional patients undergoing intrahepatic RF ablation for hepatic colorectal metastases. In these cases, remote thermometry demonstrated increases in temperature at 10 mm (62° to 72°C) and 20 mm (39° to 50°C) distances from the RF probe within 5 minutes of portal vein occlusion during constant RF application. This increase at the 20-mm distance holds particular significance as the threshold for induction of coagulation necrosis (50°C) was achieved with blood flow reduction.

In a second study, Patterson et al[48] have confirmed the strong predictive nature of hepatic blood flow on the extent of RF-induced coagulation in normal in-vivo porcine liver using a hooked electrode system. The coagulated focus created by RF during a Pringle maneuver was significantly larger in all three dimensions than coagulation with unaltered blood flow. Minimum and maximum diameters were significantly increased from 1.2 to 3.0 cm and 3.1 to 4.5 cm, respectively, when the Pringle maneuver was performed ($p = .002$). Coagulation volume was increased from 6.5 to 35.0 cm$^3$ with hepatic inflow occlusion. Additionally, the number of blood vessels within a 1-cm radius of the electrode strongly predicted minimum lesion size and lesion volume.

*Pharmacologic Modulation*

Goldberg et al[49] modulated hepatic blood flow using intraarterial vasopressin and high-dose halothane in conjunction with RF ablation in in-vivo porcine liver. Laser Doppler techniques identified a 33% increase and 66% decrease in hepatic blood flow after administration of vasopressin and halothane, respectively. Correlation of blood flow to coagulation diameter produced was excellent ($R^2 = 0.78$).

Several strategies for reducing blood flow during ablation therapy have been proposed. Total portal inflow occlusion (Pringle maneuver) has been used at open laparotomy. Angiographic balloon occlusion can be used, but may not prove adequate for intrahepatic ablation given the dual hepatic blood supply with redirection of compensated flow. Embolotherapy prior to ablation with particulates that occlude sinusoids such as Gelfoam and Lipiodol may overcome this limitation, as has been reported by Rossi et al.[50] Pharmacologic modulation of blood flow and antiangiogenesis therapy are theoretically possible, but should currently be considered experimental.

## RF Ablation in Combination with Other Therapies

The ultimate goal of tumor therapy is complete eradication of all malignant cells. Given the high likelihood of incomplete treatment by heat-based modalities alone, the case for combining thermal ablation with other therapies such as chemotherapy or chemoembolization cannot be overstated. A similar multidisciplinary approach including surgery, radiation, and chemotherapy is used for the treatment of most solid cancers. The belief that tumors can be reliably destroyed using only one technique is likely overly optimistic, given the variety of tumor types and organ sites. Combination therapy is a key avenue of current ablation research.

### RF Ablation with Adjuvant Chemotherapy

Strategies that decrease tumor tolerance to heat have been proposed, but as of yet are not well studied. Theoretically, previous insult to the tumor cells by cellular hypoxia (caused by vascular occlusion or antiangiogenesis factor therapy), or prior tumor cell damage from chemotherapy of radiation could be used to increase tumor sensitivity to heat.[9,10] Alternatively, tumor cells undergoing heat-induced reversible cell injury may demonstrate increased susceptibility to secondary chemotherapy. Synergy between chemotherapy and hyperthermic temperatures (42°–45°C) has already been established.[9,51]

In one study, Goldberg et al[52] treated 1.2- to 1.5-cm R3230 rat mammary adenocarcinoma with RF and/or intratumoral injection of doxorubicin chemotherapy. Tumors were treated with combinations of RF alone (monopolar, 70°C for 5 minutes), direct intratumoral doxorubicin injection (250 $\mu$L; 0.5 mg in total), intratumoral doxorubicin followed by RF, and no treatment. RF alone, RF with distilled water, and intratumoral doxorubicin alone produced 6.7 mm, 6.9 mm, and 2 mm of coagulation, respectively. Significantly increased coagulation occurred with combined RF and intratumoral doxorubicin (11.4 mm; $p < .001$). Additional experiments conducted to examine the effect of and timing of adminstration demonstrated greatest effect when doxorubicin was administered 30 minutes after RF application. In particular, the increased necrosis seen when the doxorubicin was injected after RF points to a potential two-hit effect, with initial reversible cell injury inflicted by sublethal doses of heat in the more peripheral ablation zone, followed by irreversible injury by doxorubicin on already susceptible cells.

Subsequently, investigators explored intravenous doxorubicin use as a means to achieve greater delivery to the zone surrounding RF-induced coagulation. Recent study has focused on the use of a commercially available, sterically stabilized liposomal preparation of doxorubicin (Doxil, Alza Pharmaceuticals). Liposomes function as delivery vehicles for a variety of chemotherapeutic agents through increased circulating time and greater tumor specificity, with the added advantage of reduced drug toxicity. Goldberg et al[53] combined RF ablation with intravenous Doxil (0.5 mL, 1.0 mg in total) in a rat mammary adenocarcinoma model. A significant increase in coagulation (13.1 mm) was seen with this particular approach compared to both RF alone (6.7 mm) and RF plus direct intratumoral free doxorubicin injection (11.4 mm) ($p < .01$).

Recently, Goldberg et al[54] conducted a pilot clinical study combining RF ablation with adjuvant Doxil therapy in 10 patients with various liver malignancies. Patients with at least one liver lesion (mean size $4.0 \pm 1.8$ cm) were randomized into two groups for treatment with RF alone ($n = 5$) and RF with pretreatment single-dose intravenous Doxil (24 hours pre-RF, 20 mg/kg). Several tumor types were treated, including primary hepatocellular carcinoma ($n = 4$), colorectal metastases ($n = 3$), neuroendocrine tumors ($n = 2$), and breast cancer metastases ($n = 1$). Patients receiving Doxil therapy with RF ablation demonstrated a 25% increase in coagulation volume 2 to 4 weeks postablation. For two Doxil/RF ablation–treated tumors, initial incomplete treatment, denoted by contrast enhancement at the periphery of the ablation zone on baseline post-RF scans, was converted to complete ablation within 4 weeks of treatment. Similar incompletely ablated tumors treated with RF alone did not show such a conversion. Additionally, in the tumors treated incompletely with combination Doxil and RF ablation, large blood vessels traversing the ablation zone were present on baseline scans, but were absent on follow-up imaging. These preliminary results highlight the potential of combining RF ablation with adjuvant liposomal chemotherapeutic agents for greater and more complete treatment.

Several separate mechanisms likely underlie this considerable synergy between RF and Doxil. Postulated reasons for this adjuvant effect can be divided into two distinct categories. The first involves increased delivery of Doxil into tumor tissue peripheral to the central RF coagulation zone. Monsky et al[55] explored intratumoral distribution using radiolabeled liposomal doxorubicin preparations identical to Doxil. They were able to visualize the distribution of liposomes within the tumor post-RF ablation, which concentrated in a thick rim of tumor surrounding the central RF zone. Quantitation of doxorubicin content of RF-treated tumors compared to untreated tumors revealed a fivefold increase in Doxil uptake ($p < .01$). Potential explanations for this increased delivery include nonspecific RF-induced inflammation in surrounding tissue leading to hyperthermic vasodilation and increased vascular permeability and increased cellular uptake and retention of doxorubicin due to disruption of cellular defense mechanisms. Kruskal et al[56] used dynamic intravital video microscopy to study microvascular and cellular alterations in normal livers of live nude mice treated with RF ablation. At temperatures well below those required for irreversible thermal damage, several distinct changes conducive to increased liposome delivery were identified beyond the central coagulation necrosis, including alterations in permeability, reversible microvascular stasis, and increased endothelial leakiness.

A second likely means of synergy between RF ablation and Doxil concerns the tumoricidal effect of both the liposome and doxorubicin components of Doxil. Interestingly, tumors treated with RF in combination with empty liposome preparations (identical formulation to Doxil without doxorubicin) also demonstrated significantly greater necrosis than RF alone (10.9 mm, $p < .01$).[53] Prior studies investigating synergy between lipid preparations and low-level hyperthermia have identified free radical generation as a cause of cellular injury.[57,58] Further research may focus on optimizing liposome structure to foster this effect for greater RF coagulation gain.

## Principles to Improve the Safety of RF Techniques

A fundamental understanding of RF principles is necessary to ensure maximal safety when performing this procedure in clinical practice. In addition to well-known complications from percutaneous needle procedures such as bleeding, infection, and pneumothorax, two broad categories of complications that are specific to this method of thermal ablation therapy—grounding pad burns and thermal damage to adjacent organs—need to be fully addressed.

### Importance of Proper System Grounding

The use of high-current RF technique has increased the risk of one significant potential complication—burns at the grounding pad site. Deleterious heating has been encountered at grounding pad sites in several cases where high current RF has been used.[59] This can be attributed to the fact (which is best illustrated by bipolar RF) that an equal amount of current is deposited at the ground as at the electrode surface. It is important to remember that energy deposited into the tissue is caused by RF waves traveling through a completed electrical circuit. For monopolar RF, grounding pads serve to complete this circuit. Since these pads meet the same impedance and energy loads, they produce an equivalent amount of heat. Hence, the return pad has been traditionally larger than the source electrode to spread the heat over a larger surface area, and has been categorized as a dispersive electrode. While previously single disposable grounding pads built for surgical electrocautery were sufficient to dissipate the short bursts of unwanted heat, the high-energy algorithms for tumor ablation (high current for many minutes) renders a small grounding pad insufficient.

Goldberg et al[60] have previously identified the factors that promote inappropriate thermal deposition at the grounding pad site during RF ablation. Temperatures were found to be nonuniform underneath the entire grounding pad surface with greatest heating at the edges of the pad. Third-degrees burns were observed when inappropriate grounding was used. All parameters studied, including the effects of surface area (one to four pads), pad orientation (horizontal, vertical, diagonal), electrode to pad distance (10–50 cm), grounding pad material (mesh or foil), RF current, and grounding pad size, had an effect on the grounding pad temperatures with the greatest thermal damage induced with the highest RF currents (2000 mA) deposited in the presence of minimum grounding pad surface area. Using four foil pads, continuous RF application of 2000 mA for 10 minutes produced minimal skin redness (42°C maximum temperature). Temperatures never exceeded 34°C when pulsed RF technique was used for up to 30 minutes of RF at 2000 mA suggesting that cooling also occurs at the grounding pad site during the 15-second periods of minimal generator output. As a result of this study, large surface

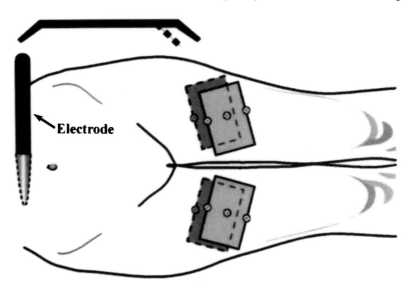

**Figure 1.6.** Proper placement of grounding pads for RF ablation. Schematic drawing depicts the placement of the grounding pads (gray rectangles) in relation to the RF electrode. To minimize grounding pad burn, multiple pads should be placed horizontally, with their long axis facing the electrode. This facilitates a more even distribution of heat dissipation minimizing untoward heating along the grounding pad surface.

area foil pads should be used and oriented to maximize the leading edge of the ground (Fig. 1.6).

### Other Safety Issues

It is important to remember that the heat that destroys tumor tissue also irreversibly coagulates adjacent structures. Several cases of untoward thermal damage to vital structures that were abutting or adjacent to a targeted lesion have been seen.[61] The gallbladder, bile ducts, and bowel are all particularly sensitive to such thermal insults. Thus, bile duct strictures, cholecystitis, and perforated bowel have been observed on occasion. As a result, careful planning to avoid these structures is essential prior to starting an RF ablation case. Additionally, large volumes of coagulation that significantly eclipse a given lesion may not always be beneficial. Such overtreatment would also be detrimental not only if surrounding structures such as the gallbladder were damaged, but also if too little normal tissue was preserved to permit adequate hepatic function (i.e., cirrhotic patients). Hence, refinement of RF ablation is desirable in an effort to permit tissue coagulation in a predictable and reproducible fashion so that the volume of induced coagulation can be appropriately matched to the tumor size and location.

## Conclusion

Preliminary clinical studies encourage optimism about the future of percutaneous minimally invasive, image-guided RF thermal ablation techniques, particularly for the treatment of hepatic neoplasms. Since adequate and total tumor eradication requires ablating the entire tumor and a 0.5- to 1.0-cm peripheral margin of grossly normal tissue, complete ablation necessitates the induction of large volumes of coagulation necrosis. Modification of RF energy delivery and/or modulation of tumor or organ biology can significantly increase the volume of induced tumor destruction, thereby enabling the attainment of the goal of adequate and predictable treatment of clinically relevant tumors. However, a fundamental understanding of the basic principles governing RF and tissue heating is essential for optimizing this process.

Recent technical innovations, including RF application to multiple and/or internally cooled electrodes, enable increased energy deposition into tissues with a resultant increase in the volume of induced coagulation necrosis. Development of strategies to reduce blood flow during RF tumor ablation may also ultimately allow for improved treatment effect, as perfusion-mediated tissue cooling limits both tissue heat deposition and the extent of coagulation necrosis induced by RF tumor ablation in vascular tissues and tumors. Synergistic combination therapies including RF and other adjuvant agents such as ethanol and doxorubicin chemotherapy will also likely receive significant attention in the near future. However, further study is necessary to determine whether any of these methods can improve patient outcomes. The answers to these questions will require substantial further research, which is ongoing at multiple tertiary centers. It is hoped that this work, and well-conducted randomized, multicenter trials will determine the proper role for this promising new paradigm of thermal ablation. Given the rapid pace of technologic development in the field, it is likely that additional innovations will be forthcoming with potential improvement in RF ablation techniques.

### References

1. Dupuy DE, Goldberg SN. Image-guided radiofrequency tumor ablation: challenges and opportunities—part II. J Vasc Intervent Radiol 2001; 12:1135–1148.
2. Pearce JA. Review of electrical field relations. In: Electrosurgery. New York: Wiley Medical Publications, 1986: 224–234.
3. Dodd GD, Soulen MC, Kane RA, et al. Minimally invasive treatment of malignant hepatic tumors: at the threshold of a major breakthrough. Radiographics 2000; 20:9–27.

4. Gazelle GS, Goldberg SN, Solbiati L, Livraghi T. Tumor ablation with radiofrequency energy. Radiology 2000; 217:6333–6346.
5. Goldberg SN, Gazelle GS, Mueller PR. Thermal ablation therapy for focal malignancy: a unified approach to underlying principles, techniques, and diagnostic imaging guidance. Am J Radiol 2000; 174:323–331.
6. McGahan JP, Dodd GD. Radiofrequency ablation of the liver: current status. Am J Radiol 2001; 176:3–16.
7. Cosman ER, Nashold BS, Ovelman-Levitt J. Theoretical aspects of radiofrequency lesions in the dorsal root entry zone. Neurosurgery 1984; 15:945–950.
8. Seegenschmiedt MH, Brady LW, Sauer R. Interstitial thermoradiotherapy: review on technical and clinical aspects. Am J Clin Oncol 1990; 13:352–363.
9. Trembley BS, Ryan TP, Strohbehn JW. Interstitial hyperthermia: physics, biology, and clinical aspects. In: Urano M, Douple E, Hyperthermia and Oncology, vol 3. Utrecht: VSP, 1992: 11–98.
10. Larson TR, Bostwick DG, Corcia A. Temperature-correlated histopathologic changes following microwave thermoablation of obstructive tissue in patients with benign prostatic hyperplasia. Urology 1996; 47:463–469.
11. Zevas NT, Kuwayama A. Pathological characteristics of experimental thermal lesions: comparison of induction heating and radiofrequency electrocoagulation. J Neurosurg 1972; 37:418–422.
12. Thomsen S. Pathologic analysis of photothermal and photomechanical effects of laser-tissue interactions. Photochem Photobiol 1991; 53:825–835.
13. Goldberg SN, Gazelle GS, Compton CC, Mueller PR, Tanabe KK. Treatment of intrahepatic malignancy with radiofrequency ablation: radiologic-pathologic correlation. Cancer 2000; 88:2452–2463.
14. Goldberg SN, Gazelle GS, Halpern EF, Rittman WJ, Mueller PR, Rosenthal DI. Radiofrequency tissue ablation: importance of local temperature along the electrode tip exposure in determining lesion shape and size. Acad Radiol 1996; 3:212–218.
15. Pennes HH. Analysis of tissue and arterial blood temperatures in the resting human forearm. J Appl Physiol 1948; 1:93–122.
16. Taha JM, Tew JM, Buncher CR. A prospective 15-year follow up of 154 consecutive patients with trigeminal neuralgia treated by percutaneous stereotactic radiofrequency thermal rhizotomy. J Neurosurg 1995; 83:989–993.
17. Van Kleef M, Liem L, Lousberg R, Barendse G, Kessels F, Sluijter M. Radiofrequency lesion adjacent to the dorsal root ganglion for cervicobrachial pain: a prospective double blind randomized study. Neurosurgery 1996; 38:1127–1151.
18. Wagshal AB, Pires LA, Huang SK. Management of cardiac arrhythmias with radiofrequency catheter ablation. Arch Intern Med 1995; 155:137–147.
19. Kay GN, Plumb VJ. The present role of radiofrequency catheter ablation in the management of cardiac arrhythmias. Am J Med 1996; 100:344–356.

20. McGahan JP, Browning PD, Brock JM, Tesluk H. Hepatic ablation using radiofrequency electrocautery. Invest Radiol 1990; 25:267–270.
21. Rossi S. Fornari F, Pathies C, Buscarini L. Thermal lesions induced by 480 kHz localized current field in guinea pig and pig liver. Tumori 1990; 76:54–57.
22. Sanchez R, Vansonenberg E, Dagostino H, Goodacre B, Esch O. Percutaneous tissue ablation by radiofrequency thermal energy as a preliminary to tumor ablation. Min Invasive Ther 1993; 2:299–305.
23. Goldberg SN, Gazelle GS, Dawson SL, Mueller PR, Rosenthal DI, Rittman W. Tissue ablation with radiofrequency: effect of probe size, ablation duration, and temperature on lesion volume. Acad Radiol 1995; 2:399–404.
24. Rossi S, DiStasi M, Buscarini E, et al. Percutaneous RF interstitial thermal ablation in the treatment of hepatic cancer. AJR 1996; 167:759–767.
25. Solbiati L, Goldberg SN, Ierace T, Livraghi T, Sironi S, Gazelle GS. Hepatic metastases: percutaneous radiofrequency ablation with cooled-tip electrodes. Radiology 1997; 205:367–374.
26. Goldberg SN, Gazelle GS, Dawson SL, Mueller PR, Rittman WJ, Rosenthal DI. Radiofrequency tissue ablation using multiprobe arrays: greater tissue destruction than multiple probes operating alone. Acad Radiol 1995; 2:670–674.
27. Rossi S, Buscarini E, Garbagnati F, et al. Percutaneous treatment of small hepatic tumors by an expandable RF needle electrode. AJR 1998; 170:1015–1022.
28. Siperstein AE, Rogers SJ, Hansen PD, Gitomirsky A. Laparoscopic thermal ablation of hepatic neuroendocrine tumor metastases. Surgery 1997; 122:1147–1155.
29. LeVeen RF. Laser hyperthermia and radiofrequency ablation of hepatic lesions. Semin Intervent Radiol 1997; 14:313–324.
30. Berber E, Flesher NL, Siperstein AE. Initial clinical evaluation of the RITA 5-centimeter radiofrequency thermal ablation catheter in the treatment of liver tumors. Cancer J 2000; 6:S319–S329.
31. de Baere T, Denys A, Wood BJ, et al. Radiofrequency liver ablation: experimental comparative study of water-cooled versus expandable systems. AJR 2001; 176:187–192.
32. McGahan JP, Wei-Zhong G, Brock JM, Tesluk H, Jones CD. Hepatic ablation using bipolar radiofrequency electrocautery. Acad Radiol 1996; 3:418–422.
33. Desinger K, Stein T, Muller G, Mack M, Vogl TJ. Interstitial bipolar RF-thermotherapy (REITT) therapy by planning by computer simulation and MRI-monitoring—a new concept for minimally invasive procedures. Proc SPIE 1999; 3249:147–160.
34. Goldberg SN, Gazelle GS, Solbiati L, Rittman WJ, Mueller PR. Radiofrequency tissue ablation: increased lesion diameter with a perfusion electrode. Acad Radiol 1996; 3:636–644.
35. Lorentzen T. A cooled needle electrode for radiofrequency tissue ablation: thermodynamic aspects of improved performance compared with conventional needle design. Acad Radiol 1996; 3:556–563.
36. Solbiati L, Ierace T, Goldberg SN, et al. Hepatic metastases: percu-

taneous radiofrequency ablation with cooled-tip electrodes. Radiology 1997; 295:367–374.

37. Goldberg SN, Solbiati L, Hahn PF, et al. Large-volume tissue ablation with radiofrequency by using a clustered, internally-cooled electrode technique: laboratory and clinical experience in liver metastases. Radiology 1998; 209:371–379.

38. Goldberg SN, Stein M, Gazelle GS, Sheiman RG, Kruskal JB, Clouse ME. Percutaneous radiofrequency tissue ablation: optimization of pulsed-RF technique to increase coagulation necrosis. J Vasc Intervent Radiol 1999; 10:907–916.

39. Arata MA, Nisenbaum HL, Clark TW, Soulen MC. Percutaneous radiofrequency ablation of liver tumors with the LeVeen probe: is roll-off predictive of response? J Vasc Intervent Radiol 2001; 12:455–458.

40. Merkle E, Goldberg SN, Boll DT, et al. Effect of supramagnetic MR contrast agents on radiofrequency induced temperature distribution: in vitro measurements in polyacrylamide phantoms and in vivo results in a rabbit liver model. Radiology 1999; 212:459–466.

41. Curley MG, Hamilton PS. Creation of large thermal lesions in liver using saline-enhanced RF ablation. Proc 19th International Conference IEEE/EMBS 1997: 2516–2519.

42. Livraghi T, Goldberg SN, Monti F, et al. Saline-enhanced radiofrequency tissue ablation in the treatment of liver metastases. Radiology 1997; 202:205–210.

43. Miao Y, Ni Y, Yu J, Zhang H, Baert A, Marchal G. An ex-vivo study on radiofrequency tissue ablation: increased lesion size by using an "expandable-wet" electrode. Eur Radiol 2001; 11:1841–1847.

44. Miao Y, Ni Y, Yu J, Marchal G. A comparative study on validation of a novel cooled-wet electrode for radiofrequency liver ablation. Invest Radiol 2000; 35:138–141.

45. Goldberg SN, Ahmed M, Gazelle GS, et al. Radiofrequency thermal ablation with adjuvant saline injection: effect of electrical conductivity on tissue heating and coagulation. Radiology 2001; 219:157–165.

46. Lobo SM, Afzal K, Ahmed M, et al. Radiofrequency ablation: modeling the enhanced temperature response of adjuvant pre-treatment. Radiology, in press.

47. Goldberg SN, Hahn PF, Tanabe KK, et al. Percutaneous radiofrequency tissue ablation: does perfusion-mediated cooling limit coagulation necrosis? J Vasc Intervent Radiol 1998; 9:101–111.

48. Patterson EJ, Scudamore CH, Owen DA, Nagy AG, Buczkowski AK. Radiofrequency ablation of porcine liver in vivo: effects of blood flow and treatment time on lesion size. Ann Surg 1998; 227:559–565.

49. Goldberg SN, Hahn PF, Halpern E, Fogle R, Gazelle GS. Radiofrequency tissue ablation: effect of pharmacologic modulation of blood flow on coagulation diameter. Radiology 1998; 209:761–769.

50. Rossi S, Garbagnati F, Lencioni R, et al. Percutaneous radiofrequency thermal ablation of nonresectable hepatocellular carcinoma after occlusion of tumor blood supply. Radiology 2000; 217:119–126.

51. Christophi C, Winkworth A, Muralihdaran V, Evans P. The treatment of malignancy by hyperthermia. Surg Oncol 1998; 7:83–90.

52. Goldberg SN, Saldinger PF, Gazelle GS, et al. Percutaneous tumor

ablation: increased coagulation necrosis with combined radiofrequency and percutaneous doxorubicin injection. Radiology 2001; 220(2):420–427.

53. Goldberg SN, Giurnan GD, Lukyanov AN, et al. Percutaneous tumor ablation: increased necrosis with combined radiofrequency and intravenous doxorubicin in a liposome carrier in a rat breast tumor model. Radiology 2002 Mar; 222(3):797–804.

54. Goldberg SN, Kamal IR, Reynolds KF, et al. Radiofrequency ablation of hepatic tumors: increased tumor destruction with adjuvant liposomal doxorubicin therapy. AJR 2002 Jul; 179:93–101.

55. Monsky WE, Goldberg SN, Lukyanov AN, et al. Radiofrequency ablation increases intratumoral liposomal doxorubicin accumulation in an animal breast tumor model. Radiology 2002 Sep; 224(3):823–829.

56. Kruskal JB, Oliver B, Huertas JC, Goldberg SN. Dynamic intrahepatic flow and cellular alterations during radiofrequency ablation of liver tissue in mice. J Vasc Intervent Radiol 2001; 12:1193–1201.

57. Kong G, Anyarambhatla G, Petros WP. Efficacy of liposomes and hyperthermia in a human tumor xenograft model: importance of triggered drug release. Cancer Res 2000; 60:6950–6957.

58. Kong G, Dewhirst MW. Hyperthermia and liposomes. Int J Hyperthermia 1999; 15:345–370.

59. Livraghi T, Solbiati L, Meloni F, Ierace T, Goldberg SN. Complications after cool-tip RF ablation of liver cancer: initial report of the Italian Multi-center Cool-tip RF Study Group [abstract]. Radiology 2000; 217(suppl):18.

60. Goldberg SN, Solbiati L, Halpern EF, Gazelle GS. Variables affecting proper system grounding for radiofrequency ablation in an animal model. J Vasc Intervent Radiol 2000; 11:1069–1075.

61. Livraghi T, Goldberg SN, Meloni F, Solbiati L, Gazelle GS. Radiofrequency ablation of large hepatocellular carcinomas. Radiology 2000; 214:761–768.

# Radiofrequency Ablation of Liver Malignancies

# 2

# Radiofrequency Ablation of Colon and Rectal Carcinoma Liver Metastases

Kenneth K. Tanabe and Michael A. Choti

Liver metastases from colon and rectal cancer are the most frequent hepatic malignancy in the United States. Although surgical resection remains the only established potentially curative option for patients with isolated hepatic metastases, most patients are not candidates for resection. Moreover, many patients experience a recurrence within the liver following resection, and few are candidates for re-resection. For these reasons, increasing interest has been focused on ablative approaches for the treatment of unresectable metastases. Radiofrequency ablation (RFA) is becoming the most commonly used and perhaps the most promising modality for tumor ablation.

One of the first clinical settings in which RFA of tissue was broadly applied was destruction of cardiac tissue to treat arrythmias. Based on several principles learned from this application, RFA was employed to manage osteomas (see Chapter 10). As a result of the successes of these initial experiences, there has been particular interest in the use of ablative therapies to treat other tumors. The application of ablative technologies to management of primary and secondary liver tumors resulted from several observations. First, existing therapies for primary and secondary liver tumors are associated with significant morbidity, mortality, and cost. Second, the only potentially curative approaches are partial liver resection or liver transplantation. Only a minority of patients have resectable tumors. In addition, a sizable portion of this patient population is afflicted with cirrhosis, such that resection is either not possible or is associated with significant risks of morbidity and mortality. Limited availability of organs and long wait-list times preclude broad application of liver transplantation. Third, nonsurgical therapies are palliative at best, and are very limited in efficacy.

Liver tumor ablation may compare favorably to surgical resection with respect to morbidity, mortality, cost, and suitability for real-time image guidance. Accordingly, patients with liver tumors are well suited for clinical trials of RFA. In the United States, the incidence of liver metastases from gastrointestinal malignancies (particularly colon and rectal cancer) is much higher than the incidence of hepatocellular carcinoma. In addition, the biology of colon and rectal carcinoma is such that these patients commonly have liver metastases in the absence of metastases in other sites. This pattern of relapse is well suited to locoregional therapies such as liver tumor ablation. Accordingly, most of the patients involved in clinical trials of liver tumor RFA in the United States have liver metastases from colon or rectal carcinoma.

This chapter presents strategies to increase the size of RFA zones that have been examined in preclinical and clinical settings, describes techniques of RFA of colon and rectal carcinoma liver metastases, and discusses clinical trials in this field.

## Strategies to Increase the Size of Ablation Zones

RFA involves placement of thin, partially insulated electrodes (14–21 gauge) into a tumor. The electrodes and grounding pads are connected to a radiofrequency generator, and during treatment 500 kHz of current travels from the uninsulated portion of the active electrode toward the grounding pads. This current produces ion agitation in the tissue surrounding the electrode, which is converted by friction into heat and induces cellular death via coagulation necrosis.[1] The tissue surrounding the electrode, rather than the electrode itself, is the primary source of heat.[2] Too much heat, however, can be counterproductive. For example, at extreme temperatures (>100°C) the tissue undergoes vaporization and carbonization, which limit electrical current and thereby limit conduction of heat into deeper tissues. This ultimately restricts the size of the zone of coagulation created by RFA.

Initial attempts at increasing the volume of coagulated tissue generated with RFA centered on increasing electrode tip length, increasing tip temperatures, and lengthening the duration of treatment.[3] With exposed electrode tips exceeding 3 cm, a greater variability in coagulation uniformity is observed, leading to unpredictable necrosis volumes. RFA with electrodes that have less than a 3-cm tip exposure and that achieve temperatures of 90° to 110°C has been the most successful in yielding reproducible uniform, coagulative necrosis. These parameters produce a predictable shape of coagulation necrosis; however, the volumes of coagulation necrosis created using single electrodes with this configuration remain too small to be clinically useful for most patients with liver tumors.

*Multielectrode Arrays*

One method for increasing energy deposition throughout the tumor lesion is the repeated insertion of the radiofrequency electrode into the tissue to increase the diameter of induced coagulation.[3,4] This approach, however, is not only time-consuming but also difficult to utilize in the clinical setting, as multiple electrodes repositionings are technically challenging, especially given the ultrasound echogenicity created during treatment. The development of deployable expandable multielectrode arrays has overcome some of these problems and has produced larger zones of necrosis in clinical trials.[5] These systems deploy an array of multiple curved stiff wires in the shape of an umbrella from a single 14- or 16-gauge cannula (Fig. 2.1). Experiments using a

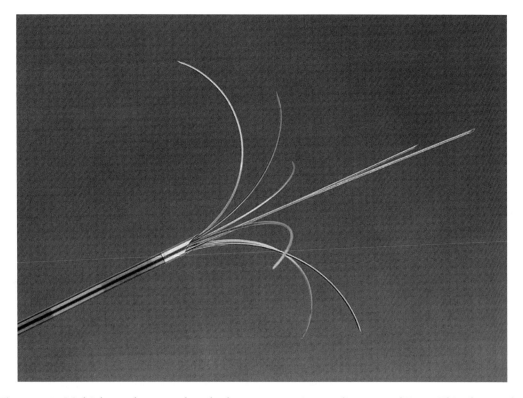

**Figure 2.1.** Multielectrode array that deploys to a maximum diameter of 7 cm. This device also incorporates hypertonic saline infusion (RITA Medical Systems StarBurst XL™).

12-hook "umbrella" array in in-vivo porcine liver have produced spherical regions of coagulation necrosis measuring up to 3.5 cm in diameter.[6] Newer multielectrode arrays have been developed that produce zones of coagulation necrosis of up to 5 to 7 cm. These newer arrays have not yet been extensively tested in clinical trials.

### Saline Infusion During Radiofrequency Ablation

The simultaneous infusion of low volumes of saline during RFA has also been used as a strategy to increase the volume of coagulation necrosis.[7–9] Either hypertonic or normal saline is infused into the tumor through tiny holes at the distal ends of the electrode during the ablation. The saline enhances thermal conduction through decreased impedance at the electrode tissue interface. In addition, the high local ion concentration produced by the saline may increase the electrode's active surface area, thus increasing the extent of the coagulation necrosis. Although initial work with this technique was hampered by the problem of producing unpredictable shapes of coagulation necrosis, more recent investigations along these lines have been promising.[10] Injection of ethanol in animal models has also been demonstrated to increase the volume of coagulation necrosis achieved by RFA.[11]

### Internally Cooled Electrodes

Another tactic to increase coagulation volumes has been the development of internally cooled radiofrequency electrodes. With internal electrode tip cooling that avoids desiccation of tissue adjacent to the electrode and increases in impedance, radiofrequency-induced coagulation necrosis is greater than that achieved with noncooled electrodes.[12] However, internally cooled electrodes generally require longer treatment times.

### Limiting Vascular Inflow

Blood flow serves as a "heat sink," such that tumors located in vascular environments are less susceptible to thermal destruction as perfusion-mediated tissue cooling reduces the extent of coagulation necrosis. Furthermore, radiofrequency-induced coagulation necrosis is often shaped in vivo by the surrounding hepatic vasculature.[13,14] Greater coagulation in porcine livers is observed in vivo when radiofrequency energy is delivered during balloon occlusion of the portal vein than when energy is delivered during normal blood flow.[15] Similarly, it has been demonstrated in clinical trials that larger zones of coagulation necrosis can be achieved with RFA with complete vascular inflow occlusion

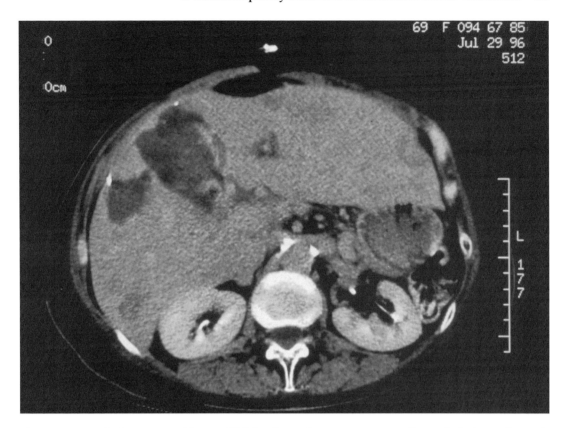

**Figure 2.2.** Radiofrequency ablation (RFA) achieved using an internally cooled electrode. Both ablation zones were created using the same amount of energy, and both colon carcinoma liver metastases measured the same size. The ablation zone located more anteriorly is significantly larger, and was created by performance of RFA during complete vascular inflow occlusion.

(achieved by a Pringle maneuver)[16] (Fig. 2.2). It is also possible to temporarily reduce hepatic venous outflow to reduce perfusion-mediated tissue cooling, and thereby create larger zones of ablation.[17]

*Pulsed Radiofrequency Ablation*

Another strategy to increase the extent of coagulation is the use of pulsed rather than of continuous currents. The concept is that by applying energy in an intermittent fashion, heat dissipation occurs between pulses thus allowing for a greater deposition of energy to tissues while preventing tissue vaporization or carbonization near the electrode.[18,19] Pulsed radiofrequency current allows deposition of a larger amount of energy while avoiding the rise in impedance seen in comparable continuous treatment applications.

## Technique of Radiofrequency Ablation During Laparotomy and Laparoscopy

One advantage of RFA over that of other ablative approaches such as cryotherapy is that it can be performed with percutaneous, open, or laparoscopic approaches. In all cases, the tumor must be clearly seen during treatment with either computed tomography (CT), magnetic resonance imaging (MRI), or ultrasound (US). Although any of these imaging modalities may be used during percutaneous RFA, intraoperative ultrasound is used for laparoscopic or open procedures. When preparing the patient, dispersive grounding electrodes are placed on the back or legs and care must be taken to assure adequate skin contact in order to avoid cutaneous burns. Large grounding pads placed on the thighs provide sufficient surface area to avoid burn injuries at the pad sites when using up to 2000 mA of current.

When performing RFA during open laparotomy, careful exploration of the abdominal cavity is first performed to exclude the presence of extrahepatic malignancy, including assessment of peritoneal surfaces and periportal nodal regions. The liver is then carefully inspected by both palpation and intraoperative US. In cases in which previous biopsy has not been obtained, core biopsy under US guidance should be considered.

Careful planning of the zone of ablation is necessary to achieve complete necrosis of the target lesion. In some cases when using an expandable multielectrode needle of sufficient size, complete ablation can be achieved with a single application, deploying the electrode from the center of the tumor. For example, a 3-cm spherical tumor and 1-cm margin can be treated with the use of a device deployed to produce a 5-cm diameter volume of necrosis. Newer electrode technology using higher energy and low-volume hypertonic saline infusion can produce zones of coagulation necrosis as large as 7 cm in diameter in some cases.

Tumor size as well as location can preclude effective RFA with curative intent. Tumor sizes larger than 4 to 5 cm are associated with an increased incidence of local recurrence.[20,21] The location of a tumor near the main portal pedicles is considered a relative contraindication to RFA. In addition to the inability to achieve an effective ablation due to the high blood flow, ablation near the porta hepatis can result in injury and stricture of a central bile duct.[22]

Once the target tumor is identified with the US transducer, the RFA electrode needle is inserted under US guidance (Fig. 2.3). Optimally, the electrode is advanced in a track parallel and within the plane of the transducer so the entire path of the needle can be visualized. When using a multielectrode needle, the array is

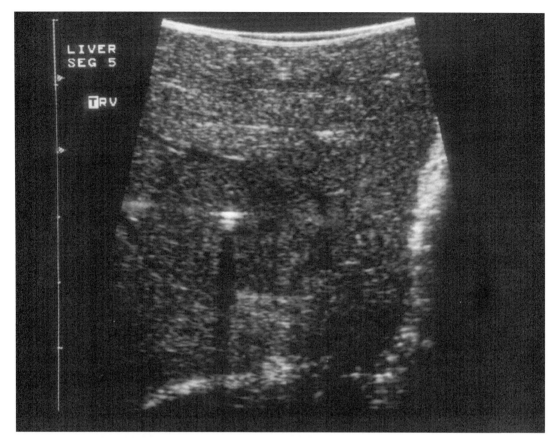

**Figure 2.3.** RFA electrode placement under real-time ultrasound guidance.

deployed within the tumor and position is confirmed ultrasonographically. With some RFA devices central ablation can first be
performed by partially deploying the array and sequentially advancing the electrodes to the desired volume.

Monitoring during thermal ablation can be performed using a
variety of methods. Some RFA devices have the capacity to measure tissue temperatures with thermistors located at the tips of
the electrodes. Alternatively, tissue impedance and current can
be monitored during treatment. With some devices, the power
output is adjusted automatically to control impedance and maintain tissue temperature between 70° and 105°C. The ablation zone
is visualized by US during treatment. Typically, local tissue
changes results in hyperechogenicity within the treated tissue
(Fig. 2.4).

In cases in which a single application is not sufficient, RFA can
be repeated to create overlapping ablation zones. Accurate placement of electrodes intraoperatively to construct overlapping ablation zones ablation can be technically challenging. There are

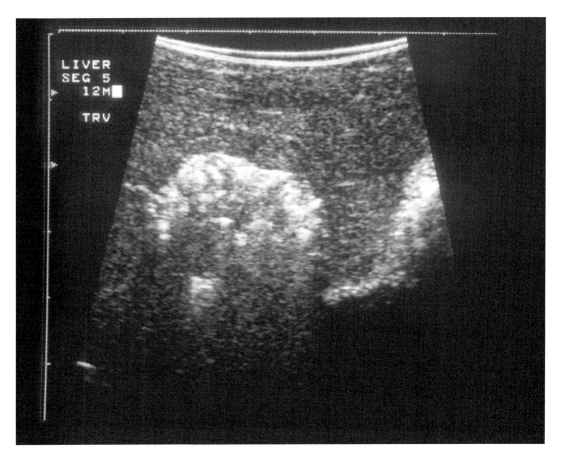

**Figure 2.4.** Ultrasongraphic image during RFA using a multielectrode array. Gas formation encompassing the zone of ablation results in hyperechoic appearance.

two methods of electrode repositioning. The first involves withdrawing the electrode along the same track before reapplication of energy to create cylindrically shaped ablation zones rather than spherical or ellipsoid zones. The second type of repositioning involves withdrawing the electrode and then reinserting it to create a series of geometrically oriented overlapping spheres. The previously ablated areas remain echogenic on ultrasound for 15 to 30 minutes, making US guidance of this type of electrode repositioning difficult. In situations where it is anticipated that overlapping treatment zones will be necessary to completely ablate a tumor, it is useful to first "map" the treatment area by inserting introducer sheaths into the precise location where electrodes will be inserted. When this maneuver is performed *before* any energy is applied to the tumor, the electrode positions can be accurately determined using US images that are not obscured by treatment-induced echogenicity. One can then more precisely map the electrode positions required to achieve overlapping cylindrically shaped ablation zones to fully ablate both the tumor and a sufficient margin.

As already described, it can be helpful intraoperatively to perform a Pringle maneuver (vascular inflow occlusion) during RFA to both shorten the time required to achieve full ablation and to increase the size of the ablation zone created with each treatment. When using overlapping ablation zones, it is also beneficial to treat areas closest to vascular heat-sinks first, as this will decrease the time required to treat the entire lesion.

Laparoscopic RFA offers the advantage of a minimally invasive procedure with the ability to visualize the abdominal cavity and perform the therapy using laparoscopic US. With this approach, patients are treated under general endotracheal anesthesia, typically in the supine position. In most cases, the procedure can be done with two or three ports.[23] The liver is typically partially mobilized, and viscera within 2 cm of the intended ablation zone are moved away. Laparoscopic cholecystectomy can be performed when a target lesion is in close proximity to the gallbladder. The RFA electrode is placed into the abdominal cavity through a percutaneous approach and does not require the placement of an additional port. An introducer sheath may be helpful to improve needle alignment and avoid abdominal wall tumor seeding. The needle is placed within the tumor under US guidance and ablation is performed and monitored as with the open technique.

## Imaging Following Radiofrequency Ablation

The optimal method for evaluating the efficacy of RFA treatment using imaging modalities is not well defined. When using intraoperative US during therapy, hyperechoic regions can be seen within the ablation zone (Fig. 2.4). However, the correlation between US appearance and outcome following RFA is generally not good.

The presence of residual viable tumor tissue after RFA can be detected using post-procedural contrast-enhanced CT or MRI, using criteria similar to those following percutaneous ethanol injection therapy. However, unlike hepatocellular carcinoma, colorectal carcinoma liver metastases are often hypovascular, and determination of postprocedure necrosis and tumor viability is difficult. Perhaps more useful in assessing the success of ablation is the size, shape, and location of the necrosis zone on postprocedural scan relative to the preprocedure images (Fig. 2.5). A contrast-enhanced CT or MRI should be performed within 1 to 7 days following RFA treatment. It is not uncommon to see an area of peripheral enhancement surrounding the treated area. This region enhances primarily on arterial phase as a result of the inflammatory reaction from the thermal injury. It is important to

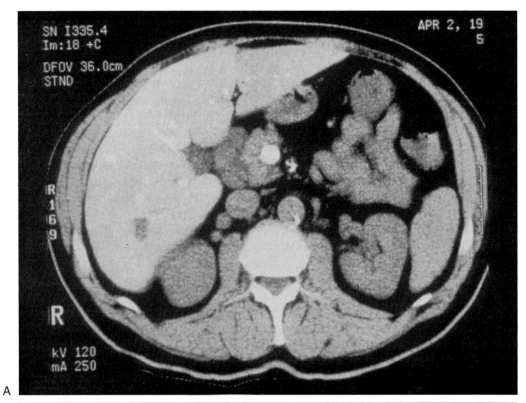

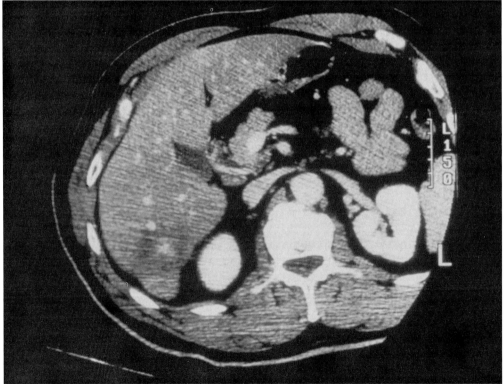

**Figure 2.5.** Computed tomography (CT) scan of colon carcinoma liver metastases prior to (A) and immediately following (B) RFA.

document that the zone of necrosis (as measured by the absence of contrast enhancement) extends beyond the original border of the tumor. Ideally, the area of coagulation necrosis should include a 0.5- to 1-cm margin in the liver parenchyma around the lesion. When concern exists over the possibility of residual untreated tumor, specific areas can be retreated percutaneously if necessary.

Serial follow-up imaging of the liver is recommended after RFA treatment. However, as with other ablative approaches, interpretation of these images can be difficult at times, as a hypoattenuated lesion may persist for months to years despite complete tumor destruction. In most cases, local recurrence is characterized by an increase in the lesion size on serial scans, or evidence of new areas of contrast enhancement.[24] CT or MRI is the most useful for follow-up imaging, emphasizing the importance of comparing images to previous ones.[25,26] The role of fluorodeoxyglucose positron emission tomography (FDG-PET) in assessing local residual or recurrent disease following RFA is yet to be defined. However, because of the biology of the disease, a careful follow-up protocol, including serum carcinoembryonic antigen (CEA) measurements and perhaps PET, is important in detecting new intrahepatic and extrahepatic metastases.

## Operative Versus Percutaneous Radiofrequency Ablation

Many of the published reports evaluating RFA of liver metastases have relied upon percutaneous electrode insertion under image guidance.[7,27,28] The principal advantage of the percutaneous approach compared to operative approaches is the lower associated morbidity and cost. A second advantage of a percutaneous approach is the ability to use US, MRI, or CT guidance, whereas imaging of RFA performed during laparotomy or laparoscopy is for the most part limited to US guidance.

However, there are several advantages to performance of ablation during laparotomy or laparoscopy. The first benefit is that of enhanced staging, as laparotomy and laparoscopy afford the opportunity to identify both hepatic and extrahepatic metastases not visualized on preoperative imaging. Ten percent to 20% of patients who undergo exploration for intent to resect colorectal liver metastases are found at laparotomy to have additional metastases that either preclude or significantly alter the planned resection. Many of these operative findings can be detected via laparoscopy as well. In addition, intraoperative ultrasound can frequently detect lesions that are not seen with transabdominal US, CT, or MRI.

Second, laparotomy affords the opportunity to combine ablation with surgical resection. It is important to point out that following ablation of tumors larger than 5 cm, the local recurrence rate is unacceptably high.[28] Accordingly, a significant fraction of patients with unresectable liver tumors can be fully treated only by the combination of resection of larger lesions and ablation of smaller lesions. For example, a patient with a 7-cm tumor occupying the left hepatic lobe and a 2-cm tumor straddling segments 6 and 7 is an ideal candidate for treatment with a combination of left hepatic lobectomy for the larger left lobe tumor and RFA of the smaller right lobe tumor.

Third, hepatic blood flow creates a "heat-sink" that reduces the efficacy of thermal ablation. Ablation during laparotomy or laparoscopy can be performed with a vascular clamp occluding hepatic arterial and portal venous blood flow. This technique has been demonstrated to safely and reproducibly increase the size of the zone of ablation.[14,16,29] Although inflow occlusion can also be accomplished using percutaneous techniques, the complexity and risk of the procedure precludes its routine use.

Fourth, laparotomy or laparoscopy affords excellent access to tumors in the dome of the liver or in other locations that are difficult to accurately target percutaneously. This location is difficult to access with precision using a path for the electrode that does not violate the pleura. In addition, motion of the liver caused by respiration creates further problems that can be better managed during an open laparotomy.

Fifth, operative approaches permit mobilization of structures away from a surface tumor that may be thermally injured during RFA. For example, the transverse colon may be adherent to a tumor in the inferior portion of the liver. Effective thermal ablation of the entire tumor would risk injury to the colon unless it were first dissected free from the tumor.

Finally, laparotomy affords the opportunity to implant a hepatic arterial infusion pump for postoperative administration of regional chemotherapy. The most common pattern of relapse following treatment of both primary and secondary hepatic malignancies is within the liver. A prospective, randomized trial comparing intravenous chemotherapy to hepatic arterial infusion chemotherapy combined with intravenous chemotherapy following curative liver resection demonstrated enhanced survival at 2 years in patients treated with the combination of hepatic arterial infusion and intravenous chemotherapy.[30] The majority of the benefit was obtained by marked reduction in hepatic recurrences observed in patients who received hepatic arterial infusion chemotherapy. Ongoing clinical trials are being conducted addressing the role of operative RFA combined with hepatic arterial infusion combined with systemic chemotherapy.

## Results of Clinical Trials

The analysis of clinical results achieved by RFA for the treatment of hepatic colorectal metastases has been hampered by the lack of appropriate controls and relatively short follow-up times. As technical improvements have occurred, investigators have used different devices and techniques. Inclusion of heterogeneous patient populations, difficulties in defining true local recurrences, and the significant impact of distant recurrence on survival have also made assessment of the efficacy of RFA challenging.

Curley et al[21] reported the largest series to date of operative RFA of unresectable primary and metastatic hepatic malignancies in 123 patients. In these patients, RFA was used to treat 169 tumors with a median diameter of 3.4 cm. Primary liver cancer was treated in 48 patients and metastatic liver tumors were treated in 75 patients. Percutaneous and intraoperative RFA was performed in 31 patients and 92 patients, respectively. No treatment-related deaths occurred and the complication rate was only 2.4%. All treated tumors were completely necrotic on imaging studies after completion of the RFA treatments. With a median follow-up of 15 months, tumor had recurred in three of 169 treated lesions (1.8%), but metastatic disease had developed at other sites in 34 patients. Based on these results, these investigators concluded that RFA is a safe, well-tolerated, and effective treatment in patients with unresectable hepatic malignancies. RFA may not cure most patients with primary or malignant metastatic disease, as witnessed by the 34 patients with disease found at extrahepatic sites, but initial disease-free rates of 20% to 50% justify continued investigation into aggressive treatment of isolated hepatic disease with a multimodality approach including RFA. Another large series was reported by Wood et al[31] in which 231 tumors in 84 patients were treated in 91 procedures. Thirty-nine procedures were performed via laparotomy and 27 were performed via laparoscopy. Of note, intraoperative ultrasound detected intrahepatic tumors that were not evident on preoperative scans in 38% of patients who underwent either laparotomy or laparoscopy. In 45% of patients, RFA was combined with resection or cryosurgical ablation. Median hospital stay overall was 3.6 days. Eight percent of patients had complications, and one patient died as a result of the procedure. With a median follow-up of 9 months, 18% of patients experienced a local recurrence at a RFA site.

In a large series from Italy, 179 liver metastases in 117 patients with colorectal cancer were treated with RFA.[28] The tumors ranged in size from 0.9 to 9.6 cm and all were percutaneously treated using internally cooled 17 gauge electrodes under image guidance. The estimated median survival was 36 months, with 1-, 2-, and 3-year survival rates of 93%, 69%, and 46%, respectively. Two thirds of patients developed recurrences at a median time of 12 months following treatment. Seventy (39%) of 179 treated lesions recurred locally, and of these recurrences, 54 were observed by 6 months and 67 by 1 year. No local recurrences were observed after 18 months, although the median follow-up time for the entire study population is not reported. As expected, the incidence of local recurrence differed by size of lesion. The local recurrence rates were 22%, 53%, and 68% for lesions measuring ≤2.5 cm, 2.6 to 4.0 cm, and ≥4.1 cm, respectively.

## Conclusion

Although surgical resection remains the "gold standard" for potentially curative therapy for colorectal carcinoma liver metastases, recent improvements in RFA technology have provided patients and physicians with a new treatment option. Advances in RFA device technology, imaging modalities, and minimally invasive tools offer the promise of a more effective and less invasive treatment in the future. The pace with which advances have been made in RFA for liver tumors has added to the excitement in the field. RFA will presumably complement established therapies, including regional and systemic chemotherapy and resection. Results of small, single-institution clinical trials evaluating RFA in this role are promising. Large-scale clinical trials and more long-term outcome data are needed to evaluate the efficacy and role of RFA for the treatment of liver metastases.

## References

1. Cosman ER, Nashold BS, Ovelman-Levitt J. Theoretical aspects of radiofrequency lesions in the dorsal root entry zone. Neurosurgery 1984; 15:945–950.
2. Organ LW. Electrophysiologic principles of radiofrequency lesion making. Appl Neurophysiol 1976; 39:69–76.
3. Goldberg SN, Gazelle GS, Dawson SL, Rittman WJ, Mueller PR, Rosenthal DI. Tissue ablation with radiofrequency using multiprobe arrays. Acad Radiol 1995; 2:670–674.
4. Rossi S, Buscarini E, Garbagnati F, et al. Percutaneous treatment of small hepatic tumors by an expandable RF needle electrode. AJR 1998; 170:1015–1022.
5. Lencioni R, Cioni D, Bartolozzi C. Percutaneous radiofrequency thermal ablation of liver malignancies: techniques, indications, imaging findings, and clinical results. Abdom Imaging 2001; 26: 345–360.
6. Siperstein AE, Rogers SJ, Hansen PD, Gitomirsky A. Laparoscopic thermal ablation of hepatic neuroendocrine tumor metastases. Surgery 1997; 122:1147–1155.

7. Livraghi T, Goldberg SN, Monti F, et al. Saline-enhanced radio-frequency tissue ablation in the treatment of liver metastases. Radiology 1997; 202:205–210.
8. Mittleman RS, Huang SK, de Guzman WT, Cuenoud H, Wagshal AB, Pires LA. Use of the saline infusion electrode catheter for improved energy delivery and increased lesion size in radiofrequency catheter ablation. Pacing Clin Electrophysiol 1995; 18:1022–1027.
9. Miao Y, Ni Y, Yu J, Zhang H, Baert A, Marchal G. An ex vivo study on radiofrequency tissue ablation: increased lesion size by using an "expandable-wet" electrode. Eur Radiol 2001; 11:1841–1847.
10. Goldberg SN, Ahmed M, Gazelle GS, et al. Radio-frequency thermal ablation with NaCl solution injection: effect of electrical conductivity on tissue heating and coagulation-phantom and porcine liver study. Radiology 2001; 219:157–165.
11. Goldberg SN, Kruskal JB, Oliver BS, Clouse ME, Gazelle GS. Percutaneous tumor ablation: increased coagulation by combining radio-frequency ablation and ethanol instillation in a rat breast tumor model. Radiology 2000; 217:827–831.
12. Lorentzen T. A cooled needle electrode for radiofrequency tissue ablation: thermodynamic aspects of improved performance compared with conventional needle design. Acad Radiol 1996; 3:556–563.
13. Rossi S, Garbagnati F, De Francesco I, et al. Relationship between the shape and size of radiofrequency induced thermal lesions and hepatic vascularization. Tumori 1999; 85:128–132.
14. Patterson EJ, Scudamore CH, Owen DA, Nagy AG, Buczkowski AK. Radiofrequency ablation of porcine liver in vivo: effects of blood flow and treatment time on lesion size. Ann Surg 1998; 227:559–565.
15. Goldberg SN, Hahn PF, Tanabe KK, et al. Percutaneous radiofrequency tissue ablation: does perfusion-mediated tissue cooling limit coagulation necrosis? J Vasc Intervent Radiol 1998; 9:101–111.
16. Goldberg SN, Gazelle GS, Compton CC, Mueller PR, Tanabe KK. Treatment of intrahepatic malignancy with radiofrequency ablation: radiologic-pathologic correlation. Cancer 2000; 88:2452–2463.
17. de Baere T, Bessoud B, Dromain C, et al. Percutaneous radiofrequency ablation of hepatic tumors during temporary venous occlusion. AJR 2002; 178:53–59.
18. Goldberg SN, Gazelle GS, Solbiati L, Mullin K. Large volume radiofrequency tissue ablation: increase coagulation with pulsed technique. Radiology 1997; 205:P258 (abstract).
19. Goldberg SN, Stein MC, Gazelle GS, Sheiman RG, Kruskal JB, Clouse ME. Percutaneous radiofrequency tissue ablation: optimization of pulsed-radiofrequency technique to increase coagulation necrosis. J Vasc Intervent Radiol 1999; 10:907–916.
20. Bowles BJ, Machi J, Limm WM, et al. Safety and efficacy of radiofrequency thermal ablation in advanced liver tumors. Arch Surg 2001; 136:864–869.
21. Curley SA, Izzo F, Delrio P, et al. Radiofrequency ablation of unresectable primary and metastatic hepatic malignancies: results in 123 patients. Ann Surg 1999; 230:1–8.
22. Dominique E, El Otmany A, Goharin A, Attalah D, de Baere T. Intraductal cooling of the main bile ducts during intraoperative radiofrequency ablation. J Surg Oncol 2001; 76:297–300.

23. Siperstein A, Garland A, Engle K, et al. Laparoscopic radiofrequency ablation of primary and metastatic liver tumors. Technical considerations. Surg Endosc 2000; 14:400–405.
24. Kuszyk BS, Choti MA, Urban BA, et al. Hepatic tumors treated by cryosurgery: normal CT appearance. AJR 1996; 166:363–368.
25. Chopra S, Dodd GD, 3rd, Chintapalli KN, Leyendecker JR, Karahan OI, Rhim H. Tumor recurrence after radiofrequency thermal ablation of hepatic tumors: spectrum of findings on dual-phase contrast-enhanced CT. AJR 2001; 177:381–387.
26. Berber E, Foroutani A, Garland AM, et al. Use of CT Hounsfield unit density to identify ablated tumor after laparoscopic radiofrequency ablation of hepatic tumors. Surg Endosc 2000; 14:799–804.
27. Solbiati L, Ierace T, Goldberg SN, et al. Percutaneous US-guided radio-frequency tissue ablation of liver metastases: treatment and follow-up in 16 patients [see comments]. Radiology 1997; 202:195–203.
28. Solbiati L, Livraghi T, Goldberg SN, et al. Percutaneous radio-frequency ablation of hepatic metastases from colorectal cancer: long-term results in 117 patients. Radiology 2001; 221:159–166.
29. Chinn SB, Lee FT Jr, Kennedy GD, et al. Effect of vascular occlusion on radiofrequency ablation of the liver: results in a porcine model. AJR 2001; 176:789–795.
30. Kemeny N, Huang Y, Cohen AM, et al. Hepatic arterial infusion of chemotherapy after resection of hepatic metastases from colorectal cancer. N Engl J Med 1999; 341:2039–2048.
31. Wood TF, Rose DM, Chung M, Allegra DP, Foshag LJ, Bilchik AJ. Radiofrequency ablation of 231 unresectable hepatic tumors: indications, limitations, and complications. Ann Surg Oncol 2000; 7:593–600.

# 3

# Combination of Radiofrequency Ablation and Intraarterial Chemotherapy for Metastatic Cancer in the Liver

Douglas L. Fraker

The variety of techniques that have been developed and utilized to treat colorectal metastases to the liver is a testimony to the fact that no single treatment is effective against this common clinical problem. If any single treatment resulted in durable responses for this disease, that approach would be modified, refined, and universally employed, much like standard adjuvant regimens for the treatment of breast cancer or other common tumors. Instead, several different approaches from various fields including medical oncology, surgical oncology, and interventional radiology have been developed and reported over the past two decades. This chapter reviews the combination of radiofrequency ablation (RFA) with intraarterial chemotherapy. To understand the potential benefit for combining these two modes of cancer treatment, the RFA procedure and the data available from intraarterial chemotherapy protocols alone (particularly adjuvant protocols) must be understood.

The various types of treatments utilized for colorectal metastases to the liver can be categorized into systemic therapies, regional therapies, or direct lesional treatments (Table 3.1). Each of these different approaches has strengths and weaknesses. The obvious benefits of systemic therapy is that it delivers a treatment

**Table 3.1 Approaches to the Treatment of Metastatic Colorectal Cancer to the Liver and Strengths and Weaknesses of Each Approach**

| Type of approach | Examples | Strengths | Weaknesses |
|---|---|---|---|
| Systemic | 5-FU + irinotecan + leucovorin | Treats entire patient | Low response rates, short duration of response |
| Vascular | Intraarterial infusion of FUDR<br>Chemoembolization<br>Isolated hepatic perfusion | Improves response rates<br>Treats entire liver | Extrahepatic recurrences<br>Moderate duration of response |
| Direct Lesional | Surgical resection<br>Cryosurgery<br>Radiofrequency ablation<br>Alcohol injection | Often complete response in lesion treated | Hepatic recurrence in residual liver<br>Systemic recurrence |

5-FU, 5-fluorouracil; FUDR, 5-fluorouracil deoxyribonucleoside.

to the entire patient. Opponents of regional cancer therapy in the medical oncology community argue that metastatic cancer is a systemic disease and requires systemic treatment approaches. The weakness of systemic therapy is the inability of currently available agents to produce significant durable responses. The best chemotherapy regimen for colorectal cancer has recently been shown to be a combination of 5-fluorouracil (5-FU), leucovorin, and irinotecan given either as the Saltz regimen[1] or the De Gramont regimen.[2] However, the maximal response rates with current combination chemotherapy still is between 28% and 37% with a median duration of response of 8 months.

Regional treatments of colorectal cancer metastatic to the liver are based on delivery of agents directly to the liver via its vasculature. The strength of regional delivery approaches is the ability to dose escalate chemotherapeutic agents within the tumor and liver microenvironment.[3] This increase in local drug concentration will theoretically lead to better response rates than can be achieved by systemic therapy. The weaknesses of regional therapeutic approaches is that they may not treat the entire patient, and micrometastatic disease located elsewhere in the body receives no therapy. Also, although the response rates may be increased by regional chemotherapy, it is not clear that the duration of response would necessarily be augmented.

The final category of treatment for colorectal metastases to the liver is direct lesional approaches. Examples of this type of treatment include surgical resection, cryosurgical ablation, RFA, and intralesional injection of alcohol or other toxic agents. The major advantage of this treatment is that there is an extremely high response rate for the specific lesion treated. Surgical resection, which is the ultimate ablative technique, produces an immediate "complete response" for a metastatic nodule successfully removed. The lesional response rate for RFA of metastatic lesions in the liver is discussed in Chapter 2. It is clear that the ability to obtain a complete response in an established tumor of the appropriate size treated by RFA far exceeds what can be achieved with systemic treatment or regional therapy. The two major disadvantages of lesional techniques are the inability to treat patients with significant disease even if it is confined to the liver, and the incidence of intrahepatic recurrences. Patients with extremely large lesions within the liver and/or a large number of metastatic lesions cannot be approached by any ablation techniques. Unfortunately, this patient population with heavy tumor burden comprises a large fraction of patients with metastatic colorectal cancer to the liver even with no extrahepatic disease. The second problem with lesional approaches is that if vascular-based therapies are criticized as regional techniques, then lesional or ablative strategies are "subregional techniques." Ablation of le-

sions within the liver not only delivers no treatment to the rest
of the patient but also does not address or deliver treatment to
other areas of the liver. Therefore, not only is no treatment delivered to extrahepatic micrometastases, but also micrometastatic disease in the liver receives no benefit from these direct ablative approaches.

The conclusion of this analysis of the strengths and weaknesses
of various treatment approaches for metastatic cancer to the liver
is that when the treatment is more focused, the response rate increases, but the potential for progressive disease elsewhere also
increases (Table 3.1). An appropriate strategy would be to combine these various strategies to capitalize on their strengths and
minimize their weaknesses. This chapter focuses on the combination of RFA with intraarterial chemotherapy for metastatic
colon cancer to the liver. Prior to evaluating the specific results
from early reports of protocols combining these treatments, it is
important to review the clinical results achieved with intraarterial therapy alone, as this would be the benchmark to assess
whether the addition of RFA to this regional treatment adds benefit for the patient.

## Treatment History

The history of the use of intraarterial chemotherapy for colorectal cancers metastatic to the liver can be divided into four stages
(Table 3.2). First, in the initial development of the technique,

Table 3.2 Phases in the Development of Intraarterial
Chemotherapy to Treat Colorectal Metastases to
the Liver

| Stage | Year | Accomplishments |
|-------|------|-----------------|
| 1 | 1975–1984 | Pharmacologic studies on drug clearance by liver<br>Demonstration of blood supply to metastases from hepatic artery<br>Development of implantable pump<br>Initial phase I/II studies |
| 2 | 1985–1994 | Phase III studies comparing intraarterial therapy to systemic |
| 3 | 1990–1995 | Phase II studies of second-generation regimen to decrease hepatic toxicity and increase response rate |
| 4 | 1976–present | Combining intraarterial chemotherapy with other modalities including surgical resection, cryosurgery, and radiofrequency ablation |

phase I and II protocols determined the appropriate infusion regimen. Second, there was validation of the optimal protocols in
phase III trials comparing intraarterial therapy with systemic
treatment. Third, there was refinement of the initial regimens in
second-generation phase II trials primarily in an attempt to decrease hepatic toxicity. Finally, the current and fourth stage explores combining this technique with various other approaches
such as surgical resection, systemic chemotherapy, and, as will
be discussed, RFA.

The initial development of intraarterial chemotherapy for metastatic disease to the liver was based on three different features
of hepatic anatomy and physiology that led to the success of this
technique. First, the liver has a dual blood supply, receiving approximately one third of its blood flow from the hepatic arterial
system, and two thirds of the blood flow from the portal venous
system. However, several studies demonstrated that 95% to
100% of blood flow to metastatic disease growing within the
liver is derived from the hepatic artery.[4] The second anatomic
vascular feature is that the hepatic arterial system is very accessible for both interventional radiologists and surgeons. The
gastroduodenal artery branches from the common hepatic artery and provides a suitable conduit for continuous infusion of
agents to the proper common hepatic artery with no other organs being perfused. The third feature of the liver that makes it
amenable to regional chemotherapy is the function of the hepatic parenchyma as the primary organ for drug metabolism.
Pharmacologic studies noted that the liver metabolizes between
95% and 98% of floxuridine (FUDR) infused into the hepatic artery during the first pass of this agent through the hepatic parenchyma.[5] These three features of the liver, combined with the
fact that metastatic colorectal cancer to the liver is a significant
clinical problem, led to the development of treatment of colorectal metastases by intraarterial infusion primarily with FUDR.
The treatment was technically possible and made sense phar-
macologically to significantly increase the drug concentration
and tumor microenvironment. The final step that allowed widespread use of this technique was the development of an im-
plantable infusion device that allowed continuous and defined
treatment.[5] Initial studies of intraarterial infusion therapy relied
on percutaneous catheters being placed, which required patients
to be at strict bed rest during the time periods of treatment.
Clearly, this percutaneous approach, although it did prove the
principle of intraarterial therapy, could not be widely used for
repetitive treatments. The development of the infusion pump
device allowed several phase II studies to be published describing response rates that could not be achieved with systemic
agents at that time.[6,7]

The initial regimen that was adopted as standard treatment using an intraarterial hepatic infusion pump was FUDR delivered at a dose of 0.30 mg/kg/day for 14 days followed by 14 days of saline infusion as a single 4-week treatment cycle. A variety of phase III trials conducted in the 1980s compared this intraarterial therapy to the best available systemic therapy, which was an intravenous 5-FU–based treatment regimen.[8–13] These randomized trials of hepatic arterial infusion have been extensively analyzed, critiqued, and discussed by both proponents of intraarterial therapy and opponents of this regional treatment.[14] The results of these trials are reported in Table 3.3.

Several conclusions can be drawn from these initial phase III studies. First, as predicted, the response rates that can be achieved by intraarterial FUDR greatly exceed what can be achieved by systemic 5-FU for colorectal metastases in the liver. The objective response rates for intraarterial therapy vary between 45% and 68%, whereas the objective response rates for systemic 5-FU regimens are between 11% and 19%.[8–13] Second, in the majority of studies there was no clear translation of this improved response rate into overall survival. Critics of intraarterial hepatic chemotherapy point out that these phase III trials were generally negative studies, and therefore the technique has been shown to have no benefit overall for the patient. The lack of survival benefits has been attributed to the fact that intraarterial therapy delivers no treatment to systemic micrometastases and because this regional treatment causes severe hepatic toxicity that either limits delivery of the treatment or in some cases may contribute to the demise of the patients.

Proponents of regional intraarterial therapy agree that the trials were generally negative in terms of a survival benefit, but attribute that to flaws in design rather than to failure of the treatment. Again, these trials have been analyzed extensively, and there are several design flaws that limit the demonstration of survival benefit. First, these were all single-institution studies and very small numbers of patients were entered, so that the trials were too underpowered to demonstrate modest improvements in survival. Second, patients in the majority of the trials who were randomized to systemic therapy, and then those who failed within the liver were allowed to "cross over" to the intraarterial pump at the time of disease progression.[9,10] By giving patients randomized to the systemic treatment arm the option to receive the experimental arm at the time of progression compromised the ability of these trials to demonstrate a survival benefit. Finally, the initial regimens of intraarterial FUDR were significantly hepatotoxic, and therefore the ability to demonstrate a survival difference was compromised by the inability to deliver the planned intraarterial treatment course. For example, in the study

**Table 3.3 Randomized Trials of Intraarterial (IA) Chemotherapy vs Systemic Chemotherapy for Colorectal Metastases to the Liver**

| Reference | Year | Objective Response Rate | | | Survival (median months) | | |
|---|---|---|---|---|---|---|---|
| | | Systemic (%) | IA (%) | $p$ | Systemic | IA | $p$ |
| 8 | 1987 | 17 | 68 | <.003 | 15 mo | 22 mo | 2-yr survival |
| 9 | 1987 | 20 | 50 | <.001 | NA—crossover | | |
| 10 | 1989 | 10 | 42 | <.0001 | NA—crossover | | |
| 11 | 1990 | 21 | 48 | <0 | 11 mo | 13 mo | N.S. |
| 12 | 1992 | 9 | 43 | NA | 11 mo | 15 mo | .025 |
| 13 | 1994 | | NA | | 7.5 mo | 13.5 mo | <.05 |

NA, not available.

at the University of California at San Francisco (UCSF),[10] the intraarterial therapy treatment was halted in the majority of the intraarterial patients due to hepatotoxicity and not due to progression of disease within the liver.

Each of these problems was addressed in a recent phase III intergroup trial that has reached its accrual goal. First, this multi-institution trial was powered to detect a smaller difference in survival by randomizing a significantly larger number of patients. Second, no crossover therapy was allowed by trial design, and this limitation was stated explicitly in the consent form of this study. Third, this trial utilized second-generation treatment regimens (discussed below), which maintain the response rates but decrease the hepatotoxicity. Again, this trial has reached its accrual goal, but the results of this study have yet to be reported.

The third phase in the development of intraarterial therapy was the refinement of the initial FUDR regimens with the primary goal of decreasing the hepatotoxicity (Table 3.4). There were two single-institution phase II regimens that were designed to address this issue. At UCSF, Stagg and Venook et al[15] made a significant modification in the regimen by significantly decreasing the FUDR dose from 0.3 to 0.1 mg/kg/day and by giving the intraarterial infusional treatment for only 1 week instead of 2 weeks. The patient also received bolus intraarterial 5-FU on days 14, 21, and 28 of a 35-day treatment cycle. The response rates with this second-generation UCSF regimen was 50%, with 0% of patients having biliary sclerosis. Kemeny and colleagues[16] at Memorial Sloan-Kettering Cancer Center modified the initial intraarterial regimen by decreasing FUDR to 0.18 mg/kg/day and

**Table 3.4 Second-Generation Phase II Intraarterial Chemotherapy Regimens for Metastatic Colorectal Cancer to the Liver**

| Regimen | Response Rate (%) | Biliary Sclerosis (%) |
|---|---|---|
| | *First-Generation Regimen* | |
| FUDR 0.3 mg/kg/d × 14 days every 4 weeks[8–13] | 42–68 | 8–50 |
| | *Second-Generation Regimen* | |
| FUDR 0.1 mg/kg/d × 7 days with bolus IA 5-FU 15 mg/kg q y days × 4[15] | 50 | 0 |
| FUDR 0.3 mg/kg/d + dexamethasone 20 mg × 14 days every 4 weeks[16] | 71 | 8 |
| FUDR 0.18 mg/kg/d + leucovorin 200 mg + dexamethasone 20 mg × 14 days every 4 weeks[16] | 75 | 3 |

adding leucovorin and 20 mg of dexamethasone. This regimen was delivered as in the initial trials for 2 weeks of continuous intraarterial infusion and then 2 weeks of heparinized saline, making it a 4-week treatment cycle. Response rates with this new phase II regimen were 78% with a 3% incidence of biliary sclerosis.[16] Even with this second-generation intraarterial protocol, hepatotoxicity was still a significant problem, and the investigators at Sloan-Kettering explained the need to follow liver function tests on a regular basis. Patients receiving either of these regimens need to have the alkaline phosphatase monitored biweekly, and if there is any increase over baseline there needs to be a dose adjustment of the infusion regimen. The vast majority of patients receiving the second generation of the Sloan-Kettering regimen will have either interruption of drug delivery or a dose reduction based on alterations of the alkaline phosphatase. It was this three-drug Sloan-Kettering regimen that was utilized in the recent intergroup study discussed above comparing this treatment to systemic 5-FU.

The fourth phase of intraarterial therapy involves combining this treatment with other categories or types of treatments for metastatic colorectal cancer to the liver. There have been recent reports of phase I and II trials combining intraarterial chemotherapy with systemic chemotherapy, particularly irinotecan.[17] There have been two important recent studies utilizing intraarterial therapy as an adjuvant therapy following surgical resection of gross disease that are discussed below.[18,19] Also, intraarterial chemotherapy has been combined with the ablative techniques of cryosurgery[20] and with the highly specialized technique of isolated hepatic perfusion.[21] Finally, there have been early reports as well as proposed multiinstitution trials combining intraarterial therapy with the relatively new ablative technique of RFA in the success seen when intraarterial therapy is combined with resection surgery.[22,23]

## Current Studies

Two recent studies have evaluated the use of intraarterial hepatic chemotherapy following surgical resection of colorectal metastases[18,19] (Table 3.5). Analyzing these studies in detail is important, as these positive results provide very clear justification of combining intraarterial therapy with the nonresective ablative technique of RFA. Several studies have reported the natural history of metastatic colorectal cancer after complete resection. These studies define the patterns of recurrence or, in other words, show where micrometastatic disease may be in this population of patients with resectable colorectal metastases. Depending on

**Table 3.5 Randomized Trial of Adjuvant Intraarterial Therapy After Hepatic Resection for Colorectal Metastases**

| | Control Arm | Intraarterial Therapy Arm |
|---|---|---|
| **Memorial Sloan-Kettering Cancer Center Trial[18]** | | |
| Regimen | 5-FU 370 mg/m² daily × 5 q 4 weeks Leucovorin 200 mg/m2 daily × 5 q 4 weeks | 5-FU 325 mg/m² + leucovorin 200 mg/m² daily × 5 q 4 weeks FUDR 0.25 mg/kg/day + dexamethasone 20 mg × 14 days q 4 weeks |
| $n$ | 82 | 74 |
| Actual 2-year survival | 72% | 86% ($p = 0.03$) |
| Hepatic 2-year disease-free survival | 60% | 90% ($p < .001$) |
| Estimated median survival | 59 mo | 72.2 mo |
| Overall disease-free survival | 42% | 57% ($p = 0.07$) |
| **Southwest Oncology Group study[19]** | | |
| Regimen | Surgery alone | 5-FU 0.1–0.2 mg/kg/d × 14 days q 4 weeks Leucovorin 200 mg/m²/d IV × 14 days q 4 weeks |
| $n$ (total) | 56 | 53 |
| $n$ (assessable) | 45 | 30 |
| 4-yr hepatic disease-free survival | 43% | 66.9% ($p = 0.03$) |
| 4-yr overall disease-free survival | 25.2% | 45.7% ($p = 0.04$) |
| 4-yr overall survival | 52.7% | 61.5% ($p = 0.06$) |

several variables such as numbers of lesions and disease-free interval, the expected 5-year disease-free survival rate after curative resection of colorectal metastases varies between 20% and 38%.[24–26] In the patients in whom recurrent disease appears, approximately half will have tumors within the liver and the other half will have extrahepatic disease in the lungs, peritoneal cavity, or nodal basins. No trial of systemic adjuvant therapy after complete resection of colorectal metastases to the liver has demonstrated a survival benefit.

Kemeny and Fong's group[18] at Sloan-Kettering randomized patients after complete hepatic resection of colorectal metastases to the liver to systemic 5-FU versus systemic 5-FU plus intraarterial FUDR. There was a significant increase in disease-free survival and overall survival in the patients who received intraarterial therapy. This benefit occurred almost entirely due to the impact of the combined therapy on micrometastatic disease in the liver, as the number of patients recurring systemically were essentially unchanged. All of the benefit in the combined therapy arm appeared to be due to a decrease in disease recurrence in the residual liver, presumably due to the effectiveness of intraarterial therapy. A second study from the Southwest Oncology Group[19] randomized patients following hepatic resection of colorectal cancer to no adjuvant treatment (which is essentially standard therapy) or to a similar experimental regimen of intraarterial FUDR plus systemic 5-FU. This trial also reported a significant improvement in overall survival due to a decrease in hepatic recurrences.

The positive results from these two studies reflects the efficacy of this treatment as well as the natural history of the disease in patients who have colorectal metastases to the liver. As described above, the hepatic intraarterial therapy has very significant response rates against bulky or gross colorectal metastases. As is common in other clinical situations, a chemotherapy regimen that is active against gross disease is often highly efficacious as an adjuvant therapy against micrometastases. The second point of analysis of this trial is the understanding that despite negative preoperative imaging studies and negative intraoperative assessment of the liver by palpation and intraoperative ultrasound, a significant proportion of patients with resectable colorectal metastases in the liver will have micrometastatic disease present in the residual liver that is undetectable. Furthermore, because these trials have shown improvement in survival, this micrometastatic disease in the liver is important in a subgroup of patients in determining their overall outcome.

Understanding the natural history of colorectal metastases to the liver and the demonstrated efficacy of intraarterial therapy for residual micrometastatic disease in the liver provide the impetus for combining RFA and intraarterial infusion regimens. It could be argued that control of hepatic recurrences in the patient population undergoing RFA is even more important than in the patient population undergoing hepatic resection for curative intent. It has been noted by several investigators that one variable that affects prognosis after hepatic resection for colorectal disease is the number of liver metastases. In the patients who are candidates for hepatic resection, some have only a single lesion, and a majority of these surgically resected patients will have less than five metastatic lesions. On the other hand, patients who are being treated currently by RFA for colorectal metastases on average have a larger number of hepatic lesions.[27] By definition, the RFA population is unresectable primarily due to the amount and distribution of colorectal metastases in the liver. The average number of lesions treated may vary between four and six, with in some cases 10 or more nodules treated. Intuitively, these patients with a large number of metastatic colon nodules within the liver would be more likely to have other micrometastases within the untreated liver than would the surgically resected population with fewer hepatic metastases. If that is the case, then effective adjuvant therapy delivered to the liver may be even more important in this situation than in patients undergoing curative resection, in which intraarterial therapy is known to improve survival as described above.

The technical aspects of RFA are also complementary to the technical aspects of placement of an intraarterial infusion pump.[28] For the majority of patients undergoing RFA for colorectal disease, because of the location and number of nodules, an open surgical technique is commonly utilized. The optimal incision to expose the amount of liver necessary for open RFA is a right subcostal incision with a possible extension to the left of midline as needed. This is also the incision that is the optimal for placement of a hepatic arterial infusion pump. The procedure for intraarterial pump insertion involves dissection of the porta hepatis and complete skeletonization of the common hepatic artery, the proper hepatic artery, and the gastroduodenal artery. A cholecystectomy is mandatory at the time of placement of the intraarterial infusion pump, as the gallbladder does not tolerate intraarterial therapy and initial studies showed severe chemical cholecystitis would occur if the gallbladder remained in place. Frequently, cholecystectomy is also needed for RFA of bilobar liver metastases, as any lesions near the gallbladder bed that need treatment require removal of the gallbladder so that no RFA injury to the gallbladder occurs.

The perioperative morbidity from each of these procedures is minimal. The RFA delivered by an open surgical technique has relatively few acute complications, as described in Chapter 8.

Similarly, placement of an intraarterial pump may have some rare vascular complications (e.g., dissection of the gastroduodenal artery) but is generally a low-risk procedure. The primary morbidity from intraarterial chemotherapy as described above is a clinical hepatitis[7,10] that may develop into biliary sclerosis in a small subset of patients later during the administration. Hepatic toxicity by RFA is extremely rare and has not been reported in the noncirrhotic patient population. Even targeting a treatment margin of normal liver tissue between 0.5- and 1.0-cm round metastatic nodules would ablate only a small proportion of the normal hepatic parenchyma.

There has been some variability among the investigators who have utilized this technique in the starting time for intraarterial therapy after RFA. When intraarterial infusion pumps are placed after major hepatic resections as described above in the adjuvant trials, intraarterial infusion does not start until 6 weeks following surgery. This allows the liver tissue to regenerate without the effects of the chemical hepatitis and intraarterial chemotherapy. In patients who undergo placement of intraarterial infusion pumps without hepatic resection, treatment can be started almost immediately upon discharge from the hospital. Combining intraarterial therapy after RFA would be somewhere in between these two situations. However, since RFA has a very minimal impact on normal hepatic parenchyma, the chemotherapy may be started relatively soon after the surgical procedure.

Both RFA of colorectal metastases and placement of intraarterial pumps with FUDR regimens are accepted nonexperimental procedures. For the various reasons described above, several institutions have initiated protocols combining these two treatment modalities. In virtually all of these cases, surgical resection either with major lobar resection or wedge resection is also allowed on these patients. In other words, the treatment strategy is to do a maximal ablation of disease within the liver using RFA and surgical resection as needed. After maximal ablation, an intraarterial infusion pump is placed. Because of the recent development of RFA, patients treated with this combined regimen have not had significant long-term follow-up to make a full assessment of results. It is clear from the early reports that there is no problem in terms of hepatic or systemic toxicity with this combination of RFA and intraarterial therapy.

To assess benefit using this combination of RFA and intraarterial therapy, it is necessary to compare results of these initial phase II trials to historical control data. There is no ideal patient population for comparison to the groups being treated with RFA and intraarterial therapy. If one utilizes the data available from systemic treatment of metastatic colorectal cancer, then there would be a significant proportion of patients with extrahepatic disease. This control population would have a greater disease burden and a lower expected survival than the population being treated in the RFA/intraarterial therapy trials. If one utilizes the historical data for patients who have undergone curative hepatic resection with no adjuvant therapy, this group would by definition have fewer lesions and would have a better prognosis than the patients who are assigned to RFA/intraarterial therapy, as these patients would have unresectable disease. Comparing RFA/intraarterial therapy patients to resected patients therefore would use a patient population that has a better prognosis than the RFA in treated patients as by definition they were resected.

Perhaps the most suitable patient population for comparison to intraarterial therapy/RFA are patients in the phase II trials[15,16] of intraarterial therapy, or patients from the phase III trials who are randomized to the intraarterial therapy group.[8-13] This provides a patient population that has disease limited to the liver from colorectal metastases but who are not resection candidates. The overall survival of these patients in the phase III trials intraarterial therapy arm is shown in Table 3.3 and there is a median survival between 13 and 22 months. Because of the early stage of development of this strategy combined with RFA plus intraarterial therapy, there are no large prospective trials with long-term follow-up to compare to this historical patient population.

There have been two early reports presented in abstract form within the past year of the initial results of combining these two modes of therapy for metastatic colorectal cancer to the liver (Tables 3.6 and 3.7). One report is from M.D. Anderson Cancer Center.[22] These investigators conducted a phase II trial in which all

**Table 3.6 Results of a Phase III Study at M.D. Anderson Combining Radiofrequency Ablation with Intraarterial Chemotherapy for the Treatment of Colorectal Metastases to the Liver[22]**

| | | |
|---|---|---|
| *n* | 31 | |
| Number of patients with a simultaneous liver resection | 17 | 55% |
| Average number of nodules | 2 | |
| Average size of nodules in cm (range) | | 1.8 (0.5–7) |
| Follow-up in months (range) | | 14 (1–31) |
| Proportion of patients: | | |
|   Alive and disease-free | 14 | 45% |
|   Alive with or without disease | 24 | 90% |
|   With recurrence of RFA treated lesion | 3 | 10% |
|   With new hepatic metastases | 11 | 35% |
|   with extrahepatic disease | 9 | 27% |

**Table 3.7 Results of a Phase II Study of the University of Pennsylvania Combining Radiofrequency Ablation and Intraarterial Chemotherapy for the Treatment of Colorectal Cancer Metastases to the Liver**

| | All Patients | Patients with Complete Ablation | Patients with Incomplete Ablation |
|---|---|---|---|
| $n$ | 43 | 23 | 20 |
| Number of nodules ablated with RFA (range) | 2.8 (1–8) | 3.0 (1–8) | 2.4 (2–7) |
| Total number of nodules | 1 to >30 | 1–8 | 2 to >30 |
| Number of patients with simultaneous liver resection | 15 (35%) | 10 (43%) | 5 (25%) |
| Follow-up in months (range) | 18 (5–40) | 18 (5–37) | 18 (6–40) |
| Median survival | 22.3 | 22.3 | 18.4 |

patients had metastatic colon cancer to the liver with no evidence of extrahepatic disease. There was a maximum of six nodules allowed for entry to the trial. Patients underwent exploratory laparotomy and ablation and/or resection of all lesions. Postoperatively, the patients received intraarterial FUDR at a relatively modest dose utilizing the UCSF regimen of 0.1 mg/kg/day for 7 days infusional FUDR followed by bolus 5-FU again at a modest dose of 12.5 mg/kg on days 15, 22, and 29 of the treatment cycle. This bolus dose is 17% less than what was utilized in the phase II study at UCSF. Thirty-one patients were treated, of whom 17 had resection in addition to ablation. The median follow-up was 14 months. The results show that 45% of the patients had no active disease (NAD) at the time of the report, and 10% of patients died from progressive disease during the follow-up (Table 3.6). The authors reported that 10% of the patients had local recurrence of the radiofrequency-treated lesion, which is higher than this same group as reported in terms of local recurrence rate for patients who receive RFA alone without intraarterial infusion. The remainder of the recurrent disease is split between elsewhere in the liver and systemic recurrences.

A similar trial was conducted at the University of Pennsylvania.[23] In this study, there was no maximal limit of number of lesions, but patients who entered the trial were thought able to be fully ablated of gross disease with a combination of RFA and resection based on their preoperative imaging scans. Because the number of nodules was not limited, a large number of patients were found at laparotomy to have relatively diffuse disease that was not possible to completely debulk. Twenty-three patients had complete ablation or resection, and 20 patients had incomplete ablation or resection. As with the M.D. Anderson series, a large number of these patients did have liver resection in conjunction with their ablation treatment. The follow-up was somewhat longer; the median survival of the entire population was 22 months, and the median survival of the patients who had complete ablation was 22.3 months. Patients with incomplete ablation, not surprisingly, had a median survival of 18.4 months. Both of these studies showed relatively low toxicity rates, although these were not discussed in detail.

When these reports are compared to the intraarterial infusion arm from the randomized phase II trials of the late 1980s, the median survival of 22 months in the University of Pennsylvania trial compares favorably to the majority of the reports that have median survivals in the range of 13 to 15 months. It certainly compares favorably to the median survival that is achieved with current systemic chemotherapy. The M.D. Anderson report did not distinctly state a median survival time, but with a median follow-up of 14 months and 90% of the patients still alive, including 45% of the patients who were disease free, one would anticipate the median survival will be well more than 20 months. It will be important for these types of trials to mature and to provide baseline data to plan future phase III studies.

Currently, there are two multiinstitution phase II studies combining RFA plus intraarterial therapy that are similar to the single-institution studies discussed above. Although there will be several single-institution studies from centers with a major interest in treatment of colorectal metastases to the liver that will mature earlier than these multiinstitution studies, these initial phase II efforts are important in describing the toxicity of these regimens when they are widely used in patients at institutions without highly specialized expertise in these areas. One study that is open is an industry-sponsored trial by McMasters in Louisville, Kentucky. In this study, patients must have fewer than 10 separate lesions and must be completely ablated and/or resected in terms of gross disease. A patient will postoperatively receive intraarterial therapy with FUDR using the second-generation Sloan-Kettering regimen. A second study proposed by Tanabe in the American College of Surgeons Oncology group targets a similar patient population, limiting the number of lesions to fewer than six. In contrast to the McMasters study, the study by Tanabe utilizes not only intraarterial FUDR but also systemic irinotecan.

## Phase III Trials

To understand the contribution from either RFA or intraarterial therapy, phase III trials will be needed. The design of these trials is difficult for two major reasons. First, patients who are eligible for these studies have frequently been pretreated with currently available systemic regimens of 5-FU and irinotecan. This variability in pretreatment regimens makes it difficult to plan a control treatment arm or even an experimental treatment arm as patients may have been exposed to and failed the agents in that regimen. The second problem in trial design is the overall issue of whether the hypothesis is to prove the benefit of adding RFA to intraarterial therapy or the benefit of adding intraarterial therapy to RFA ablation techniques. An optimal strategy would be to treat patients with liver-directed therapy with RFA alone, intraarterial therapy alone, and RFA plus intraarterial therapy. The problem with the RFA-alone arm as described above is that there are often minimal opportunities to add meaningful systemic treatment as many of the patients have failed all available systemic agents at the time of registration to this type of protocol. The problem with the intraarterial arm is that RFA is so minimally morbid that many investigators feel that it is irresponsible not to ablate disease during placement of an infusion pump if it can ablate all gross disease. However, to determine the final benefit of these two modalities and how they should be utilized in this large patient population with metastatic colorectal trial will require appropriately designed phase III studies.

## References

1. Saltz LB, Cox JV, Blanke C, et al. Irinotecan plus fluorouracil and leucovorin for metastatic colorectal cancer. N Engl J Med 2000; 343:905–914.
2. Douillard JY, Cunningham D, Roth AD, et al. Irinotecan combined with fluorouracil compared with fluorouracil alone as first-line treatment for metastatic colorectal cancer: a multicentre randomized trial. Lancet 2000; 355:1041–1047.
3. Fraker DL. Regional therapies of cancer. In: Norton JA, Bolinger RR, Chang AE, et al., eds. Surgery: Scientific Basis and Current Practice. New York: Springer-Verlag, 2001:1863–1880.
4. Sigurdson ER, Ridge JA, Kemeny N, Daly JM. Tumor and liver drug uptake following hepatic artery and portal vein infusion in man. J Clin Oncol 1987; 5:1836–1840.
5. Collins JM. Pharmacologic rationale for hepatic arterial therapy. Recent Results Cancer Res 1986; 100:140–147.
6. Neiderhuber JE, Ensminger W, Gyves J, Thrall J, Walker S, Cozzi E. Regional chemotherapy of colorectal cancer metastatic to the liver. Cancer 1984; 53:1336–1343.
7. Venook AP, Warren RS. Regional chemotherapy approaches for primary and metastatic liver tumors. Surg Oncol Clin North Am 1996; 5:411–427.
8. Chang A, Schneider PD, Sugarbaker PH, et al. A prospective randomized trial of regional versus systemic continuous 5-fluorodeoxyuridine chemotherapy in the treatment of colorectal metastases. Ann Surg 1987; 206:685–693.
9. Kemeny N, Daly J, Reichman B, Geller N, Botet J. Oderman P. Intrahepatic or systemic infusion of fluorodeoxyuridine in patients with liver metastases from colorectal carcinoma. Ann Intern Med 1987; 107:459–465.
10. Hohn DC, Stagg RJ, Friedman MA, et al. A randomized trial of continuous intravenous versus hepatic intra-arterial floxuridine in patients with colorectal cancer metastatic to the liver: the Northern California Oncology Group Trial. J Clin Oncol 1989; 7:1646–1654.
11. Martin J, O'Connell M, Wieand H, et al. Intra-arterial floxuridine versus systemic fluorouracil for hepatic metastases from colorectal cancer: a randomized trial. Arch Surg 1990; 125:1022–1027.
12. Rougler PH, Laplanche A, Huguier M, et al. Hepatic arterial infusion of floxuridine in patients with liver metastases from colorectal

carcinoma: long-term results of a prospective randomized trial. J Clin Oncol 1992; 10:1112–1118.

13. Allen-Mersh TG, Earlam S, Fordy C. Quality of life and survival with continuous hepatic artery infusion for colorectal liver metastases. Lancet 1994; 344:1255–1260.

14. Patt YZ. Regional hepatic arterial chemotherapy for colorectal cancer metastatic to the liver: the controversy continues. J Clin Oncol 1993; 11:815–819.

15. Stagg R, Venook A, Chase J, et al. Alternating hepatic intraarterial floxuridine and fluorouracil: a less toxic regimen for treatments of liver metastases from colorectal cancer. J Natl Cancer Inst 1991; 83:423–428.

16. Kemeny N, Conti J, Cohen A, et al. A phase II study of hepatic arterial FUDR, leucovorin, and dexamethasone for unresectable liver metastases from colorectal carcinoma. J Clin Oncol 1994; 12:2288–2295.

17. Kemeny N, Gonen M, Sullivan D, et al. Phase I study of hepatic arterial infusion of floxuridine and dexamethasone with systemic irinotecan for unresectable hepatic metastases from colorectal cancer. J Clin Oncol 2001; 19:2687–2695.

18. Kemeny N, Huang Y, Cohen AM, et al. Hepatic arterial infusion of chemotherapoy after resection of hepatic metastases from colorectal cancer. N Engl J Med 1999; 34:2039–2048.

19. Kemeny MM, Adak S, Gray B, et al. Combined-modality treatment for resectable metastatic colorectal carcinoma to the liver: surgical resection of hepatic metastases in combination with continuous infusion of chemotherapy—an intergroup study. J Clin Oncol 2002; 20:1499–1505.

20. Stubbs RS, Alwan MH, Booth MW. Hepatic cryotherapy and subsequent hepatic arterial chemotherapy for colorectal metastases to the liver. Hepatic Pancreatobiliary Surg 1998; 11(2):97–104.

21. Alexander HR, Bartlett DL, Libutti SK, Fraker DL, Moser T, Rosenberg SA. Isolated hepatic perfusion with tumor necrosis factor and melphalan for unresectable cancers confined to the liver. J Clin Oncol 1998; 16:1479–1489.

22. Scaife CL, Cutley SA, Patt Y, et al. Feasibility of adjuvant hepatic arterial infusion (HAI) of chemotherapy following radiofrequency ablation (RFA) +/− resection in patients with hepatic metastasis from colorectal cancer. Ann Surg Oncol 2002; 9(11):526.

23. Kesmodel SB, Canter RJ, Raz DJ, Bauer TW, Spitz FR, Fraker DL. Survival following regional treatment for metastatic colorectal cancer to the liver using radiofrequency ablation and hepatic artery infusion pump placement. Ann Surg Oncol 2002; 9(11):568.

24. Hughes KS, Simon R, Songhorabodi S, et al. Resection of the liver for colorectal carcinoma metastases: a multi-institutional study of patterns of recurrence. Surgery 1986; 100:278–284.

25. Gayowski TJ, Iwatsuki S, Madariaga JR, et al. Experience in hepatic resection for metastatic colorectal cancer: analysis of clinical and pathological risk factors. Surgery 1994; 116:703–711.

26. Fong Y, Fortner JG, Sun R, Brennan MF, Blumgart LH. Clinical score for predicting recurrence after hepatic resection for metastatic colo-

rectal cancer. Analysis of 1001 consecutive cases. Ann Surg 1999; 230:309–321.

27. Curley SA, Izzo F, Delrio P, et al. Radiofrequency ablation of unresectable primary and metastatic hepatic malignancies: results in 123 patients. Ann Surg 1999; 230:1–8.

28. Fraker DL. Radiofrequency ablation of colorectal metastases to the liver. In: Saltz L, ed. Colorectal Cancer: Multimodality Management. Totowa, NJ: Humana Press, 2002:437–454.

# 4

# Deciding When to Use Resection or Radiofrequency Ablation in the Treatment of Hepatic Malignancies

Mark S. Roh

Malignant involvement in the liver remains the primary determinant of survival in patients suffering from cancer. Adequate control of the hepatic malignancy can prolong survival, and in an increasing number of cases offer the chance for cure. Hepatic resection remains the best chance for cure with 5-year survival rates for colorectal liver metastases of 25% to 40%.[1,2] In patients with metastases, hepatic involvement is a manifestation of systemic disease, and resection represents a regional therapy. Success occurs only when the resection eliminates the last remnant of disease. Persistence of disease upon completion of hepatic resection indicates a failure to provide benefit. The risks of hepatic resection continue to decrease and currently the operative mortality is significantly <5% and morbidity is <15%.[3] Unfortunately, only 10% to 20% of patients are candidates for hepatic resection.[1] The rest are treated with various therapies that do not offer a realistic chance for cure.[4] Increasing the number of patients eligible for surgical management will enhance survival.

Radiofrequency ablation (RFA) is a relatively new treatment modality for hepatic malignancies and is capable of increasing the number of patients undergoing surgical therapy.[5] The indications for utilizing RFA alone in the treatment of hepatic malignancies are not well established and are dependent on the perspective of individual hepatic surgeons. Likewise, the role of RFA in combination with hepatic resection remains to be determined.

Hepatic resection is the gold standard for the treatment of hepatic malignancies, and its indications and results are reviewed here. Proposed indications for the use of RFA alone and in conjunction with other modalities are also discussed. These recommendations have been developed from personal experience but are controversial.

## Hepatic Resection

### Indications

Currently, the indications for hepatic resection are undergoing a critical reassessment. Clinical findings that were previously considered to be contraindications to hepatic resection are being challenged. The indications are categorized as basic, extended, and evolving (Table 4.1). Basic indications are those that are well established and have proven over time to be associated with the best chance for cure. The extended indications represent clinical situations in which adverse prognostic findings are present but a resection is technically feasible. The evolving indications are clinical findings that historically, and in the opinion of the majority of liver surgeons, are still considered contraindications. However, evidence is accumulating that aggressive surgical management has the potential to provide long-term survival.[6–13]

**Table 4.1  Indications for Hepatic Resection**

Basic
  Colorectal primary malignancy
  Solitary metastases
  Unilobar disease
  Tumor <8 cm in diameter
  Location and size permits >1-cm margin
  Normal liver function
  >1-year disease-free interval from primary resection
  CEA <100 ng/mL

Extended
  Noncolorectal primary malignancy
  Multifocal
  Bilobar
  Synchronous metastases
  Location necessitates removal of 80% of liver
  Direct extension into adjacent organs

Evolving
  Presence of resectable extrahepatic disease
  Resection requires reconstruction of vital structures

CEA, carcinoembryonic antigen.

The ultimate success of all oncologic therapy is dependent on the biology of the malignancy. Specific clinical factors can provide insight into the nature of the disease and often predict the likelihood of successful treatment. The majority of patients with a solitary colorectal liver metastasis and a greater than 1 year disease-free interval from the primary resection can be cured of their disease with hepatic resection.[1,2,14,15] The size and location of the metastasis must allow for a tumor-free resection and preservation of an adequate hepatic remnant.[16] Additional favorable factors include the absence of extrahepatic disease, a preoperative carcinoembryonic antigen (CEA) <50 ng/mL, tumor <8 cm, and normal hepatic function.[2,3]

Patients with hepatocellular carcinoma, cholangiocarcinoma, or metastases from other primary sites may also be candidates for hepatic resection, but the success is less certain.[17] Hepatocellular carcinoma in cirrhotic patients has a poorer prognosis due to the high incidence of recurrence and postoperative morbidity. Frequently, the underlying cirrhosis limits the volume of liver that can be safely resected.[12,18–21] These tumors often invade the portal and/or hepatic veins, which adversely affects the chance for cure after hepatic resection. Metastases from other primary sites (breast, lung, stomach, neuroendocrine pancreas, sarcoma) are a manifestation of a systemic disease, and hepatic resection is potentially beneficial only when no other evidence of disease is present.[22–32] Direct extension of a hepatic malignancy into adjacent structures (diaphragm, pericardium, stomach, colon, pancreas) reflects a strategically located tumor with aggressive biology. Tumors may be located within the liver that require resection of 80% of the parenchyma in order to achieve a tumor-free margin. This extensive resection increases the incidence of a positive margin, postoperative hepatic failure, and other postoperative complications.[33]

The presence of extrahepatic disease is an extremely poor prognostic finding and is frequently considered a distinct contraindication. Recent reports have shown that an R0 resection (complete treatment of all visible tumor with an adequate margin) of the extrahepatic disease in conjunction with hepatic resection can provide survival benefit.[34] Strategically located tumors may necessitate resection of vital structures (inferior vena cava, all of the hepatic veins, portal vein) to achieve a tumor-free margin.[6–8,10,12] Reconstruction of the structures increases the morbidity and mortality of the resection.

### Results

Patients with the basic indications for hepatic resection have the best chance for cure following surgery. Patients with metachronous colorectal metastases from a node-negative primary have a

5-year survival of 71%.[2] The survival decreases progressively as the number of metastases increases.[1] Patients with extended indications have a less favorable outcome yet may achieve prolonged survival with resection. Although the majority of these patients are not cured of their disease, significant prolongation of survival can be achieved.[6–8,24] Since alternative therapies have little chance to impact favorably on survival, aggressive surgical treatment is warranted.[4]

## Radiofrequency Ablation

Over the years numerous ablative therapies have been developed to provide local treatment for hepatic malignancies. Most were greeted with initial enthusiasm and eventually were used sporadically after they had been tested further and/or new technologies became available. For many years RFA has been used to treat aberrant cardiac arrhythmias, and within the past 10 years it has been used to treat hepatic malignancies. This technology has essentially replaced cryoablation as the optimal ablative therapy. The operative time is shorter, morbidity is significantly reduced, and the success is equivalent. In addition, RFA can be administered either percutaneously or via a laparoscope. Percutaneous RFA should be used in patients with significant comorbid disease or recurrent or progressive disease.

### Indications

The indications for RFA have not been well established and are still evolving (Table 4.2). The goal is to achieve complete local control of all of the disease within the liver. The ablation must include the entire tumor and surrounding hepatic parenchyma. Incomplete ablation will fail to provide benefit.[35] RFA can be utilized as the primary treatment or in combination with hepatic resection. RFA should also be considered in patients undergoing a

**Table 4.2 Indications for Radiofrequency Ablation**

Unresectable disease

Simultaneous extrahepatic resection

Hepatocellular carcinoma

Absence of vascular invasion

Colorectal liver metastases

Noncolorectal liver metastases

Liver dominant disease

Recurrent disease

simultaneous extrahepatic resection (e.g., colorectal resection, pancreaticoduodenectomy for neuroendocrine tumor, nephrectomy, pelvic exenteration) in order to achieve complete curative therapy.

All patients, regardless of primary diagnosis, should be considered for RFA. The specific diagnosis directly affects how the RFA should be administered. Patients with metastatic disease from noncolorectal primary sites (breast, lung, esophagus, stomach, pancreas, small bowel, etc.) that are not usually considered for operative intervention should still be evaluated for RFA.[36] In these cases, minimally invasive approaches (percutaneous, laparoscopic) can be used to achieve local control of the hepatic disease.[37–40] The risks are minimal and control of the metastases will reduce the tumor burden and may provide benefit.

Patients with unresectable hepatocellular carcinoma due to underlying cirrhosis can benefit from RFA.[41–48] The lesions can be effectively treated despite the presence of portal hypertension and thrombocytopenia. Patients with significant cardiac or pulmonary disease should be evaluated for percutaneous RFA. Other indications are patients with liver disease that is amenable to RFA and patients with minimal extrahepatic disease. Likewise, patients with recurrent hepatic malignancy that is not amenable to resection should be considered for RFA.

The number of metastatic deposits is an important determinant of the eventual success of RFA. All of the disease must be treated, and the greater the number of lesions the higher the likelihood of incomplete therapy. In my opinion, the majority of patients with more than four metastases will have additional disease that is occult and will become evident with time. These patients should undergo chemotherapy or other nonsurgical therapy and be reevaluated in 3 months. If no other hepatic disease can be documented, then RFA should be considered, as long as all of the disease can be treated.

The diameter of the lesions is a critical factor in achieving a successful ablation. Tumors ≤3 cm can be consistently treated with a percutaneous approach. Lesions ≥3 cm require overlapping ablations and an increased chance for incomplete treatment. Lesions ≤5 cm can be effectively ablated when treated at laparotomy. As larger arrays become available, these recommendations are subject to change. RFA can be enhanced by the temporary occlusion of the hepatic vein and/or portal pedicle during treatment. This maneuver reduces the blood flow and eliminates the "heat sink" effect.[49]

The location of the tumors determines the best approach to apply RFA. Malignancies in certain strategic areas of the liver are difficult to access and are inadequately treated by the percutaneous approach. Tumors in segments 1, 2, 4A, and 8 are challenging to accurately localize from a percutaneous perspective. In these instances, RFA should be performed from a laparoscopic or open approach. Lesions located adjacent to the base of the gallbladder should not be ablated as thermal injury to the biliary tract can occur. Tumors near the surface that are adherent to adjacent intestine should not be ablated percutaneously.

## RFA in Conjunction with Hepatic Resection

Proper use of RFA increases the number of patients that are eligible for surgical treatment of the hepatic disease. Deciding how each lesion should be treated remains to be defined. The strengths of each modality should be used to provide maximal benefit to the patient. Number and location of the tumors often limit the opportunity for hepatic resection, but in many cases these limitations do not apply to RFA. Patients with multiple, bilobar disease are unresectable by classic techniques but can be resected when treated in conjunction with RFA. Certain locations (i.e., between right and left/middle hepatic vein, adjacent to anterior/posterior division of the right portal vein with bilobar disease) cannot be resected yet can be effectively treated with RFA.

The decision whether to resect or ablate the disease is based on many factors (Fig. 4.1). Detailed preoperative imaging is mandatory to assess the extent of disease and to design the operative strategy. Whenever possible, all of the liver metastases should be resected. If all of the disease cannot be resected, then the largest and strategically located lesions should be extirpated. Tumors ≥5 cm are optimally treated with resection, as RFA may be inadequate. Adequate hepatic remnant must remain prior to proceeding with a resection. If the remnant is inadequate, then no ablation or resection should be performed. In patients with colorectal liver metastases, a hepatic intraarterial catheter should be inserted into the gastroduodenal artery for regional chemotherapy.

Lesions ≤5 cm in diameter can be effectively ablated provided they are located >5 mm from vital intrahepatic structures. Frequently, multiple overlapping ablations are required to ensure a complete destruction of the tumor and a margin of uninvolved parenchyma. This may still hold true with the use of larger arrays as tumors do not always form in the shape of a sphere. Ablation of tumors located <5 mm from vascular structures (portal and/or hepatic vein) will frequently be incomplete. Vessels adjacent to the treatment area act as a "heat sink" by not allowing the temperature to reach cyctotoxic levels. Significant blood flow compromises the ablation due to an inadequate temperature at the tumor–vessel interface. Tumors located <5 mm from vascu-

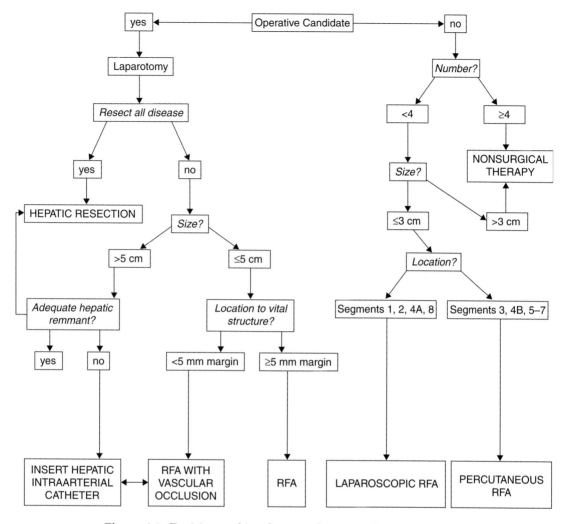

**Figure 4.1.** Decision-making factors when considering ablation.

lar structures can still be effectively treated with RFA in conjunction with vascular occlusion. Interruption of blood flow increases the volume of necrosis and enhances the therapeutic impact. Vascular structures can tolerate extreme temperatures without permanent sequelae. Tumors that are adjacent to major biliary structures should not be ablated due to the high incidence of biliary fistula. Unlike the vascular structures, the bile ducts are unable to tolerate elevated temperatures and will become necrotic.

The long-term effects of RFA are not yet available. With more experience, the indications for using RFA will become apparent. Although beneficial, local tumor control will not be sufficient for long-term survival and will require multimodality therapies.

## References

1.  Fong Y, Cohen A, Fortner J, et al. Liver resection for colorectal metastases. J Clin Oncol 1997; 15(3):938–946.
2.  Scheele J, Stang R, Altendorf-Hofmann A, Paul M. Resection of colorectal liver metastases. World J Surg 1995; 19(1):59–71.
3.  Fong Y, Fortner J, Sun R, et al. Clinical score for predicting recurrence after hepatic resection for metastatic colorectal cancer: analysis of 1001 consecutive cases. Ann Surg 1999;230(3):309–318; discussion 318–321.
4.  Simmonds P. Palliative chemotherapy for advanced colorectal cancer: systematic review and meta-analysis. Colorectal Cancer Collaborative Group. BMJ 2000; 321:521–522.
5.  Elias D, Debaere T, Muttillo I, et al. Intraoperative use of radiofrequency treatment allows an increase in the rate of curative liver resection. J Surg Oncol 1998; 67(3):190–191.
6.  Madariaga J, Fung J, Gutierrez J, et al. Liver resection combined with excision of vena cava. J Am Coll Surg 2000; 191(3):244–250.
7.  Lodge J, Ammori B, Prasad K, Bellamy M. Ex vivo and in situ resection of inferior vena cava with hepatectomy for colorectal metastases. Ann Surg 2000; 231(4):471–479.
8.  Hemming A, Langham M, Reed A, et al. Resection of the inferior vena cava for hepatic malignancy. Am Surg 2001; 67(11):1081–1087; discussion 1087–1088.
9.  Habib N, Michail N, Boyle T, Bean A. Resection of the inferior vena cava during hepatectomy for liver tumours. Br J Surg 1994; 81(7):1023–1024.
10. Hardwigsen J, Baque P, Crespy B, et al. Resection of the inferior vena cava for neoplasms with or without prosthetic replacement: a 14-patient series. Ann Surg 2001; 233(2):242–249.
11. Melendez J, Ferri E, Zwillman M, et al. Extended hepatic resection: a 6-year retrospective study of risk factors for perioperative mortality. J Am Coll Surg 2001; 192(1):47–53.
12. Wu C, Hsieh S, Chen J, et al. An appraisal of liver and portal vein resection for hepatocellular carcinoma with tumor thrombi extending to portal bifurcation. Arch Surg 2000; 135(11):1273–1279.
13. Nakagohri T, Konishi M, Inoue K, et al. Extended right hepatic lobectomy with resection of inferior vena cava and portal vein for intrahepatic cholangiocarcinoma. J Hepatobiliary Pancreat Surg 2000; 7(6):599–602.
14. Sato T, Konshi K, Yabushita K, et al. The time interval between primary colorectal carcinoma resection to occurrence of liver metastases is the most important factor for hepatic resection. Analysis of total course following primary resection of colorectal cancer. Int Surg 1998; 83(4):340–342.
15. Scheele J, Altendorf-Hofmann A, Grube T, et al. Resection of colorectal liver metastases. What prognostic factors determine patient selection? Chirurg, 2001; 72(5):547–560.
16. Seiler C, Redaelli C, Schmied B, et al. Liver resection for liver metastases—1998 Bern Symposium. Swiss Surg 2000; 6(4):164–168.
17. Gouillat C, Manganas D, Saguier G, et al. Resection of hepatocellu-

lar carcinoma in cirrhotic patients: long-term results of a prospective study. J Am Coll Surg 1999; 189(3):282–290.

18. Okusaka T, Okada S, Nose H, et al. The prognosis of patients with hepatocellular carcinoma of multicentric origin. Hepatogastroenterology 1996; 43(10):919–925.

19. Matsuda M, Fujii H, Kono H, Matsumoto Y. Surgical treatment of recurrent hepatocellular carcinoma based on the mode of recurrence: repeat hepatic resection or ablation are good choices for patients with recurrent multicentric cancer. J Hepatobiliary Pancreat Surg 2001;8(4):353–359.

20. Lise M, Bacchetti S, Da Plan P, et al. Prognostic factors affecting long term outcome after liver resection for hepatocellular carcinoma: results in a series of 100 Italian patients. Cancer 1998; 82(6):1028–1036.

21. Abdel-Wahab M, Sultan A, el-Ghawalby A, et al. Is resection for large hepatocellular carcinoma in cirrhotic patients beneficial? Study of 38 cases. Hepatogastroenterology 2001; 48(39):757–761.

22. Selzner M, Morse M, Vredenburgh J, et al. Liver metastases from breast cancer: long-term survival after curative resection. Surgery 2000; 127(4):383–389.

23. Seifert J, Weigel T, Gonner U, et al. Liver resection for breast cancer metastases. Hepatogastroenterology 1999; 46(29):2935–2940.

24. Pocard M, Pouillart P, Asselain B, Salmon R. Hepatic resection in metastatic breast cancer: results and prognostic factors. Eur J Surg Oncol 2000; 26(2):155–159.

25. Ochiai T, Sasako M, Mizuno S, et al. Hepatic resection for metastatic tumours from gastric cancer: analysis of prognostic factors. Br J Surg 1994; 81(8):1175–1178.

26. Maksan S, Lehnert T, Bastert G, Herfarth C. Curative liver resection for metastatic breast cancer. Eur J Surg Oncol 2000; 26(3):209–212.

27. Lang H, Nussbaum K, Kaudel P, et al. Hepatic metastases from leiomyosarcoma: a single-center experience with 34 liver resections during a 15-year period. Ann Surg 2000; 231(4):500–505.

28. Karavias D, Tepetes K, Karatzas T, et al. Liver resection for metastatic non-colorectal non-neuroendocrine hepatic neoplasms. Eur J Surg Oncol 2002; 28(2):135–139.

29. Kalil A, de Lourdes Pereira B, Brenner M, Pereira-Lima L. Liver resections for metastases from intraabdominal leiomyosarcoma. HPB Surg 1999; 11(4):261–264.

30. Grazi G, Cescon M, Pierangeli F, et al. Highly aggressive policy of hepatic resections for neuroendocrine liver metastases. Hepatogastroenterology 2000; 47(32):481–486.

31. Elias D, Lasser P, Montrucolli D, et al. Hepatectomy for liver metastases from breast cancer. Eur J Surg Oncol 1995; 21(5):510–513.

32. De Matteo R, Shah A, Fong Y, et al. Results of hepatic resection for sarcoma metastatic to liver. Ann Surg 2001; 234(4):540–547; discussion 547–548.

33. Scheele J, Rudroff C, Altendorf-Hofmann A. Resection of colorectal liver metastases revisited. J Gastrointest Surg 1997; 1:408–422.

34. Jaeck D, Nakano H, Bachellier P, et al. Significance of hepatic pedicle lymph node involvement in patients with colorectal liver metastases: a prospective study. Ann Surg Oncol 2002. 9:430–438.

35. Siperstein A, Garland A, Engle K, et al. Local recurrence after laparoscopic radiofrequency thermal ablation of hepatic tumors. Ann Surg Oncol 2000; 7(2):106–113.

36. Iannitti D, Dupuy D, Mayo-Smith W, Murphy B. Hepatic radiofrequency ablation. Arch Surg 2002; 137(4):422–426; discussion 427.

37. Chung M, Wood T, Tsioulias G, et al. Laparoscopic radiofrequency ablation of unresectable hepatic malignancies. A phase 2 trial. Surg Endosc 2001; 15(9):1020–1026.

38. Iannitti D, Dupuy D. Minimally invasive management of hepatic metastases. Semin Laparosc Surg 2000; 7(2):118–128.

39. Livraghi T, Goldberg S, Solbiati L, et al. Percutaneous radiofrequency ablation of liver metastases from breast cancer: initial experience in 24 patients. Radiology 2001; 220(1):145–149.

40. Wood T, Rose D, Chung M, et al. Radiofrequency ablation of 231 unresectable hepatic tumors: indications, limitations, and complications. Ann Surg Oncol 2000; 7(8):593–600.

41. Buscarini L, Buscarini E, Di Stasi M, et al. Percutaneous radiofrequency ablation of small hepatocellular carcinoma: long-term results. Eur Radiol 2001; 11(6):914–921.

42. Curley S, Izzo F, Delrio P, et al. Radiofrequency ablation of unresectable primary and metastatic hepatic malignancies: results in 123 patients. Ann Surg 1999; 230(1):1–8.

43. Curley S, Izzo F, Ellis L, et al. Radiofrequency ablation of hepatocellular cancer in 110 patients with cirrhosis. Ann Surg 2000; 232(3): 381–391.

44. Lencioni R, Cioni D, Bartolozzi C. Percutaneous radiofrequency thermal ablation of liver malignancies: techniques, indications, imaging findings, and clinical results. Abdom Imaging 2001; 26:345–360.

45. Montorsi M, Santambrogio R, Bianchi P, et al. Laparoscopic radiofrequency of hepatocellular carcinoma (HCC) in liver cirrhosis. Hepatogastroenterology 2001; 48(37):41–45.

46. Nicoli N, Casaril A, Marchiori L, et al. Treatment of recurrent hepatocellular carcinoma by radiofrequency thermal ablation. J Hepatobiliary Pancreat Surg 2001; 8(5):417–421.

47. Podnos Y, Henry G, Ortiz J, et al. Laparoscopic ultrasound with radiofrequency ablation in cirrhotic patients with hepatocellular carcinoma: technique and technical considerations. Am Surg 2001; 67(12):1181–1184.

48. Poggi G, Gatti C, Cupella F, et al. Percutaneous US-guided radiofrequency ablation of hepatocellular carcinomas: results in 15 patients. Anticancer Res 2001; 21(1B):739–742.

49. Moriyasu F. Radiofrequency ablation therapy and blood flow in hepatocellular carcinoma. Cancer J 2000; 6:S351–355.

# 5

# Laparoscopic Radiofrequency Ablation of Liver Tumors

Eren Berber and Allan E. Siperstein

The management of primary and metastatic tumors of the liver continues to be a challenge for physicians. Primary liver cancer is rare in the United States, whereas colorectal cancer is responsible for up to 75% of liver metastases. Of 160,000 new cases of colorectal carcinoma in the U.S. each year, approximately 40,000 will develop liver metastases. Liver metastases develop in 5% to 90% of patients with neuroendocrine tumors that, in contrast to most metastatic adenocarcinomas, have an indolent course, which may be dominated by symptoms related to the hormonal activity.[1–3]

Although surgery is the "gold standard" for treating liver tumors, most of these patients are excluded from resectional therapy due either to bilobar or multifocal disease within the liver, or to the presence of extrahepatic disease. Since medical therapy has a limited benefit, regional treatment methods have emerged as alternative treatment options. Radiofrequency ablation (RFA) is indicated for (1) unresectable primary or metastatic liver tumors; (2) predominant liver disease with minor additional extrahepatic disease; and (3) enlarging liver lesions, worsening of symptoms, or failure to respond to other treatment modalities. We use the following criteria to select the patients for RFA: (1) not more than eight liver lesions, (2) less than 20% of total liver volume replaced with tumor, (3) largest lesion smaller than 8 cm in diameter, and (4) normal biliary ductal diameters.

## Technique

Laparoscopic RFA is performed under general endotracheal anesthesia. Cefazolin 1 g is used for surgical prophylaxis. The patient is positioned supine on the operating table; however, the left decubitis position, with the table slightly flexed, is used in selected patients with disease limited to the posterior segments of the right lobe. Two 11-mm trocars are placed beneath the right costal margin for the laparoscope and the laparoscopic ultrasound transducer (Fig. 5.1). The abdominal cavity is entered under direct view using an optical access trocar.[4] It is not necessary to take down the falciform, triangular, or coronary ligaments; however, perihepatic adhesions from prior abdominal surgeries need to be taken down using endoscissors or the ultrasonic scalpel. Any adherent viscera that may be close to the zone of ablation should also be identified, and dissected away from the liver if necessary. If lesions encroach upon the gallbladder fossa, the gallbladder should also be removed prior to ablation, so as to avoid thermal injury to the wall of the gallbladder with delayed bile leakage.

First, diagnostic laparoscopy is performed to rule out widespread abdominal carcinomatosis that would be a contraindication for the procedure. The diaphragm, abdominal wall, omen-

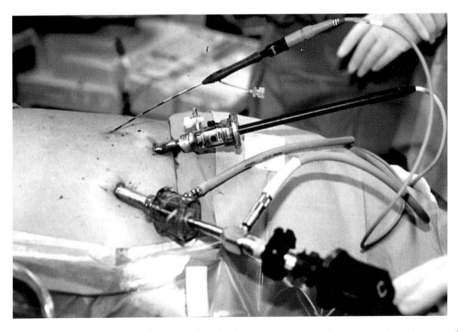

**Figure 5.1.** Placement of subcostal trocars for the laparoscope and laparoscopic ultrasound transducer. The radiofrequency ablation catheter is placed through a separate percutaneous puncture.

tum, viscera, and pelvic cavity are inspected for the presence of metastases not evident on preoperative imaging studies. For some tumor types, the finding of limited amounts of extrahepatic disease is not a contraindication to proceed with ablation.

Next, laparoscopic ultrasonography of the liver is performed using a high-frequency laparoscopic transducer. We prefer a 10-mm rigid, linear, side-viewing transducer. The liver parenchyma is scanned by moving the transducer linearly from the cephalad to caudad aspects of the liver and the lesions are mapped out. Contact scanning is usually adequate to scan the liver without using any intermediate medium. However, if the curvature at the dome does not allow for adequate contact between the transducer and the liver parenchyma, the use of saline as a stand-off medium can be helpful to characterize the superficial lesions at these locations. Each lesion is thus assigned a liver segment by tracing the portal and hepatic vein branches. The use of a picture-in-picture box to superimpose a quarter-sized laparoscopic image over the full-sized ultrasound image is helpful to coordinate the movement of the laparoscopic ultrasound transducer with the laparoscopic image. Once the lesions are identified, core biopsies of representative lesions are obtained with an 18-gauge spring-loaded biopsy gun with an echogenic needle tip using the free-hand technique. Tissue diagnosis is confirmed via frozen section. It is most useful to insert the biopsy needle in parallel and within the plane of the ultrasound transducer, so that the entire path of the needle can be visualized as it traverses the liver parenchyma. Adjustment of the angle of insertion is done if the needle is off target. Before proceeding with ablation, the lesion sizes are measured and tumor vascularity is assessed using Doppler color flow.

Initially, we used the first-generation RFA technology, which consisted of the RITA Medical Systems (Mountainview, CA) model 500 generator and the model 30 (four-prong) or model 70 (seven-prong) 3-cm-diameter thermal ablation catheters with thermocouples at the tip of the prongs. This technology allowed for the ablation of 3.5- to 4-cm-diameter spherical tumor tissue per cycle by running the radiofrequency (RF) generator in a temperature-controlled mode with an average target temperature of 105°C and maximum power of 50 W. Once the catheter tip was positioned at the center of the intended ablation zone, curved prongs were deployed that deliver RF electrical energy to the tissues and affix the catheter in place (Fig. 5.2). Thermocouples mounted within the tips of the deployed prongs are used to monitor tissue temperature as the ablation proceeds, and these readings are also used to regulate the amount of energy delivered via the catheter. With this setup, each cycle of ablation was maintained for a period of 5 minutes, with the overall ablation cycle

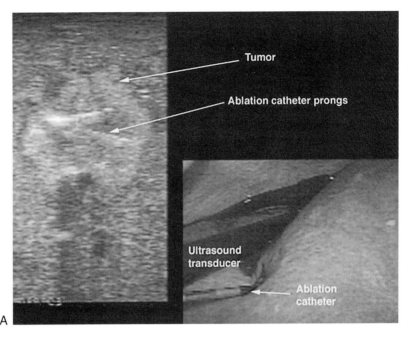

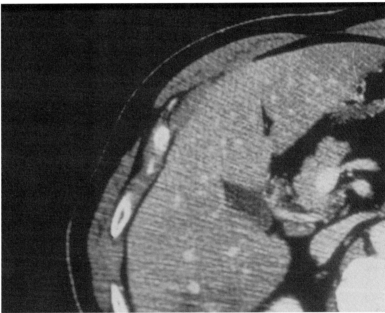

**Figure 5.2.** A picture-in-picture box is useful to show the laparoscopic and the ultrasound image on the same screen. (A) This intraoperative capture demonstrates the deployment of the ablation catheter inside the tumor under laparoscopic ultrasound guidance. (B) Then ablation is started and nitrogen outgassing is seen within the tumor treated. This hypoechoic image thus obtained can be used to assess the ablation margins around the tumor.

taking between 7 and 10 minutes. A single cycle of ablation was adequate for tumors ≤3 cm in diameter; however, for tumors >3 cm in diameter, multiple overlapping thermal ablation zones were required to achieve an adequate tissue margin.

In patients with large tumors, this technique was cumbersome, in that surgery was lengthy and exquisite skill was required during catheter repositionings to encompass all tumor margins. Since 2000, we have used the second-generation RFA technology: a 5-cm, nine-array ablation catheter with a 150-W generator (RITA Medical Systems, Mountainview, CA; StarBurst™ XL thermal ablation catheter, and the model 1500 generator). The catheter consists of a 14-gauge needle, 25 cm in length. The catheter deploys one straight prong along the axis of the catheter, four curved prongs around the "equator," and four curved prongs around the "northern hemisphere." The prong at the center and the four prongs going to the equator have thermocouples at the tips for monitoring temperature during ablation for feedback control of power delivery, and after power has been turned off to measure the actual temperature in the ablated tissues. The catheter is targeted into the center of the tumor through a skin puncture without using an additional trocar. The generator is run at the "average temperature" mode with the target temperature set to 105°C. Different sizes of ablation zones are obtained by starting with an initial catheter deployment (e.g., 2 or 3 cm), advancing the catheter to the desired size, and maintaining ablation for a certain time at each deployment length. For a 5-cm ablation, the time at target temperature ranges between 14 and 20 minutes in various ablation algorithms (Fig. 5.3). Once the programmed ablation time is over, the power is turned off to determine the tissue temperature with the continued monitoring of the thermocouples. In the first 10 to 20 seconds, the temperature of the metal prongs decreases rapidly by 20° to 30°C to equilibrate with the surrounding tissue. This decrease in temperature then proceeds at a slower rate as heat is dissipated from the zone of ablation. Thermocouple temperatures in the 60° to 70°C range 1 minute after the ablation process has ceased indicates that a successful ablation has been performed. Tumors ≤3 cm are ablated with a single 3-cm ablation, and those between 3 and 4 cm with a single 4-cm ablation cycle. Tumors <5 cm are treated with one cycle of a 5-cm ablation and larger tumors may require two to four cycles of ablation to obtain adequate margins.

The ablation process is assessed in three ways. The first and most crucial is monitoring of thermocouple temperatures during and after the ablation process. The second is the observation of outgassing of dissolved nitrogen into the heating tissues (Fig. 5.2). As the tissues are heated, the solubility of dissolved nitro-

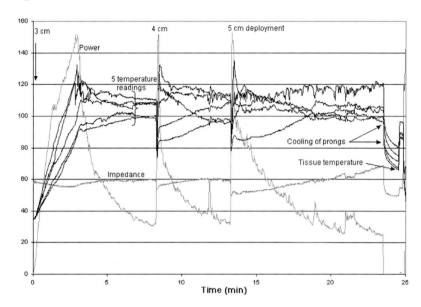

**Figure 5.3.** Line graph showing the temperature (black lines), power (gray line), and impedance (gray line) profiles during the ablation process. The generator has a computer connection that allows for the display of the power (in watts), impedance (in ohms), and temperature at the tip of the prongs (in degrees Celsius) on the computer screen. The current graph shows the data during a 5-cm ablation cycle. When the catheter is deployed to 3 cm initially, the maximum power of 150 W and the average target temperature of 105°C are reached in a few minutes, and then the power starts to decrease. After 5 minutes, the prongs are deployed to 4 cm without changing the original position of the catheter, and the power automatially increases to 150 W again. After another 5 minutes, the catheter is deployed to 5 cm, which causes the power to again increase to 150 W to attain the target temperature. The ablation is continued at this position for 10 to 15 minutes. At the end of this time period, the power is turned off, allowing the prongs to cool down and equilibriate with the tissue temperature. In this case, the tissue temperature is read to be above 60°C, which is above the lethal range.

gen decreases, resulting in microbubble formation within the tissue. This appears as an echogenic blush that enlarges to encompass the zone of ablation. In those tumors that demonstrate tumor flow preablation, color flow Doppler is repeated postablation to demonstrate the absence of blood flow within the ablated zones.

Two grounding pads on the anterior aspect of the right and left thigh are used during the procedure. Skin temperature under one of the grounding pads is monitored via a temperature sensor placed under the leading edge of the pad. If the temperature goes above 40°C, the delivered power is decreased to 100 W for that cycle or the ablation cycle is interrupted for a couple of minutes until the temperature cools down. Bleeding from the needle track is rarely a problem on withdrawal of the needle. Nevertheless, the needle track may be coagulated with 20 to 30 W of power during withdrawal of the needle. Important ablation parameters (the maximum power, time on target temperature, total ablation time, impedance, and the temperatures at the tip of the five thermocouples) are displayed on the front panel of the generator. These data are also displayed graphically on a laptop screen using a special software enabling real-time monitorization of the ablation.

Now available are 7-cm ablation catheters that work on a somewhat different principle in that hypertonic saline is infused in the active prongs into the tissues. This improves the conductance of electricity into the tissues by two means. First the local cooling effect of the solvent prevents desiccation around the electrode, allowing higher power (200 W) to be used. Second, the ionic nature of the hypertonic saline diffusing locally around the metal electrodes increases the virtual surface area of the electrode, again allowing more power and larger lesions to be formed. For this device, additional "passive" prongs that do not deliver electricity are used to monitor temperature at the periphery of the ablated zone.

Informed consent is obtained before the procedure. Patients require only routine care in the postoperative period without any requirement for narcotics in most. Those patients not undergoing a concomitant surgical procedure are discharged within 24 hours. In our series, laparoscopic thermal ablation was performed on all identified lesions, and this treatment did not preclude any subsequent chemotherapy or other treatment modalities. In a number of patients who developed new or recurrent liver disease in follow-up, laparoscopic RFA was applied repeatedly (up to three times in one patient with neuroendocrine liver metastases) to maintain local tumor control in the liver.

Laboratory studies consist of a complete blood count (CBC), renal panel, liver function panel, serum albumin, prothrombin time (PT), partial thromboplastin time (PTT), and tumor markers obtained preoperation, postoperation, and 1 week after the operation. Quality of life is assessed using the SF-36 questionnaire. Radiologic studies include plain chest films and triphasic (noncontrast, arterial, and portal-venous) computed tomography (CT) scans obtained 1 week before and 1 week after the thermal ablation procedure (Fig. 5.4). The patients were followed up by repeating the questionaire and the laboratory and radiologic studies every 3 months.

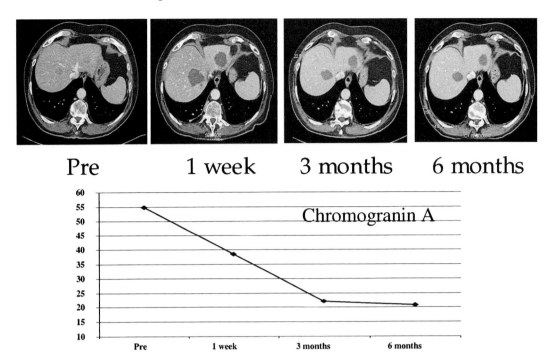

**Figure 5.4.** Figure showing the computed tomography (CT) and tumor marker response of a 72-year-old man with two carcinoid liver metastases. CT scans demonstrate an ablated area larger than the original tumors in the postoperative 1 week scan due to ablation of a rim of normal tissue around the tumors. In serial follow-up scans, the lesions show a reduction in tumor size and volume, accompanied by a dramatic decrease in serum chromogranin A levels.

## Results

Between January 1996 and December 2001, 254 patients (159 men and 95 women) with 913 liver primary and secondary tumors underwent laparoscopic RFA. Patient age, mean ± standard deviation (SD), was 58 ± 14 years. Laparoscopic radiofrequency thermal ablation was successfully completed in all patients. Thirty-six patients (14%) with 62 lesions (7%) had primary liver cancer and 218 patients with 851 lesions had metastatic liver cancer. The majority (110 patients, 43%) had colorectal liver metastases. Other types of metastases included neuroendocrine tumors in 51 patients (20%), and various types of adenocarcinoma and sarcoma in 38 (15%) and 18 (7%) patients, respectively (Fig. 5.5). Twenty percent of patients had one or more lesions seen by laparoscopic ultrasound, but not seen by preoperative triphasic CT scans. The average number of lesions treated per patient was 3.6 and ranged from 1 to 16. Tumor diameter, mean ± standard error of the mean (SEM), was 2.6 ± 0.2 cm (range 0.5–10.2 cm).

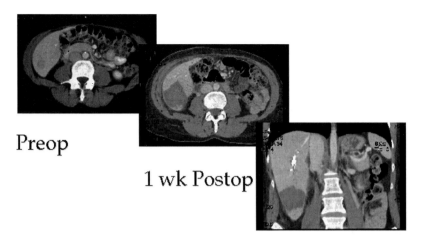

Preop

1 wk Postop

**Figure 5.5.** Computed tomography (CT) scans of a patient who underwent radiofrequency thermal ablation of a single 2-cm liver metastasis from colon adenocarcinoma in segment VI. CT scans obtained 1 week after the procedure showed an ablation zone of 5.6 cm. The CT reconstructions made in the coronal plane demonstrated the spherical nature of the ablation zone. The clips seen within the liver are from a prior bilobar resection.

With a 3-, 4-, and 5-cm deployment, the 1 week postablation maximum lesion CT diameter was found to be $3.5 \pm 0.1$ cm (mean $\pm$ SEM), $4.2 \pm 0.2$ cm, and $5.3 \pm 0.1$ cm, respectively. Ninety-six percent of the lesions were larger in the postablation CT scans compared to the preablation scans (mean lesion diameter 4.1 cm versus 2.2 cm, respectively) due to the ablation of a rim of normal liver tissue around them. A progressive decline in lesion size was seen in 88% of the lesions followed for at least 3 months (mean 13.9 months, range 4.9–37.8 months) suggesting resorption of the ablated tissue. At a mean follow-up of 12 months, there was a 12% local failure rate with larger adenocarcinomas and sarcomas at greatest risk. Failures occurred early in follow-up, with most occurring by 6 months. Predictors of failure included a lack of increased lesion size at 1 week, adenocarcinoma or sarcoma, larger tumors (failures, 18 cm$^3$, versus successes, 7 cm$^3$), and vascular invasion on laparoscopic ultrasound.

In neuroendocrine patients, amelioration of symptoms was obtained in 95% with significant or complete symptom control in 80% for a mean of 10+ months (range 6–24 months). Survival after diagnosis of primary disease, detection of liver metastases, and performance of RFA was $5.5 \pm 0.8$ years (mean $\pm$ SEM), $3.0 \pm 0.3$ years, and $1.6 \pm 0.2$ years, respectively. Sixty-five percent of the patients demonstrated a partial or significant decrease in their tumor markers in follow-up.

There was no mortality. Complications were observed in seven patients (2.8%) including liver abscess in two patients (treated with percutaneous drainage in one and antibiotics in the other), and transient atrial fibrillation, pulmonary embolism, postprocedure pain requiring admission, angioedema-urticaria, and recurrent ascites in one patient each.[5–9]

In 16% of the patients, RFA was performed in combination with other procedures including laparoscopic cholecystectomy, colon and small bowel resections, open liver resections, ventral hernia repairs, and various oncologic minor procedures. The morbidity was not increased in these procedures, and recovery was determined by the convalescence from the concomitant procedure. Although patients undergoing laparoscopic RFA in combination with a clean-contaminated procedure could be at high risk for secondary infection of ablated foci, this was not observed.[10]

## Identifying Ablated Tumor in Postablation CT Scans

Often the interpretation of the postablation CT scans is difficult because the actual lesion remains in place. At times the change in morphology is quite subtle, particularly if the tumor is hypodense compared to the liver parenchyma before any ablative therapy. The density of the tissues on a CT image is measured in Hounsfield units (HU), which represent an arbitrary scale with air at $-1000$ units, water at 0, and bone at $+1000$ to $+2000$ units. A lack of increase in HU density with contrast injection indicates necrotic tissue, whereas perfused tissue shows an increase in HU density. We previously reported that the liver parenchyma shows a similar amount of enhancement with contrast injection compared to the noncontrast phase in both pre- and postablation CT scans (mean $\pm$ SEM 56.4 $\pm$ 2.4 vs 57.1 $\pm$ 2.4 HU, respectively, $p =$ .3). In contrast, ablated liver lesions show a preablation enhancement of 45.7 $\pm$ 3.4 HU with contrast injection but only a minimal step-up of 6.6 $\pm$ 0.7 HU ($p < .0001$) in postablation triphasic CT scans. This is an objective means of identifying ablated tissue after the procedure.[11]

## Discussion

Laparoscopic RFA is a promising safe and effective treatment modality for patients with primary and metastatic liver malignancies. It provides excellent local tumor control with overnight hospitalization and low morbidity for otherwise untreatable lesions. Laparoscopic ultrasonography is a critical part of the procedure, as it enables identification and targeting of the lesions, and monitorization of the ablation process. Technically, it is the most chal-

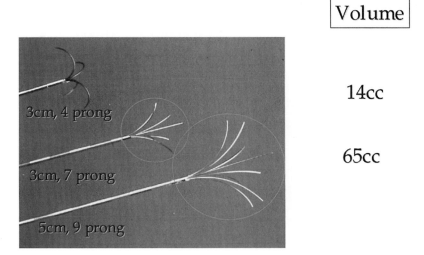

Figure 5.6. Radiofrequency thermal ablation catheters. The first-generation catheters could deploy out to 3 cm and had four or seven prongs. The second-generation catheters have nine prongs and can deploy out to 5 cm. An increase in the catheter deployment from 3 to 5 cm causes the ablation volume to increase dramatically from 14 to 65 cc (4.6-fold).

lenging part of the procedure. With the development of larger ablation catheters (Fig. 5.6) and more powerful RF generators, it has been possible to ablate large sizes of tumors with a decreased need for overlapping ablations, theoretically decreasing the risk of local recurrence. In fact, using the newer technology, 87% of the lesions in our series were ablated with a single ablation cycle. Still, the general principles of RFA should be followed, and lesions near the major bile ducts in the porta hepatis should be approached with caution to avoid a possible bile duct injury. Triphasic CT scans are essential for documenting objective tumor responses, and can also objectively identify ablated tumor with the use of HU density measurements.

It is very important that the radiofrequency thermal ablation procedure be done with minimal morbidity in these advanced-stage cancer patients with already depressed immune systems. In this regard, laparoscopic surgery is superior to open surgery as it is associated with a lesser degree of immune suppression,[12] shorter hospital stay, and faster recovery. Compared to percutaneous RFA, the laparoscopic approach enables the imaging of the entire liver, more precise targeting, abdominal staging, and treatment of peripheral tumors.

Radiofrequency ablation technology is rapidly evolving. The determinance of long-term survival and performance of randomized clinical studies will better establish the role of RFA in the treatment of liver tumors. In our experience, the application of laparoscopic RFA with a debulking intent in a large number of patients resulted in significant palliation of symptoms, especially in neuroendocrine liver metastases, and also rendered the other types of metastasis more susceptible to other treatment modalities such as systemic chemotherapy. These results underscore the concept of palliative liver ablation for patients with liver metastases who are not a candidate for surgical resection. Our patient population and results also support RFA of liver tumors as a palliative liver surgery model. Another important advantage of laparoscopic RFA is that it can be applied multiple times during the disease course, analogous to chemotherapy, to obtain local tumor control without increasing the morbidity of the procedure.

## References

1. Berber E. Liver cancer and resection. In: Ponsky J, ed. The Cleveland Clinic Guide to Surgical Patient Management. St. Louis: Mosby, 2001:151–158.
2. Siperstein AE, Berber E. Cryoablation, percutaneous alcohol injection, and radiofrequency ablation for treatment of neuroendocrine liver metastases. World J Surg 2001; 25(6):693–696.
3. Silverberg E, Boring CC, Squires TS. Cancer statistics, 1990 [see comments]. CA Cancer J Clin 1990; 40(1):9–26.
4. String A, Berber E, Foroutani A, Macho JR, Pearl JM, Siperstein AE. The use of the optical access trocar for safe and rapid entry in various laparoscopic procedures. Surg Endosc 2000; 14(S1):S220.
5. Foroutani A, Garland AM, Berber E, et al. Laparoscopic ultrasound vs triphasic computed tomography for detecting liver tumors. Arch Surg 2000; 135(8):933–938.
6. Berber E, Flesher NL, Siperstein AE. Initial clinical evaluation of the RITA 5-centimeter radiofrequency thermal ablation catheter in the treatment of liver tumors. Cancer J 2000; 6(S4):S319–329.
7. Siperstein A, Garland A, Engle K, et al. Local recurrence after laparoscopic radiofrequency thermal ablation of hepatic tumors. Ann Surg Oncol 2000; 7(2):106–113.
8. Siperstein A, Garland A, Engle K, et al. Laparoscopic radiofrequency ablation of primary and metastatic liver tumors. Technical considerations. Surg Endosc 2000; 14(4):400–405.
9. Berber E, Flesher NL, Siperstein AE. Laparoscopic radiofrequency ablation of neuroendocrine liver metastases. World J Surg 2002; 26(8):985–990.
10. Berber E, Senagore A, Rogers AM, Herceg N, Costa N, Siperstein AE. Laparoscopic radiofrequency ablation of liver tumors combined with other surgical procedures (abstract). 8th World Congress of Endoscopic Surgery, March 13–16, 2002, New York.
11. Berber E, Foroutani A, Garland AM, et al. Use of CT Hounsfield unit density to identify ablated tumor after laparoscopic radiofrequency ablation of hepatic tumors. Surg Endosc 2000; 14(9):799–804.
12. Vittimberga FJ Jr, Foley DP, Meyers WC, Callery MP. Laparoscopic surgery and the systemic immune response. Ann Surg 1998; 227(3):326–334.

# 6

# Radiofrequency Ablation of Hepatocellular Carcinoma

Steven A. Curley and Francesco Izzo

Local control of primary hepatic malignancies in patients with only liver disease is an ongoing quest for surgeons and oncologists. Treatment of primary hepatic malignancies with systemic or regional chemotherapy rarely results in a durable complete response, and the toxicities of these treatments and adverse impact on the patients' quality of life can be substantial. Surgical resection or complete tumor ablation still provides patients with the best opportunity for long-term disease-free and overall survival.

Hepatocellular carcinoma (HCC) is one of the most common solid cancers in the world, with an annual incidence estimated to be at least one million new patients.[1] Surgical resection of HCC can result in significant long-term survival benefit in 20% to 35% of patients.[2,3] Unfortunately, only 5% to 15% of newly diagnosed HCC patients undergo a potentially curative resection.[2,3] Patients with disease confined to the liver may not be candidates for resection because of multifocal disease, proximity of tumor to key vascular or biliary structures that precludes a margin-negative resection, potentially unfavorable biology with the presence of multiple liver metastases, or inadequate functional hepatic reserve related to coexistent cirrhosis. Thus, for the majority of patients with primary hepatic malignancies confined to the liver who are not candidates for surgical resection, novel treatment approaches to control and potentially cure the liver disease must be explored.

Localized application of thermal energy produces destruction of tumor cells. When tumor cells are heated above 45° to 50°C, intracellular proteins are denatured and cell membranes are destroyed through dissolution and melting of lipid bilayers.[4,5] Radiofrequency ablation (RFA) is a localized thermal treatment technique designed to produce tumor destruction by heating tumor tissue to temperatures that exceed 60°C.

## Background and Basics of Radiofrequency Tissue Ablation

The earliest recorded use of heat to treat tumors comes from Egyptian and early Greek descriptions of medical practice when superficial tumors were subjected to cautery.[6] In general, thermal injury to cells begins at 42°C, with the exposure times to low-level hyperthermia needed to achieve cell death ranging from 3 to 50 hours depending on the tissue type and conditions.[7] As one increases the temperature above 42°C, there is an exponential decrease in the exposure time necessary for a cytodestructive response. For example, only 8 minutes at 46°C is needed to kill malignant cells, and 51°C can be lethal after only 2 minutes.[8,9] At temperatures above 60°C, intracellular proteins become denatured, lipid bilayers melt, and cell death is inevitable.[10] Interestingly, malignant cells are more resistant to lethal damage from freezing compared to normal cells, but are more sensitive to hyperthermic damage than normal cells.[11,12]

The use of radiofrequency (RF) energy to produce thermal tissue destruction has been the focus of increasing research and practice for the past several years.[13–18] During the application of RF energy, a high-frequency alternating current moves from the tip of an electrode into the tissue surrounding that electrode. As the ions within the tissue attempt to follow the change in the direction of the alternating current, their movement results in frictional heating of the tissue (Fig. 6.1). As the temperature within the tissue becomes elevated beyond 60°C, cells begin to die, resulting in a region of necrosis surrounding the electrode.[19] A typical RFA treatment results in local tissue temperatures that exceed 100°C, which produces coagulative necrosis of the tumor tissue and surrounding hepatic parenchyma. The tissue microvasculature is completely destroyed, and thrombosis of hepatic arterial, portal venous, or hepatic venous branches <3 mm in diameter occurs. Only tissue through which RF electrical current passes directly is heated above a cytotoxic temperature. The geometry of the RF current pathway around the ablation electrode creates a relatively uniform zone of radiant/conductive heat within the first few millimeters of electrode–tissue interface. The conductive heat emitted from the tissue radiates out from the electrode, and if the tissue impedance is relatively low, a dynamic expanding zone of ablated tissue is created. The final size

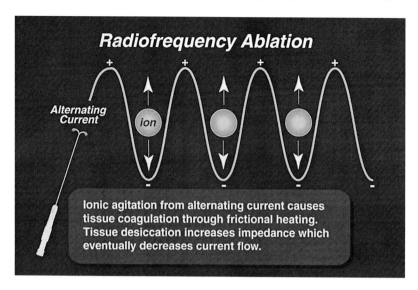

**Figure 6.1.** An alternating electrical current is passed across the electrode array at the tip of a radiofrequency needle (lower left), resulting in ionic agitation and heating in the tissue surrounding the electrode array. As coagulative necrosis gradually develops in the tissue, tissue impedance rises, leading to reduction and eventual cessation in current flow from the radiofrequency generator.

of the region of heat-ablated tissue is proportional to the square of the RF current, also known as the RF power density. The RF power/current delivered via a monopolar electrode decreases in proportion to the square of the distance for the electrode. Therefore, the tissue temperature falls rapidly with increasing distance away from the electrode.

The decrease in tissue heating with increasing distance away from the electrode results in only 1.0- to 1.5-cm cylindrically shaped zones of coagulative necrosis of tissue when using monopolar simple needle electrodes. New needles (13- to 15-gauge diameter) have been developed with multiple array hook electrodes (Fig. 6.2). The insulated needle electrode shaft is placed into the tumor with the array retracted. Using real-time ultrasound guidance, the array is then deployed from the needle tip into the tumor. These deployed multiple array hooks create a series of electrodes with a diameter of 2.0 to 5.0 cm, across which the RF current can be passed. The multiple array electrode is a technologic innovation that permits ablation of much larger zones of tissue compared to simple needle electrodes.

An RF needle electrode is advanced into the unresectable liver tumor via a percutaneous, laparoscopic, or open (laparotomy) route. The needle electrode we have used most frequently is a 14-gauge, 15 to 25 cm long insulated cannula containing 12 individual hook-shaped electrode arms or tines with a maximum

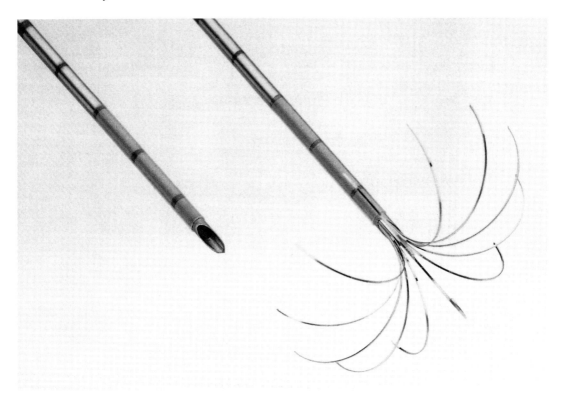

**Figure 6.2.** Insulated shaft 14-gauge radiofrequency needle electrodes showing the multiple array retracted into the needle sheath (left) and fully deployed from the needle tip (right). The 10 individual tines of the multiple array are clearly seen with the array deployed to the full 4.0-cm diameter.

diameter of 4.0 cm when completely deployed. Using transcutaneous or intraoperative ultrasonography to guide placement, the needle electrode is advanced to the targeted area of the tumor and then the individual wires or tines of the electrode are deployed into the tissues. Once the tines have been deployed, the needle electrode is attached to an RF generator, and two dispersive electrodes (return or grounding pads) are placed on the patient, one on each thigh (Fig. 6.3). The RF energy is then applied following an established treatment algorithm (Fig. 6.4). Tumors less than 2.5 cm in their greatest diameter can be ablated with the placement of a needle electrode with an array diameter of 3.5 to 4.0 cm when the electrode is positioned in the center of the tumor. Tumors larger than 2.5 cm require more than one deployment of the needle electrode. For larger tumors, multiple placements and deployments of the electrode array may be necessary to completely destroy the tumor (Fig. 6.5). Treatment is planned such that the zones of coagulative necrosis overlap to ensure complete destruction of the tumor. Typically, the array is first placed at the most posterior interface between the tumor and nondiseased liver parenchyma, and then the needle is repositioned and

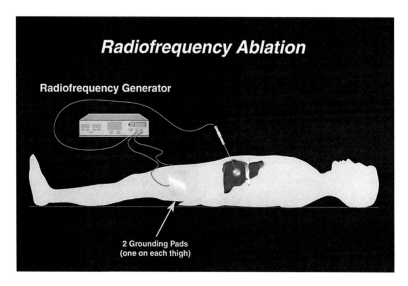

**Figure 6.3.** A schematic diagram showing a radiofrequency needle electrode with the multiple array deployed in a liver tumor. The white area represents the tumor, and the surrounding gray zone represents the larger area of coagulative necrosis produced by the radiofrequency energy transmitted from the generator. Grounding pads are placed on both thighs of the patient, which allows the alternating current of radiofrequency energy to move between the needle electrode and the grounding pads. The resulting ionic stimulation produces frictional heating and coagulative necrosis of the tumor and tissue surrounding the needle electrode.

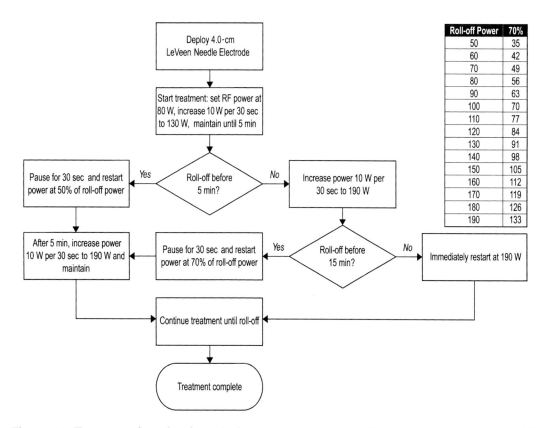

**Figure 6.4.** Treatment algorithm for radiofrequency ablation of malignant liver tumors using a 4.0-cm-diameter LeVeen multiple array needle electrode and a 200-W radiofrequency (RF) generator.

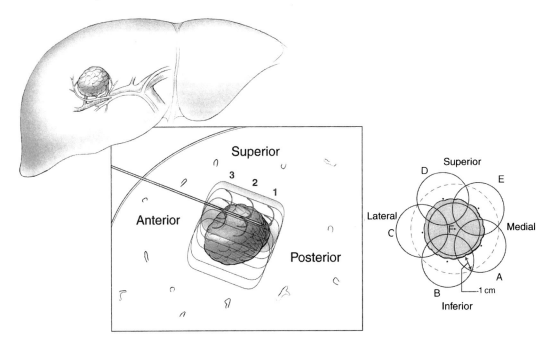

**Figure 6.5.** A schematic illustration of a 5-cm-diameter malignant tumor in the right lobe of the liver. The upper illustration shows the tumor in relation to the portal venous and hepatic arterial inflow blood supply to the tumor and the surrounding hepatic parenchyma. The inset illustration is a sagittal view showing the multiple overlapping cylinders of radiofrequency (RF)-induced thermal ablation that must be created to assure complete destruction of the tumor and a surrounding zone of normal hepatic parenchyma. The first areas treated are the more medial aspects of the tumor (A and B in far right illustration, superior view) to destroy this region of the tumor and its inflow blood supply. The needle electrode is placed sequentially at the margin of the tumor in the normal parenchyma so that part of the secondary multiple array is opened within the tumor and part is in the surrounding hepatic parenchyma. As demonstrated in the central inset illustration, the needle is first placed at the posterior interface of tumor and normal parenchyma (area 1). After this area has been completely treated, the array is retracted and the needle is pulled back to area 2, and the array is deployed and treatment performed. Finally, the more anterior or superficial interface between tumor and parenchyma is treated (area 3) to produce a cylinder-shaped zone of coagulative necrosis. The far right illustration shows an idealized view looking directly down on the tumor to emphasize the RF treatment planning. Overlapping cylinders of thermal ablation are created to destroy the entire tumor and a 1-cm zone of surrounding hepatic parenchyma. Included is the sequence of needle electrode placements (A–F); treat first the aspects of the tumor adjacent to its inflow blood supply (A, B).

the array is redeployed anteriorly at 2.0- to 2.5-cm intervals within the tissue. To mimic a surgical margin in these unresectable tumors, the needle electrode is used to produce a thermal lesion that incorporates not only the tumor but also nonmalignant liver parenchyma in a zone 1 cm wide surrounding the tumor (Figs. 6.3 and 6.5). Computed tomography (CT) scans performed after RFA of primary or metastatic liver tumors initially demonstrate a cystic-density lesion larger than the original tumor (Fig. 6.6); the size of this cystic area decreases slightly over time.

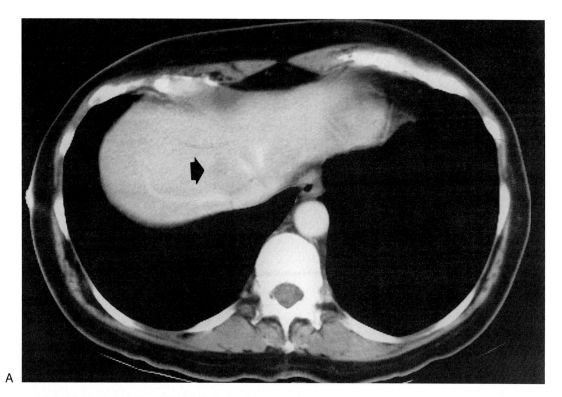

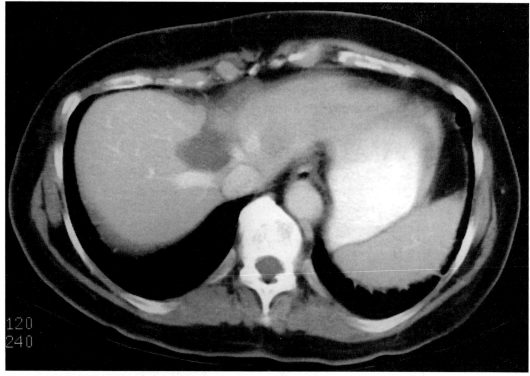

**Figure 6.6.** (A) Computed tomography (CT) scan of a patient with hepatocellular cancer (arrow) and Childs's class B cirrhosis secondary to chronic hepatitis C virus infection. (B) CT scan performed 3 months after radiofrequency ablation shows the size of the zone of thermal ablation to be larger than the original tumor.

## Indications for Radiofrequency Ablation of HCC

Radiofrequency energy to produce coagulative necrosis in hepatic malignancies has been used in patients who did not meet the criteria for resectability of HCC and yet were candidates for a liver-directed procedure based on the presence of liver-only disease.[13–18,20] The selection of patients to be treated with RFA is based on rational principles and goals. Any local therapy for malignant hepatic tumors, be it surgical resection, RFA, or some other tumor ablative technique, is generally performed with curative intent, but a significant proportion of patients subsequently develop clinically detectable hepatic or extrahepatic recurrence from their coexistent micrometastatic disease. Thus, we perform RFA only in patients with no preoperative or intraoperative evidence of extrahepatic disease. From a tumor biology and behavior perspective, it is unlikely that RFA of more than three or four HCC tumors will result in a survival benefit for the patient, so we do not treat patients with ultrasonographically discrete tumors exceeding these numbers. Finally, RFA can be used to treat patients with a solitary HCC in a location that precludes a margin-negative hepatic resection, such as a tumor nestled between the inferior vena cava (IVC) and the entrance of the three hepatic veins into the IVC (Fig. 6.7). Our group has successfully treated tumors abutting major hepatic or portal vein branches because the blood flow acts as a heat sink that protects the vascular endothelium from thermal injury while allowing complete coagulative of tissue immediately surrounding the blood vessel wall.[21] The only area of the liver we avoid treating with RFA is the hilar plate where the portal vein and hepatic arterial branches enter the liver. While these blood vessels can tolerate the RFA treatment, the large bile ducts coursing with them do not tolerate heat and biliary fistulae or strictures would occur after RFA. RFA-induced biliary injury can be avoided by excluding patients with tumors involving the perihilar region.

Given the limitations of currently available RFA equipment, we do not recommend RF treatment for tumors >6.0 cm in diameter. The local recurrence rate in larger tumors is much higher and represents incomplete coagulative necrosis of malignant cells near the tumor periphery. New RFA equipment is being developed to treat larger hepatic tumors. This equipment must be assessed over time to determine the adequacy of treatment.

When considering patients for a combined approach of liver resection of large tumors and RFA of smaller lesions in the opposite lobe, standard surgical considerations apply. Thus, an adequate volume of perfused, functional hepatic parenchyma must remain to avoid postoperative liver failure. The volume of liver that must remain varies from patient to patient, depending on

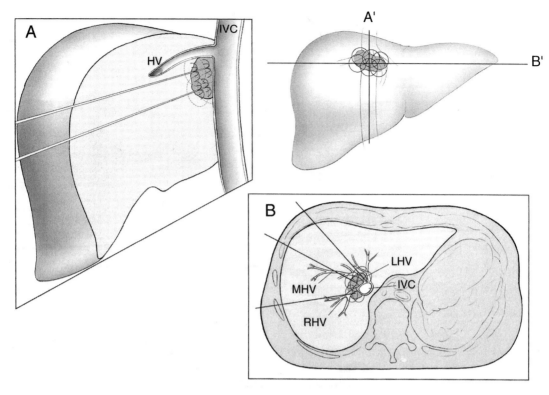

**Figure 6.7.** Illustration of a malignant hepatic tumor abutting the inferior vena cava (IVC) and nestled under the right, middle, and left hepatic veins (RHV, MHV, LHV). (A) Sagittal section. (B) Axial section. (A) Sagittal view of the tumor lying on the IVC and abutting a hepatic vein. Multiple insertions of the radiofrequency (RF) ablation needle electrode are required with the secondary multiple array opened just outside the IVC first, and then sequentially withdrawn to treat the more anterior aspects of tumor. (B) Axial view, with lines indicating the multiple placements of the RF needle electrode to produce thermal ablation of the entire tumor and a surrounding zone of hepatic parenchyma. Blood flow in the IVC and hepatic veins prevents thermal destruction or thrombosis of these major vessels.

the presence of normal liver versus diseased liver related to chronic hepatitis virus infection, ethanol abuse, or some other cause of chronic hepatic inflammation leading to cirrhosis. RFA does not replace standard hepatic resection in patients wtih resectable disease. Rather, RFA expands the population of patients who may be treated with aggressive liver-directed therapy in attempts to improve survival, quality of life, and/or palliation. Some patients who heretofore were not candidates for surgical therapy because of bilobar liver tumors now can be treated with a combination of liver resection and RFA. Other patients with tumor(s) inopportunely located at an unresectable site involving major blood vessels in the liver may be candidates for RFA. RFA is also ideally suited to treat small HCCs in cirrhotic patients who may not be candidates for resection based on the severity of their liver dysfunction.[22] We are currently conducting a randomized, prospective trial comparing resection, RFA, and percutaneous ethanol injection in cirrhotic HCC patients to determine the efficacy, safety, and long-term survival rate after treatment with these three techniques.

## Radiofrequency Ablation Treatment Approaches

Radiofrequency ablation of liver tumors can be performed percutaneously, using laparoscopic guidance, or as part of an open surgical procedure. The choice of treatment approach is individualized in any given patient. In general, patients with one to three small (<3.0 cm diameter) cancers located in the periphery of the liver are considered for ultrasound-guided percutaneous RFA. Lesions located high in the dome of the liver near the diaphragm are not always accessible by a percutaneous approach. Furthermore, general anesthesia or monitored sedation is required for most patients treated percutaneously because of pain associated with the heating of tissue near the liver capsule. Patients treated percutaneously are usually discharged within 24 hours of their RFA. A percutaneous approach has been most commonly used in our patients with small, early-stage HCC with coexistent cirrhosis.

A laparoscopic approach offers the advantages of laparoscopic ultrasonography, which provides better resolution of the number and location of liver tumors, and a visual survey of the peritoneal cavity to exclude the presence of extrahepatic disease. Using laparoscopic ultrasound guidance, the RFA needle electrode is advanced percutaneously into the target tumor(s) for treatment. The laparoscopic ultrasound permits more precise positioning of the RF needle multiple array near major blood vessels. Our group uses a laparoscopic approach for patients with no prior history of extensive abdominal operations, and one or two liver tumors <4.0 cm in diameter located centrally in the liver near major intrahepatic blood vessels.

The majority of patients in our studies underwent RFA of hepatic tumors during an open surgical procedure.[17,20] This is our preferred approach in patients with large tumors (>4.0- to 5.0-cm diameter), multiple tumors, if tumor abuts a major intrahepatic blood vessel, or if a laparoscopic approach is impractical because of dense postsurgical adhesions. In contrast to percutaneous RFA treatments, it is possible to perform temporary occlusion of hepatic inflow during the intraoperative RFA procedure. Hepatic inflow occlusion facilitates RFA of large or hypervascular tumors, such as HCCs and tumors near blood vessels. The amount of blood flow to a tumor is known to be a critical determinant of temperature response to a given increment of heat.[23,24] Because heat loss or cooling effect is principally dependent on blood circulation in a given area, temperature response and blood flow are inversely related. By temporarily occluding hepatic inflow during RFA, the cooling effect of blood flow on perivascular tumor cells is minimized.[25] The inflow occlusion increases the size of the zone of coagulative necrosis and enhances the likelihood of complete tumor cell kill, even if the tumor abuts a major intrahepatic blood vessel. Our previous preclinical work demonstrated that RFA treatment combined with vascular inflow occlusion can produce complete circumferential necrosis of tissue around major portal or hepatic vein branches without damaging the integrity of the vessel wall.[21] Another reason we frequently choose an open approach is the ability to combine resection of tumors too large to ablate in one lobe with RFA of smaller tumors in the opposite lobe.

## Radiofrequency Ablation of Primary Liver Tumors

The use of RFA to treat primary and metastatic liver tumors in patients from the University of Texas M.D. Anderson Cancer Center in Houston, Texas, and the G. Pascale National Cancer Institute in Naples, Italy, has been reported recently.[17,22] The sizes of HCCs addressed in this patient population ranged from 1 to 7 cm in their greatest dimension (Table 6.1). As the size of the tumor increased, the number of deployments of the needle electrode and the total time of applying RF energy increased (Table 6.1). Primary liver tumors tend to be highly vascular, so a vas-

**Table 6.1 The Number of Deployments of a Radiofrequency Ablation (RFA) Multiple Array Needle Electrode and Total Elapsed Time to Achieve Complete Tumor Ablation in Patients with Hepatocellular Carcinomas (HCCs) of Varying Diameters[21]**

| Greatest Diameter of Liver Tumor (cm) | No. of Tumors Treated | Mean Number of Deployments of the Needle Electrode Array | Mean Elapsed Time to System-wide Impedance[b] (minutes) |
|---|---|---|---|
| 0.1 to 1.0 | 2 | (1 to 2)[a] | 13 (8 to 20) |
| 1.1 to 2.0 | 14 | (2 to 4) | 19 (15 to 33) |
| 2.1 to 3.0 | 14 | (2 to 5) | 27 (17 to 35) |
| 3.1 to 4.0 | 17 | (4 to 8) | 49 (36 to 71) |
| 4.1 to 5.0 | 7 | (5 to 9) | 83 (47 to 95) |
| >5.0 | 3 | (6 to 12) | 94 (56 to 110) |

[a]Values in parentheses are ranges of the measurements.
[b]Total time needed to complete radiofrequency ablation of tumor.

cular heat sink phenomenon may contribute to the extended ablation times.

All 110 HCC patients in our recent study have been followed for a minimum of 12 months after RFA; the median follow-up is 19 months.[22] Percutaneous or intraoperative RFA was performed in 76 (69%) and 34 patients (31%), respectively. A total of 149 discrete HCC tumor nodules were treated with RFA. Median diameter of tumors treated percutaneously (2.8 cm) was smaller than that of lesions treated during laparotomy (4.6 cm), $p < .01$. Local tumor recurrence at the RFA site developed in four patients (3.6%); all four subsequently developed recurrent HCC in other areas of the liver. New liver tumors or extrahepatic metastases developed in 50 patients (45.5%), but 56 patients (50.9%) have no evidence of recurrence.

Procedure-related complications were minimal in patients with HCC. There were no treatment-related deaths, but complications developed in 12.7% of the HCC patients.[22] These complications included symptomatic pleural effusion, fever, pain, subcutaneous hematoma, subcapsular liver hematoma, and ventricular fibrillation. In addition, one patient (with Childs's class B cirrhosis) developed ascites, and another class B cirrhotic patient developed bleeding in the ablated tumor 4 days after RFA, requiring hepatic arterial embolization and transfusion of two units of packed red blood cells. All patient events resolved with appropriate clinical management within 1 week following the RFA procedure, with the exception of the development of ascites, which resolved with use of diuretics within 3 weeks of the RFA treatment. No patient developed thermal injury to adjacent organs or structures, hepatic insufficiency, renal insufficiency, or coagulopathy following the application of RF energy into the target tumors. The overall complication rate following RFA of HCCs was low, which is particularly notable because there were 50 Childs's class A, 31 class B, and 29 class C cirrhotic patients treated.

For HCC patients, serum liver function tests (e.g., alanine aminotransferase, aspartate aminotransferase, and γ-glutamyltransferase) were elevated two- to fourfold above baseline values immediately following the procedure, but for most patients these values returned to baseline levels within 7 days, and for all patients the values returned to baseline within 1 month after the procedure. The serum tumor marker $\alpha$-fetoprotein (AFP) was elevated in 71% of the patients prior to the application of RF energy, but 1 month later it was noted to have returned to normal levels in 66% of the patients. All but one of the patients in whom these markers did not decrease after the procedure eventually developed new clinically detectable metastases in other regions of the liver or at distant organ sites, demonstrating the high incidence of multifocality and intrahepatic subclinical metastases in HCC patients.

## Radiofrequency Ablation Compared to Other Local Ablation Techniques

Cryoablation has been used to treat otherwise unresectable primary liver cancers. Studies have demonstrated that liver tumors must be cooled to at least $-35°C$ throughout the entire tumor to achieve a reliable tumor cell kill.[26,27] Tumor cell death is not a direct consequence of lowering tissue temperature, but rather is caused by ice crystal formation during rapid freezing, with resultant destruction of normal cellular structures. To ensure adequate cryoablation, most tumors are treated with two freeze/thaw cycles to maximize this mechanical disruption of tumor cells. The low temperature necessary for tumor cell destruction with cryoablation is difficult to achieve at the periphery of tumors larger than 5 to 6 cm in diameter, when the tumor abuts a major intrahepatic branch of the portal or hepatic veins, or if it lies near the inferior vena cava.

Complications described after hepatic cryoablation include a mortality rate of 1.6%, significant intraoperative hemorrhage, cold injury in adjacent organs, biliary fistulae, coagulopathy, thrombocytopenia, myoglobinuria, acute renal failure, intrahepatic abscess in the cryolesion, and symptomatic pleural effusions.[26–29] The overall reported complication rates after cryoablation range from 15% to 60%, with an average of 45%.[29] We have compared treatment-related serious complications in patients treated with hepatic tumor cryoablation or RFA.[30] Clinically significant RFA treatment-related complications developed in <4% of our patients, and while there were no deaths at the time of that report, we have now had a single RFA-related death (mortality rate 0.3%). There were no episodes of heat injury to adjacent organs, renal failure, coagulopathy, intrahepatic abscess, symptomatic pleural effusion, or intraoperative bleeding. In contrast, we noted a 2% mortality rate and a 41% clinically significant complication rate in our patients treated with cryoablation.[30] These complications included renal failure requiring dialysis, abscess in the cryoablated tumor, symptomatic pleural effusion, and postoperative coagulopathy.

The small diameter of the RFA needle electrodes and the treatment-induced tissue coagulation explains the minimal, if any, bleeding associated with this treatment. In contrast, the mean blood loss reported during cryoablation operations is up to 750 ml, and as many as one third of patients require blood transfusions.[27,31,32] Intraoperative hemorrhage may occur from the 3- to 15-mm-diameter cryoprobe track or from liver surface cracking during thawing of the iceball.[27,33–35] Liver suturing or packing is required to control hemorrhage in most of these cases. Thrombocytopenia and consumptive coagulopathy are not uncommon after hepatic cryoablation and can be the cause of delayed hemorrhage in the treated lesion or at distant sites.[27,33,35] Thrombocytopenia or coagulopathy did not develop in any of our RFA patients. The complete coagulation of tumor and the surrounding hepatic microvasculature by RFA seems to prevent the rapid release of necrotic cellular products into the circulation, and thus explains the absence in our RFA patients of myoglobinuria, tumor lysis syndrome, and renal dysfunction that has been reported after cryoablation.[27–29,34] An abscess has been reported to develop in the necrotic, cryoablated liver tumor in 3% to 20% of the treated lesions.[29,35–37] In contrast, we have had a single abscess develop in an RFA-treated tumor (in a patient with an indwelling biliary endostent) with a total experience of over 600 tumors treated with RFA (0.2% incidence rate).

The largest published series using cryotherapy to treat HCC in 235 patients reported that there were no treatment-related deaths, but complications and local recurrence in the cryoablated tumors was not reported.[38] This study is also difficult to interpret because cryotherapy alone was used in only 78 patients (33.2%). The majority of patients were treated with cryotherapy plus hepatic artery ligation, transarterial chemoembolization, hepatic artery infusion chemotherapy, or resection of the frozen tumor. Our group has abandoned cryotherapy to treat primary or metastatic liver tumors based on our finding of a significantly higher local tumor recurrence rate with cryoablation compared with RFA (13.6% vs. 2.2%, respectively, $p < .01$) and a much higher complication rate following cryoablation (40.7% vs. 3.3%, respectively, $p < .001$).[30]

Other local therapies have been employed to treat HCC. Direct image-guided intratumoral injection of absolute ethanol has been used extensively around the world. Percutaneous ethanol injection (PEI) is usually performed with transabdominal ultrasonographic guidance with the tumor injected with 5 to 10 mL of ethanol twice a week. The volume of ethanol required to ablate the tumor is estimated based on the diameter of the HCC. For tumors less than 2 cm in size, three to five injection sessions are required, while five to eight sessions are necessary for tumors 2 to 3 cm in diameter.[39] A study of 207 HCC patients with tumors less than 5 cm in diameter treated with PEI was performed in Italy.[40] The HCC was solitary in 162 patients and multiple in 45 patients. In the 162 patients with solitary tumors, the 1-year survival rate following PEI was 90%, and the 3-year survival rate was 63%. In contrast, the 3-year survival rate in patients with multiple tumors injected with ethanol was only 31%. Patient compliance with PEI has been a problem because of the multiple injections required and the pain associated with the treatment, but serious complications such as intraperitoneal hemorrhage, hepatic insufficiency, bile duct necrosis or biliary fistula, hepatic infarction, and hypotension occur in less than 5% of patients.[41] Local recurrence rates have been reported infrequently in most studies of PEI. Most reports mention that local recurrence is common in tumors greater than 5 cm in diameter and recommend that PEI not be used to treat such large HCCs.[39–41] Furthermore, a recent report of PEI in HCC patients with tumors less than 3 cm in diameter found a local recurrence rate of 38%.[42] After a 3-year follow-up of all patients, HCCs had recurred locally or at other intrahepatic sites in 81% of the patients.[42] Because PEI required multiple treatment sessions and was associated with a high local recurrence rate, the authors recommended that PEI be considered only for tumors less than 1.5 cm in diameter and that all other patients with small HCCs be treated with resection or other definitive, single-treatment ablation techniques, like RFA.

Heat ablation of liver tumors can also be performed using microwave coagulation therapy or laser-induced thermotherapy.[43–45] Like RFA, these procedures can be performed during an open laparotomy, with laparoscopic or thoracoscopic guidance, or percutaneously. The effectiveness of these treatments is currently limited by the small zones of necrosis achieved with the rapid heating and desiccation of the tissue around the microwave or laser probes. Multiple insertions of the probes are required to treat tumors more than 1 cm in diameter with microwave coagulation therapy, or more than 2 cm in diameter with laser-induced thermal ablation.[43–45] Currently, the treatment complexity of placing multiple intratumoral probes and the cost for these microwave or laser systems (at least 10 times higher than RF generators and needle electrodes) is limiting the clinical utility of these alternative thermal ablation techniques.

## Summary

The use of RF energy to treat unresectable liver tumors is unlikely to be curative for most patients; however, a subset of patients treated with RFA may achieve long-term disease-free survival. Longer follow-up of hepatic tumor patients treated with RFA is needed to determine long-term disease-free and overall survival rates. New metastatic tumors develop in many of these patients at an incidence rate comparable with those treated with surgical resection or cryoablation. Surgical resection remains the gold standard for treating primary liver tumors; however, few patients are candidates for hepatic resection because of tumor size, number, location, or the presence of cirrhosis too severe to permit liver resection. Cryoablation of unresectable tumors has been an option for several years, but complications associated with the freezing of tissue can be problematic. RFA of unresectable liver tumors provides a relatively safe, highly effective method to achieve local disease control in some liver cancer patients who are not candidates for liver resection. Ongoing research and refinements in RF techniques and equipment may permit effective treatment of larger liver tumors and of malignant tumors at other body sites. Combining RFA of liver tumors with regional and/or systemic adjuvant treatments is being studied in attempts to reduce the incidence of development of new metastases, and thus improve the overall survival rates of these patients.

## References

1. Di Bisceglie A, Rustgi V, Hoofnagle J, et al. NIH conference on hepatocellular carcinoma. Ann Intern Med 1988; 108:390–401.
2. Liver Cancer Study Group of Japan. Primary liver cancer in Japan: clinicopathologic features and results of surgical treatment. Ann Surg 1990; 211:277–284.
3. Nagorney DM, van Heerden JA, Ilstrup DM, et al. Primary hepatic malignancy: surgical management and determinants of survival. Surgery 1989; 106:740–748.
4. McGahan JP, Browning PD, Brock JM, et al. Hepatic ablation using radiofrequency electrocautery. Invest Radiol 1990; 25:267–270.
5. Lounsberry W, Goldschmidt V, Linke C. The early histologic changes following electrocoagulation. Gastrointest Endosc 1995; 41:68–70.
6. LeVeen RF. Laser hyperthermia and radiofrequency ablation of hepatic lesions. Semin Intervent Radiol 1997; 14(3):313–324.
7. Dickson JA, Calderwood SK. Temperature range and selective sensitivity of tumors to hyperthermia: a critical review. Ann NY Acad Sci 1980; 335:180–205.
8. Hill RP, Hunt JW. Hyperthermia. In: Tannock IF, Hill RP, eds. The Basic Science of Oncology. New York: Pergamon Press, 1987: 337–357.
9. Haines DE, Watson DD, Halperin C. Characteristics of heat transfer and determination of temperature gradient and viability threshold during radiofrequency fulguration of isolated perfused canine right ventricle. Circulation 1987; 76:278–283.
10. Grundfest WS, Litvack FI, Doyle DL, et al. Laser-tissue interactions: considerations for cardiovascular applications. In: White RA, Grundfest WS, eds. Lasers in Cardiovascular Disease. Chicago: Yearbook Medical Publishers, 1987: 32–43.
11. Bischof J, Christov K, Rubinsky B. A morphological study of cooling rate response in normal and noeplastic human liver tissue: cryosurgical implications. Cryobiology 1993; 30:482–492.
12. Steeves RA. Hyperthermia in cancer therapy: Where are we today and where are we going? Bull N Y Acad Med 1992; 68:341–350.
13. Siperstein AE, Rogers SJ, Hansen PD, et al. Laparoscopic thermal ablation of hepatic neuroendocrine tumor metastases. Surgery 1997; 122:1147–1155.

14. Goldburg SN, Gazelle GS, Solbiati L, et al. Ablation of liver tumors using percutaneous RF therapy. Am J Res 1998; 170:1023–1028.
15. Lencioni R, Goletti O, Armillotta N, et al. Radio-frequency thermal ablation of liver metastases with a cooled-tip electrode needle: results of a pilot clinical trial. Eur Radiol 1998; 8(7):1205–1211.
16. Nagata Y, Hiraoka M, Nishimura Y, et al. Clinical results of radiofrequency hyperthermia for malignant liver tumors. Int J Radiat Oncol Biol Phys 1997; 38(2):359–365.
17. Curley SA, Izzo F, Delrio P, et al. Radiofrequency ablation of unresectable primary and metastatic hepatic malignancies: results in 123 patients. Ann Surg 1999; 230(1):1–8.
18. Wood TF, Rose DM, Chung M, et al. Radiofrequency ablation of 231 unresectable hepatic tumors: indications, limitations, and complications. Ann Surg Oncol 2000; 7(8):593–600.
19. McGahan JP, Brock JM, Tesluk H, et al. Hepatic ablation with use of radio-frequency electrocautery in the animal model. J Vasc Intervent Radiol 1992;3:291–297.
20. Curley SA, Izzo F, Ellis L, et al. Radiofrequency ablation of malignant liver tumors in 304 patients. Proceedings ASCO 2000; 19:248a.
21. Curley SA, Davidson BS, Fleming RYD, et al. Laparoscopically guided bipolar radiofrequency ablation of areas of porcine liver. Surg Endosc 1997; 11:729–733.
22. Curley SA, Izzo F, Ellis LM, et al. Radiofrequency ablation of hepatocellular cancer in 110 cirrhotic patients. Ann Surg 2000; 232:381–391.
23. Patterson J, Strang R. The role of blood flow in hyperthermia. Int J Radiat Oncol Biol Phys 1979; 5:235–242.
24. Kolios MC, Sherar MD, Hunt JW. Large blood vessel cooling in heated tissues: a numerical study. Phys Med Biol 1995; 40:477–494.
25. Sturesson C, Liu DL, Stenram U, et al. Hepatic inflow occlusion increases the efficacy of interstitial laser-induced thermotherapy in rats. J Surg Res 1997; 71:67–72.
26. Quebbeman EJ, Wallace JR. Cryosurgery for hepatic metastases. In: Condon RE, ed. Current Techniques in General Surgery. New York: Mosby, 1997: 1–75.
27. Gagne DJ, Roh MS. Cryosurgery for hepatic malignancies. In: Curley SA, ed. Liver Cancer. New York: Springer-Verlag, 1998: 173–200.
28. McCarty TM, Kuhn JA. Cryotherapy for liver tumors. Oncology 1998; 12(7):979–987.
29. Seifert JK, Morris DL. World survey on the complication of hepatic and prostate cryotherapy. World J Surg 1999; 23(2):109–113.
30. Pearson AS, Izzo F, Fleming RYD, et al. Intraoperative radiofrequency ablation or cryoablation for hepatic malignancies. Am J Surg 1999; 178:592–599.
31. Ross WB, Horton M, Bertolino P, et al. Cryotherapy of liver tumours: a practical guide. HPB Surg 1995; 8:167–173.
32. Morris DL, Ross WB. Australian experience of cryoablation of liver tumors. Surg Oncol Clin North Am 1996; 52:391–397.
33. Cuschieri A, Crosthwaite G, Shimi S, et al. Hepatic cryotherapy for liver tumors. Surg Endosc 1995; 9:483–489.

34. Cozzi PJ, Stewart GJ, Morris DL. Thrombocytopenia after cryotherapy for colorectal metastases: correlates with hepatocellular injury. World J Surg 1994; 18:774–776.
35. Shafir M, Shapiro R, Sung M. Cryoablation of unresectable malignant liver tumors. Am J Surg 1996; 171:27–31.
36. Sarantou T, Bilchik A, Ramming KP. Complications of hepatic cryosurgery. Semin Surg Oncol 1998; 14(2):156–162.
37. Riley DK, Babinchak TJ, Zemel R, et al. Infection complications of hepatic cryosurgery. Clin Infect Dis 1997; 24:1001–1003.
38. Zhou XD, Tang ZY. Cryotherapy for primary liver cancer. Semin Surg Oncol 1998; 14:171–174.
39. Lin DY, Lin SM, Liaw YF. Non-surgical treatment of hepatocellular carcinoma. J Gastroenterol Hepatol 1997; 12:S319–S328.
40. Livraghi T, Bolondi L, Lazzaroni S, et al. Percutaneous ethanol injection in the treatment of hepatocellular carcinoma in cirrhosis. A study on 207 patients. Cancer 1992; 69:925–929.
41. Fujimoto T. The experimental and clinical studies of percutaneous ethanol injection therapy (PEIT) under ultrasonography for small hepatocellular carcinoma. Acta Hepatol Jpn 1988; 29:52–56.
42. Hasegawa S, Yamaski N, Hiwaki T, et al. Factors that predict intrahepatic recurrence of hepatocellular carcinoma in 81 patients initially treated by percutaneous ethanol injection. Cancer 1999; 86:1682–1690.
43. Seki T, Wakabayashi M, Nakagawa T, et al. Percutaneous microwave coagulation therapy for solitary metastatic liver tumors from colorectal cancer: a pilot clinical study. Am J Gastroenterol 1999; 94:322–327.
44. Yamashita Y, Sakai T, Maekawa T, et al. Thoracoscopic transdiaphragmatic microwave coagulation therapy for a liver tumor. Surg Endosc 1998; 12:1254–1258.
45. Vogl TJ, Mack MG, Roggan A, et al. Internally cooled power laser for MR-guided interstitial laser-induced thermotherapy of liver lesions: initial clinical results. Radiology 1998; 209:381–385.

# 7

# Radiofrequency Ablation of Carcinoid and Sarcoma Liver Metastases

Alexander A. Parikh, Bruno Fornage, Steven A. Curley, and Lee M. Ellis

The relative safety of radiofrequency ablation for malignant tumors has increased the indications for its use in the therapy of metastatic disease. Although tumor debulking has been considered inappropriate oncologic therapy in the past due to the associated complications and lack of clinical benefit, with safer techniques we are now able to determine if destroying most of the tumor mass in the liver can translate into improved palliation or even improved survival in patients with diseases considered inoperable in the past.

## Radiofrequency Ablation (RFA) of Hepatic Metastases from Carcinoid Tumors

Carcinoid tumors belong to the family of neuroendocrine tumors and are the most frequent gastrointestinal endocrine tumors (55%). They are still relatively rare, representing only 10% of small bowel tumors and 2% of all gastrointestinal malignancies.[1,2] The overall incidence is reported to be between 1 and 2/100,000 per year.[3–5] Carcinoid tumors have traditionally been classified according to their embryologic derivation. Foregut carcinoids comprise 20% of all carcinoid tumors and include thymic, lung, gastric, and duodenal tumors. Hindgut carcinoids constitute 15% of all carcinoid tumors and commonly originate from the colon or rectum. Midgut carcinoids arise from the small bowel, appendix, and proximal colon, and make up 40% of carcinoid tumors.[4,5] The most common gastrointestinal site of origin is the appendix, followed by the small intestine and rectum. Carcinoid tumors produce a variety of biologically active hormones depending on their site of origin. The best characterized of these substances is serotonin, but they have also been found to produce and secrete adrenocorticotropic hormone (ACTH), gastrin, histamine, dopamine, substance P, chromogranin A, neurotensin, prostaglandins, and others.[4,5]

Although generally indolent in their growth and progression, carcinoid tumors are the most frequent neuroendocrine tumors to metastasize to the liver.[6] In fact a majority of patients present with disseminated disease and involvement of the liver at the time of diagnosis. These patients usually have primary and metastatic carcinoid tumors that remain asymptomatic until their hepatic tumor burden overtakes the liver's ability to metabolize active hormones produced by these tumors, resulting in carcinoid syndrome. This severe endocrinopathy is characterized by flushing, diarrhea, cardiac valvular damage, bronchoconstriction, and asthma.[2,4,5,7] The incidence of carcinoid syndrome, caused by metastases to the liver is about 0.5/100,000, and most are associated with primary tumors of the small intestine.[8]

Patients in whom metastatic disease is suspected should be evaluated by abdominal imaging, including ultrasound, computed tomography (CT), CT-angioportography, magnetic resonance imaging (MRI), or octreotide scintigraphy to rule out liver metastases.[1] Liver function tests are usually unreliable for screening for metastasis, as they are only elevated when there is a large burden of tumor in the liver.[5] Carcinoid metastases are usually hypervascular. Thus when utilizing CT for imaging (Fig. 7.1), the images should be obtained before and after administration of intravenous contrast.[1] Measurement of 24-hour urine 5-hydroxy-indoleacetic acid (5-HIAA; serotonin metabolite) and serum chromogranin may also be useful in confirming and, more importantly, in subsequently monitoring metastatic disease and the adequacy of therapy.[5]

The treatment of patients with carcinoid tumor metastases to the liver presents a continuing challenge to the clinician. Although these tumors are generally indolent and slow growing in nature, hormone secretion from these metastases can cause significant morbidity in patients.[9] Patients with hepatic carcinoid metastases usually succumb from complications related to excess hormone secretion, with 5-year survival in the range of 11% to 40%.[10,11] In contrast, the cause of death from most other hepatic metastases is usually related to liver failure from diffuse hepatic replacement.

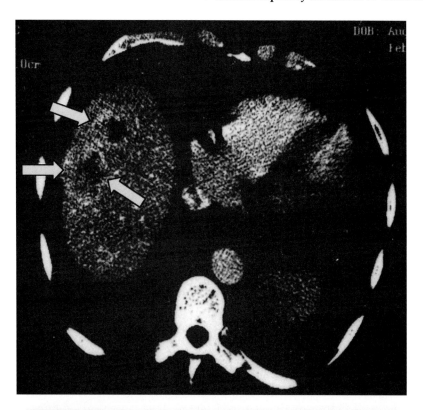

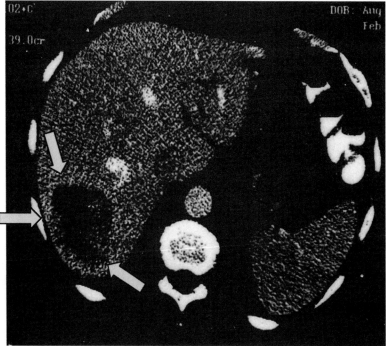

**Figure 7.1.** Computed tomography (CT) appearance of a carcinoid metastasis to the liver showing characteristic hypervascular rims (arrows).

No general agreement has been reached about when or if systemic chemotherapy should be given to patients with metastatic carcinoid. Single- or multiple-agent chemotherapy yields low response rates ranging from 0% to 30% and is particularly poor with midgut carcinoids. Overall 5-year survival for all patients with carcinoid liver metastases usually does not exceed 20% to 40%.[3,12,13] Considering the toxicity, the poor response rates, as well as the indolent nature of the tumor allowing some patients to live a long time without therapy, chemotherapy is usually reserved for selected cases only.[4,5]

Resection of isolated hepatic metastases may be beneficial in selected patients. Overall 5-year survival rates after hepatic resection range from 45% to 50%, but rises to 60% to 86% after successful curative (R0) resection. Relief of clinical symptoms is achieved in an even higher number of patients.[9,13–15] This high rate of clinical benefit may actually be a function of patient selection, however, rather than success of surgical therapy. Moreover, most patients present with multiple metastatic foci within the liver or with significant extrahepatic disease and only a minority (<10%) are therefore candidates for curative surgical resection.[9,14–16]

The role of cytoreductive or debulking surgery in patients in whom the entire tumor cannot be removed is less clear. Proponents of cytoreductive surgery argue that resection of hepatic metastases may relieve clinical endocrinopathies, and the symptomatic response may last several months. It has been recommended that if greater than 80% to 90% of the tumor can be removed, resection should be considered.[9,14,17] Although no prospective trials have been performed, retrospective analyses have suggested that surgical debulking of metastatic carcinoid tumors is safe and can provide temporary relief of symptoms.[9,14,17] Palliative resection may also allow other therapies to be utilized (by decreasing overall tumor burden) and may result in a discontinuation or reduction of medication requirements.

Hepatic resection, even when palliative, may still not be possible for technical reasons. Patients with multiple metastases involving both lobes, patients with metastatic lesions in proximity to major blood vessels and biliary structures, and patients without adequate hepatic reserve have in the past been considered to have unresectable disease. The resulting small number of patients eligible for curative surgery together with the limited value of chemotherapy and the long, indolent course and importance of palliation in these patients has led to the development of several alternative treatment modalities including hepatic artery embolization/chemoembolization, alcohol injection, biotherapy, orthotopic liver transplant, and ablative therapies including alcohol injection, cryotherapy, and RFA.

The role of liver transplantation is still unclear, and the number of patients in whom this has been attempted is small. Although 5-year survival of nearly 70% has been observed in selected patients,[18] the overall morbidity and mortality of the procedure, the poor results observed with other tumors, and the shortage of donors has limited the utilization of liver transplant for metastatic carcinoid. Biotherapy using somatostatin analogues has presented a breakthrough in the treatment of patients with carcinoid tumors. Three times daily administration can result in a reduction of hormonal symptoms in nearly 90%, but treatment is cumbersome and tumor shrinkage rare.[7,19] Overall 5-year survival when liver metastases are present is still only 20%, with a 2-year median survival.[4] Long-acting formulations of somatostatin analogues are less cumbersome to use and preferred by patients, but appear to be no more effective than shorter-acting agents as far as symptom and biochemical control are concerned. In addition, no results regarding tumor shrinkage or survival have been reported.[20,21] Interferon-$\alpha$ has also been used alone or in combination with somatostatin analogues. Although it is also effective in relieving symptoms, the low rate of tumor regression and the high incidence of side effects including fever, fatigue, anorexia, and weight loss often limits its use.[7]

Since carcinoid liver metastases obtain most of their blood supply from the hepatic artery, embolization of the hepatic artery with an embolizing agent or with a chemotherapeutic agent (chemoembolization) has also been utilized. Several studies have shown a reduction of hormonal symptoms as well as tumor burden in 50% to 70% of patients.[22–24] This procedure can be associated with substantial side effects, however, including fever, nausea, pain, and even the hepatorenal syndrome.[5,12,23,25] Furthermore, the duration of the response after hepatic artery occlusion or embolization is usually between 6 and 12 months, and new or refractory metastases often do not respond to additional embolization due to the development of collateral nutrient vessels.[5,6]

Radiofrequency ablation may provide a viable therapeutic option for both surgical candidates (resectable) and those traditionally considered unresectable (Fig. 7.2). The physics of RFA and the approaches are described elsewhere in this book. Although most reports of RFA in the treatment of liver metastases include a variety of different lesions, particularly colorectal metastases, a few studies involving neuroendocrine metastatic lesions have been reported. Siperstein et al[26] reported on six patients with 13 neuroendocrine tumors metastatic to the liver, including islet cell, carcinoid, and medullary thyroid cancers. They were treated with laparoscopic ultrasound and RFA using the multiprobe array electrode. The lesions ranged in size from 1.5

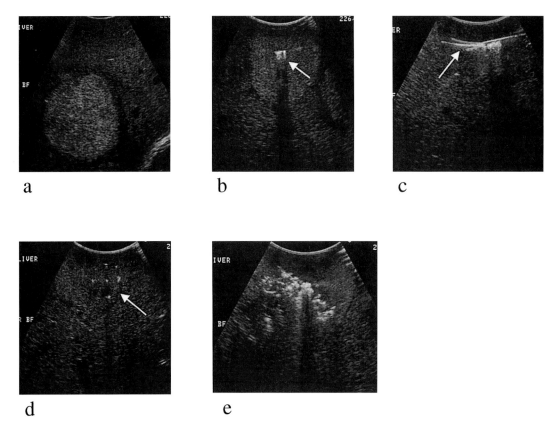

**Figure 7.2.** Ultrasound-guided radiofrequency ablation (RFA) of a carcinoid hepatic metastasis. (A) Lesion prior to RFA. (B) Coronal view of the RFA multiprobe array being inserted into the lesion. (C,D) Tangential and coronal views of the deployed multiprobe array (decreased magnification). (E) Appearance of the lesion following RFA.

to 7 cm in diameter, and up to four lesions were ablated per patient without any major complications. Technical success was noted in all lesions by CT scan at 1 week and in all evaluable patients at 3 months. Although there was a relatively short follow-up, no local recurrences were noted and most of the patients noted improvement in their symptoms. In a recent update of their series, 18 patients with 115 neuroendocrine tumors were ablated with RFA. The mean lesion size was 3.2 cm (range 1.3–10 cm), and the average number of lesions ablated per patient was six (range 1–14). There were two complications, atrial fibrillation in one patient and an upper GI hemorrhage in another. Fifteen patients (83%) harboring a total of 100 lesions were followed for a mean of 12.1 months (range 3–35 months). Local recurrence was detected in three patients (20%) and three patients died during follow-up. The data regarding potential symptom improvement were not reported, however.[11]

Wessels and Schell[6] reported on 13 patients with unresectable bilobar carcinoid metastases that were treated with hepatic artery embolization. Three patients developed refractory symptoms and new hepatic lesions and subsequently underwent RFA. At a follow-up of 3 to 6 months, all three patients experienced improvement in symptoms and required less octreotide support. There were no complications related to RFA, although one patient eventually died of systemic disease.

These studies, although small, suggest that RFA may be effective in diminishing symptoms associated with metastatic neuroendocrine tumors in those patients who are eligible for surgical resection or debulking.

Our group has noted similar results for patients with neuroendocrine liver metastasis. Over a 4-year period, 11 patients with liver metastases from carcinoid tumors have been treated with RFA. The size of the lesions have ranged from 0.5 to 6.5 cm in diameter, and between one and 12 lesions were ablated at each session. At the time of this report, follow-up is available on 10 patients. All of them are alive, but seven of these patients have either recurred or have disseminated disease. In one patient with active carcinoid syndrome from multiple hepatic lesions, we measured serum serotonin levels pre-RFA, during the procedure, and 1 hour post-RFA. In this patient, the pre-RFA serum serotonin level was 971 mg/mL, compared to 975 and 803 mg/mL during and after the RFA procedure, respectively. Thus the procedure itself did not cause any increase in circulating serum serotonin and the patient remained hemodynamically stable throughout the procedure and the postoperative period. In addition, his 24-hour urine 5-HIAA excretion was 123 mg, which decreased to 44 mg post-RFA. The patient's symptoms resolved following this procedure, which has typically been the case in our experience with patients who undergo RFA for symptomatic carcinoid tumor metastatic to the liver.

In those patients who are scheduled to undergo RFA liver metastases, it is critical to treat them preoperatively to try to prevent the carcinoid crisis. This is more likely to occur in those patients with the carcinoid syndrome but can also occur in asymptomatic patients. To avoid any complications associated with release of hormones during RFA, patients should be blocked preoperatively with octreotide. Many patients will present preoperatively already being treated with long-acting octreotide. However, we recommend additional treatment with 100 $\mu$g of octreotide subcutaneously twice a day for the 5 days prior to surgery. Although there is no evidence to support such use, the risk of adverse affects from this regimen is low, as patients are likely to have previously received octreotide therapy. In addition, the development of the carcinoid crisis during surgery is associated with an extremely high mortality and thus one should be conservative about approaching these patients with any surgical modality.

### Summary

Carcinoid metastasis to the liver remains uncommon and although it is usually slow growing and indolent, significant morbidity is present in the patients due to hormone overproduction. Curative hepatic resection appears to be effective in relieving symptoms and can lead to increased survival, although only a minority of patients are candidates. Although few patients with metastatic carcinoid tumors can be cured of their disease, carcinoid metastases are unique in that significant palliation may be afforded by cytoreductive measures. RFA has been shown to be well tolerated in patients with carcinoid metastases and has the advantage of being less invasive and associated with fewer side effects as compared to other ablative techniques. Preliminary evidence suggests that RFA may be effective in treating hepatic metastases from carcinoid tumors with low recurrence rates and symptomatic improvement. For patients with carcinoid syndrome or for those with progressive disease despite hormonal blockade and chemotherapy. RFA is a viable and attractive therapeutic option. Evaluation of a larger group of patients over a longer time period will be necessary to further determine the role of RFA in the treatment of carcinoid tumors metastatic to the liver. The use of RFA in combination with multimodality therapy, including long-acting somatostatin analogues, is particularly attractive and remains to be evaluated.

### Sarcoma

Soft tissue sarcomas represent about 1% of all malignancies, and experience with hepatic metastases is rare. Synchronous liver involvement has been reported in 1% to 20% of patients with soft tissue sarcoma depending on the primary origin.[27,28] Metastases to the liver as a component of recurrence have been reported in as high as 86% of patients, however.[28–30] Liver involvement by soft tissue sarcoma usually results from primary visceral and retroperitoneal tumors rather than from extremity sarcomas. In a large study from Memorial Sloan-Kettering Cancer Center (MSKCC), liver metastases were 75 times less common than lung metastases from extremity sarcomas, but were 1.5 times more common than lung metastases for retroperitoneal sarcomas and 10 times more common than lung metastases for sarcomas of visceral origin. In that study of nearly 1000 patients, 0.5% of patients with extremity sarcoma had liver metastases versus 16% of patients with retroperitoneal sarcomas and 62% of patients with visceral sarcomas.[30]

Leiomyosarcomas tend to be the most common histology, and 90% of liver metastases are high-grade lesions.[28,31] Unfortunately, most patients have extensive hepatic or extrahepatic disease precluding hepatic resection. In published series, between 17% and 22% of patients with hepatic metastases from sarcoma are reported to be resectable. For those patients who undergo surgical resection, median survival has been reported to be between 11 and 54 months, compared to 6 to 20 months for patients with unresectable disease. Due to the small numbers of patients, however, the increase in median survival has not reached statistical significance. Overall 5-year survival after hepatic resection for soft tissue sarcoma remains dismal, between 0% and 11% in reported series.[28–30,32]

Chemotherapy remains the standard palliative therapy for metastatic soft tissue sarcoma. Although response rates between 18% and 44% from doxorubicin-based single- or combination-agent therapy have been noted, the efficacy in the treatment of hepatic metastases is unclear. In the series from MSKCC, 80% of the patients with hepatic metastases received chemotherapy, the majority doxorubicin-based, with only a 6% partial response rate. No complete responses were noted and no responses were noted in 32 patients undergoing a second round of chemotherapy as salvage treatment. Univariate analysis failed to show any improvement in survival with chemotherapy for hepatic metastases from soft tissue sarcoma.[30]

Radiofrequency ablation is an attractive option for patients with hepatic metastases from soft tissue sarcoma for several reasons (Fig. 7.3). Since patients appear to do somewhat better when their disease is resectable, RFA alone or in combination with hepatic resection may be able to increase the number of patients amen-able to surgical resection. For palliative therapy, RFA has the distinct advantage of being the least invasive technique with minimal morbidity. Considering the poor results of chemotherapy alone in the treatment of patients with hepatic metastases from sarcoma, RFA combined with systemic therapy may also have some potential therapeutic value.

The use of RFA in the treatment of hepatic metastases has been reported only as part of larger series of patients encompassing a variety of different primary cancers. In these series, only a few patients had soft tissue sarcoma as their primary cancer.[33–38] Although none of the reports had mentioned a difference in efficacy or survival for patients with sarcoma metastases, the numbers are too small to draw any general conclusions.

At our institution, 20 patients with hepatic metastases from sarcoma over the past $3^1/_2$ years have undergone RFA. The lesions

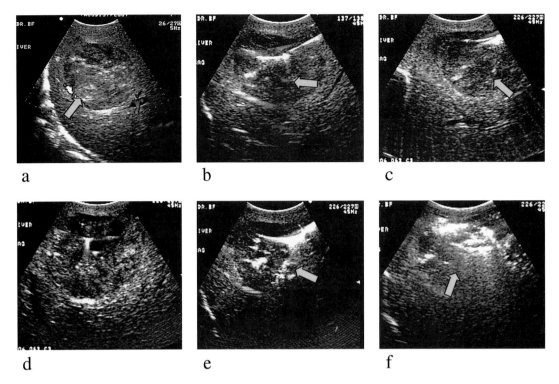

**Figure 7.3.** Ultrasound-guided RFA of a sarcoma Gastrointestinal Stroma Tumor (GIST) hepatic metastasis. (A) Lesion prior to RFA. (B) RFA multiprobe array inserted into lesion. (C,D) Appearance of lesion during the RFA procedure. (E) RFA multiprobe array being removed. (F) Appearance of lesion following RFA.

ranged from 0.5 to 7 cm in diameter and leiomyosarcoma was the histologic type in 16 of the 20 patients. RFA was performed on one to six lesions per patient. At the time of this report, follow-up is available on 16 patients; only two patients are alive without evidence of disease, three have died, eight have locally recurred, and three have metastatic disease elsewhere.

*Summary*

Hepatic metastases from soft tissue sarcomas are rare and usually are associated with advanced and disseminated disease with a poor overall prognosis. Although complete hepatic resection may provide an increase in survival, most patients are unresectable. Given the lack of effective systemic therapy, RFA may have a role in the treatment of sarcoma metastases. Although experience is limited, RFA does appear to be well tolerated and initially effective. Local recurrence remains a problem, although the ability to repeat the ablative procedure is a distinct advantage. The use of RFA with hepatic resection and or systemic therapy remains to be evaluated but may potentially increase palliation and even long-term survival in these patients.

## References

1. Wallace S, Ajani JA, Charnsangavej C, et al. Carcinoid tumors: imaging procedures and interventional radiology. World J Surg 1996; 20(2):147–156.
2. Therasse E, Breittmayer F, Roche A, et al. Transcatheter chemoembolization of progressive carcinoid liver metastasis. Radiology 1993; 189(2):541–547.
3. Modlin IM, Sandor A. An analysis of 8305 cases of carcinoid tumors. Cancer 1997; 79(4):813–829.
4. Oberg K. Carcinoid tumors: current concepts in diagnosis and treatment. Oncologist 1998; 3(5):339–345.
5. Kulke MH, Mayer RJ. Carcinoid tumors. N Engl J Med 1999; 340(11):858–868.
6. Wessels FJ, Schell SR. Radiofrequency ablation treatment of refractory carcinoid hepatic metastases. J Surg Res 2001; 95(1):8–12.
7. Oberg K. Neuroendocrine gastrointestinal tumors—a condensed overview of diagnosis and treatment. Ann Oncol 1999; 10(suppl 2):S3–8.
8. Norheim I, Oberg K, Theodorsson-Norheim E, et al. Malignant carcinoid tumors. An analysis of 103 patients with regard to tumor localization, hormone production, and survival. Ann Surg 1987; 206(2):115–125.
9. McEntee GP, Nagorney DM, Kvols LK, et al. Cytoreductive hepatic surgery for neuroendocrine tumors. Surgery 1990; 108(6):1091–1096.
10. Oberg K. The use of chemotherapy in the management of neuroendocrine tumors. Endocrinol Metab Clin North Am 1993;22(4): 941–952.
11. Siperstein AE, Berber E. Cryoablation, percutaneous alcohol injection, and radiofrequency ablation for treatment of neuroendocrine liver metastases. World J Surg 2001; 25(6):693–696.
12. Ruszniewski P, Rougier P, Roche A, et al. Hepatic arterial chemoembolization in patients with liver metastases of endocrine tumors. A prospective phase II study in 24 patients. Cancer 1993; 71(8):2624–2630.
13. Dousset B, Saint-Marc O, Pitre J, et al. Metastatic endocrine tumors: medical treatment, surgical resection, or liver transplantation. World J Surg 1996; 20(7):908–914; discussion 914–905.
14. Nave H, Mossinger E, Feist H, et al. Surgery as primary treatment in patients with liver metastases from carcinoid tumors: a retrospective, unicentric study over 13 years. Surgery 2001; 129(2):170–175.
15. Que FG, Nagorney DM, Batts KP, et al. Hepatic resection for metastatic neuroendocrine carcinomas. Am J Surg 1995; 169(1):36–42.
16. Ihse I, Persson B, Tibblin S. Neuroendocrine metastases of the liver. World J Surg 1995; 19(1):76–82.
17. Drougas JG, Anthony LB, Blair TK, et al. Hepatic artery chemoembolization for management of patients with advanced metastatic carcinoid tumors. Am J Surg 1998; 175(5):408–412.

18. Le Treut YP, Delpero JR, Dousset B, et al. Results of liver transplantation in the treatment of metastatic neuroendocrine tumors. A 31-case French multicentric report. Ann Surg 1997; 225(4):355–364.

19. Hajarizadeh H, Ivancev K, Mueller CR, et al. Effective palliative treatment of metastatic carcinoid tumors with intra-arterial chemotherapy/chemoembolization combined with octreotide acetate. Am J Surg 1992; 163(5):479–483.

20. Rubin J, Ajani J, Schirmer W, et al. Octreotide acetate long-acting formulation versus open-label subcutaneous octreotide acetate in malignant carcinoid syndrome. J Clin Oncol 1999;17(2):600–606.

21. O'Toole D, Ducreux M, Bommelaer G, et al. Treatment of carcinoid syndrome: a prospective crossover evaluation of lanreotide versus octreotide in terms of efficacy, patient acceptability, and tolerance. Cancer 2000; 88(4):770–776.

22. Brown KT, Koh BY, Brody LA, et al. Particle embolization of hepatic neuroendocrine metastases for control of pain and hormonal symptoms. J Vasc Intervent Radiol 1999; 10(4):397–403.

23. Clouse ME, Perry L, Stuart K, et al. Hepatic arterial chemoembolization for metastatic neuroendocrine tumors. Digestion 1994; 55(suppl 3):92–97.

24. Marlink RG, Lokich JJ, Robins JR, et al. Hepatic arterial embolization for metastatic hormone-secreting tumors. Technique, effectiveness, and complications. Cancer 1990; 65(10):2227–2232.

25. Eriksson BK, Larsson EG, Skogseid BM, et al. Liver embolizations of patients with malignant neuroendocrine gastrointestinal tumors. Cancer 1998; 83(11):2293–2301.

26. Siperstein AE, Rogers SJ, Hansen PD, et al. Laparoscopic thermal ablation of hepatic neuroendocrine tumor metastases. Surgery 1997; 122(6):1147–1154; discussion 1154–1155.

27. Lawrence W Jr, Neifeld JP. Soft tissue sarcomas. Curr Probl Surg 1989; 26(11):753–827.

28. Hafner GH, Rao U, Karakousis CP. Liver metastases from soft tissue sarcomas. J Surg Oncol 1995; 58(1):12–16.

29. Merimsky O, Terrier P, Stanca A, et al. Liver metastases from extremity soft tissue sarcoma. Am J Clin Oncol 1999; 22(1):70–72.

30. Jaques DP, Coit DG, Casper ES, et al. Hepatic metastases from soft-tissue sarcoma. Ann Surg 1995; 221(4):392–397.

31. Torosian MH, Friedrich C, Godbold J, et al. Soft-tissue sarcoma: initial characteristics and prognostic factors in patients with and without metastatic disease. Semin Surg Oncol 1988; 4(1):13–19.

32. Foster JH. Survival after liver resection for secondary tumors. Am J Surg 1978; 135(3):389–394.

33. de Baere T, Elias D, Dromain C, et al. Radiofrequency ablation of 100 hepatic metastases with a mean follow-up of more than 1 year. AJR 2000; 175(6):1619–1625.

34. Wood TF, Rose DM, Chung M, et al. Radiofrequency ablation of 231 unresectable hepatic tumors: indications, limitations, and complications. Ann Surg Oncol 2000; 78(8):593–600.

35. Rossi S, Buscarini E, Garbagnati F, et al. Percutaneous treatment of small hepatic tumors by an expandable RF needle electrode. AJR 1998; 170(4):1015–1022.

36. Rossi S, Di Stasi M, Buscarini E, et al. Percutaneous RF interstitial thermal ablation in the treatment of hepatic cancer. AJR 1996; 167(3):759–768.
37. Solbiati L, Ierace T, Goldberg SN, et al. Percutaneous US-guided radio-frequency tissue ablation of liver metastases: treatment and follow-up in 16 patients. Radiology 1997; 202(1):195–203.
38. Pearson AS, Izzo F, Fleming RY, et al. Intraoperative radiofrequency ablation or cryoablation for hepatic malignancies. Am J Surg 1999; 178(6):592–599.

# 8

# Complications of Hepatic Radiofrequency Ablation: Lessons Learned

Richard J. Bleicher and Anton J. Bilchik

Radiofrequency ablation (RFA) was first utilized in the 1980s for the ablation of aberrant conduction pathways in the heart.[1] At that time, there was concern that ventricular dysrhythmias would be associated with its use, but this complication was infrequent. With only a 3% to 5% overall complication rate for cardiac ablation,[2] RFA was deemed safe and its use became widespread. RFA has since been applied to unresectable hepatic primary and metastatic malignancies.[3] While resection remains the gold standard for liver tumors, two thirds of these tumors are found to be unresectable at operation after preoperative screening.[4] Therefore, RFA has become a useful alternative or adjunct to excision.[5] It must be stressed, however, that this technology is not a replacement for hepatectomy.

The prevalence of RFA is rapidly increasing because of its safety and versatility. It has been effectively performed by surgeons via an open approach (laparotomy) or through a laparoscope. More recently, percutaneous ablations are being performed by radiologists under ultrasound or computed tomography (CT) guidance. Each of these three approaches has unique advantages as well as associated morbidities and complications. When defined as individual complications per patient, overall complication rates vary from 0% in a study of 10 patients with hepatocellular carcinoma,[6] to 31.6% in a much larger heterogeneous series.[7]

This chapter discusses the potential problems that may arise as a result of RFA, and describes perioperative steps that may minimize risk in some patients. We have classified the complications both by their etiology and by their association with the various RFA approaches.

## Preoperative Risk Minimization

As with any operative procedure, a comprehensive history and physical examination is crucial to evaluate a patient's candidacy for RFA and to plan the most appropriate RFA approach. Patients with an extensive surgical history are more likely to have intraperitoneal adhesions and may not be ideal candidates for laparoscopic RFA. The physician must use this information as well as the location of the lesions to decide which RFA method (open, laparoscopic, or percutaneous) is most likely to prove safe and effective. A previous laparotomy may also increase the risk of a percutaneous approach due to the increased likelihood of adhesions. Resection may alter a patient's anatomy, making radiologic imaging more difficult to interpret. Because this modality relies solely on CT or ultrasound guidance for probe placement, the interventionalist must be supplied with the details of prior procedures to appropriately target the lesion to be ablated.

The medical condition and immune function of the patient are also important considerations because the destroyed tissue left in situ is an ideal nidus for infection. In fact, infection remains the most frequent complication in these patients, accounting for up to 5.7% of complications in the literature[8] and 7.2% of complications in the John Wayne Cancer Institute experience to date.[8A] Clinical assessment of the patient's medical status is therefore mandatory, and historical findings such as familial history of immunologic impairment, or risk factors for human immunodeficiency virus (HIV) should prompt further assessment of immune function. Preoperative evaluation should also rule out any current evidence of infection. Pulmonary, gastrointestinal, and indwelling vascular and Foley catheter–related sepsis that could seed the coagulum must be treated prior to any ablative procedure.

Because RFA is most frequently performed on hepatic malignancies, particularly hepatocellular carcinoma, liver function and volume relative to tumor burden should be assessed preoperatively by CT or magnetic resonance imaging (MRI). While current standards dictate that all but 20% of the liver parenchyma may be resected,[9] poor liver function, prior resection, and surgeon judgment may dictate otherwise. There have been several cases of postablation hepatic failure/insufficiency noted (Table 8.1). Anatomic variance between patients may also affect the eval-

**Table 8.1 Complications from RFA in Recent Series**

| Complication | Curley et al[10] | Jiao et al[8] | Yamasaki et al[6] | Wood et al[11] | Curley et al[12] | de Baere et al[13] | Bowles et al[7] | Bleicher et al[8A] |
|---|---|---|---|---|---|---|---|---|
| Total patients | 123 | 35 | 10[a] | 84 | 110 | 68 | 76 | 152[b] |
| Overall complication rate (incidents/patient) | 2.4% | 2.3% | 0% | 9.5% | 12.7% | 7.4% | 31.6% | 23.7% |
| Visceral damage | | 1* | | | | | | |
| Hemorrhage: hepatic/into ablation site/subcapsular | 1* | 1* | | 1 lap | 2 perc | | 1* | 2 perc 1 lap |
| Hemorrhage: abdominal wall/subcutaneous | | | | | 1 perc 1 open | | | |
| Hepatic vascular damage | | 1 open | | | | | | |
| Biliary injury (leak/obstruction/stricture) | | | | | | 1 perc | 5* | 4 perc 1 open |
| Hematobilia with obstruction | | | | | | | | 1 perc |
| Hepatic insufficiency | | | | 1 open | 1 open | | 1* | 1 open |
| Ascites | | | | | 2 open 2 perc | | 1* | |
| Pneumothorax | | | | | | | | 1 perc |
| Hydropneumothorax | | | | | 1 perc | | | |
| Symptomatic pleural effusion | | | | | 2 perc | | | |
| Persistent fever, infection, sepsis | | 1 open | | | 1 perc | | 2* | 2 perc |
| Discrete abscess | 2 open[c] | 1* | | 2 perc 1 open | | 2 perc | | 5 perc 4 open |

(continued)

**Table 8.1 Continued**

| Complication | Curley et al[10] | Jiao et al[8] | Yamasaki et al[6] | Wood et al[11] | Curley et al[12] | de Baere et al[13] | Bowles et al[7] | Bleicher et al[8A] |
|---|---|---|---|---|---|---|---|---|
| Thrombocytopenia | | | | | | | 4* | |
| Fistula | | | | | | | | 3 perc |
| Pseudoaneurysm | | | | | | | | 2 perc |
| Ureteral stricture | | | | | | | | 1 perc |
| Myoglobinuria | | | | | | | 5* | |
| Thermal injury: skin/ abdominal wall | | | | 1 perc | | | 1* | 1 perc |
| Thermal injury: diaphragm | | | | 1 perc | | | | 1 perc |
| Thermal injury: stomach | | | | | | | | 1 perc 1 open |
| Thermal injury: Grounding pad | | | | | | 2* | 1* | |
| Pain requiring aborting procedure | | 3 perc | | | | | | 1 perc |
| Brachial plexopathy | | | | | | | | 2 perc |
| Pacemaker malfunction | | | | | | | 1* | |
| Ventricular fibrillation | | | | | 1 perc | | | |
| Myocardial infarction/ congestive heart failure | | | | 1 open | | | 2* | 1 open |

[a]No major complications.
[b]Some patients experienced >1 complication.
[c]These two patients' abscesses were perihepatic; not at the RFA sites.
*Modality not indicated.
JWCI, John Wayne Cancer Institute; perc, percutaneous; lap, laparoscopic.

**Table 8.2  Preoperative Considerations for RFA Candidates**

Prior surgical procedures

Operative (medical) candidacy

Immune function

Concurrent infection

Liver function

Tumor burden

Liver volume

uation of hepatic reserve; a Riedel's lobe may increase the amount of tissue that can be ablated, and an aplastic lobe may decrease the patient's tolerance for RFA. General preoperative assessment parameters are summarized in Table 8.2.

## Radiofrequency Ablation–Specific Complications

Radiofrequency ablation–specific complications can generally be attributed to the form and function of the probe, the applied current and generated heat, and/or necrotic tissue that remains in situ.

### Probe Design and Function

Currently used probes include the umbrella-shaped Starburst™ XL with retractable tines (RITA Medical Systems, Mountain View, CA), the similarly retractable LeVeen Needle Electrode (Radiotherapeutics, Mountain View, CA), and the straight cooled Cool-Tip (Radionics, Burlington, MA). The designs vary somewhat, but most complications that arise are applicable to all probe types. All probes have a rigid stem and use transcapsular and intraparenchymal penetration to reach their target. Percutaneous and laparoscopic approaches often require a stab wound through the skin. As with any procedure involving parenchymal disruption or skin penetration, bleeding is possible. At the John Wayne Cancer Institute, the incidence of combined intrahepatic, intrabiliary, and subcutaneous hemorrhage is 2%, while in the literature, the reported incidence ranges from 0.8% to 5.7%.[7,8,10–13]

Scirrhous tumors can make extension of probe tines more difficult and occasionally bend them to prevent optimal ablation and tumor coverage. No probe breakage has yet been reported as a consequence, but if tine advancement is distorted and unrecognized, the effectiveness of the ablation may be limited. For this reason, complete visualization of the probe stem during insertion and of prong extension during placement and ablation is crucial under ultrasound or CT.

### Heat and Current

Because the heat generated during ablation can denature protein, any structure in proximity to the ablation field is at risk for thermal or current-related injury. Usually, ablation of a tissue margin surrounding a tumor is of no consequence if no vital structures are present. However, significant skin burns have been noted in abdominal and breast procedures,[14] and one case of RFA-induced diaphragmatic necrosis following ablation of a large tumor on the dome of the liver was noted at the John Wayne Cancer Institute.[8A] Within this series, the bowel and stomach were found to be particularly at risk, with two gastric burns requiring local resection (Fig. 8.1) and three fistulae to date. Bowles et al[7] also noted one abdominal wall burn, and two studies have documented burns at the grounding pad site.[7,13]

Liver tumors often arise adjacent to branches of the portal vein. Because of continuous blood flow within these large tributaries, heat is carried away from the vein adjacent to the ablation site and no thermal injury to the vein is noted. Some devices give real-time readings of the wattage of each tine. Lower values of

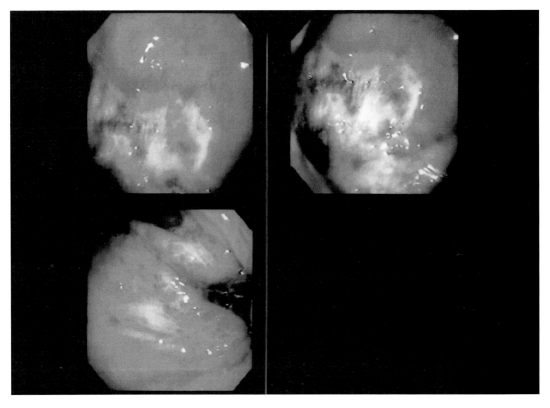

**Figure 8.1.** Severe full-thickness gastric burns seen via esophagogastroduodenoscopy, after percutaneous radiofrequency ablation of metastatic breast carcinoma. This patient subsequently underwent resection of the thermally damaged gastric wall.

those prongs adjacent to venous channels reflect this diffusion of perivenous heat. Arteries are more susceptible to injury from RFA, likely because of their thick muscular wall. Destruction of tissue may lead to pseudoaneurysms requiring embolization. This has occurred twice in our experience after percutaneous RFA (Fig. 8.2).[15] The biliary system is similar, since lesions in proximity to the porta hepatis are at risk for bile duct injuries resulting in obstruction, leak, and stricture. Such injuries are seen in up to 6.6% of patients[7] and may require stenting or definitive repair. Because of this, lesions in close proximity to the bile ducts are seen as a relative contraindication to RFA.

While upper abdominal procedures are not considered dangerous, thoracic complications may occur even if the thorax is not entered. Pleural effusions[12] underscore that some ablations are in close proximity to the diaphragm, and may result in a thoracic inflammatory reaction. Other nonpenetrating complications within the chest, such as dysrhythmias, can also occur. One large series by Curley et al[12] noted induction of ventricular fibrillation. While the precise etiology is unclear, current-induced dysrhythmias are plausible with the proximity of some ablation fields to the heart. Patients with pacemakers and internal defibrillators pose unique challenges due to implanted conduction wire and electrical sensitivity. When electrocautery is allowed to arc between instruments en route to the patient, it demodulates, causing frequency fluctuation.[16] Such variation can enter into the frequency detection and operational range of pacemakers and implanted cardiac devices (ICDs) causing dysfunction. While no data on RFA and implanted cardiac devices exists, certain precautions are advisable (Table 8.3).

Clearance from other structures is also vital, either manually or by a nonconductant retractor. If lesions are near the surface of the liver, surrounding organs should be displaced from the field of ablation. If adjacent structures cannot be easily displaced, moist laparotomy pads may be used as a heat sink to protect them. One advantage of open or laparoscopic approaches to RFA is the ability to insulate viscera in close proximity to the tumor. This is one important consideration when deciding which approach to use.

## Coagulation

Radiofrequency ablation leaves a coagulum of necrotic tissue in situ. Even with the most sterile technique, this environment is ideal for bacterial growth and abscess formation. A discrete abscess requiring intervention and treatment is the most common individual complication to date as noted in Table 8.1. The reported incidence of sepsis and idiopathic persistent fever ranges from 0.9% to 2.9%.[7,8,12] If, after several days, a patient remains

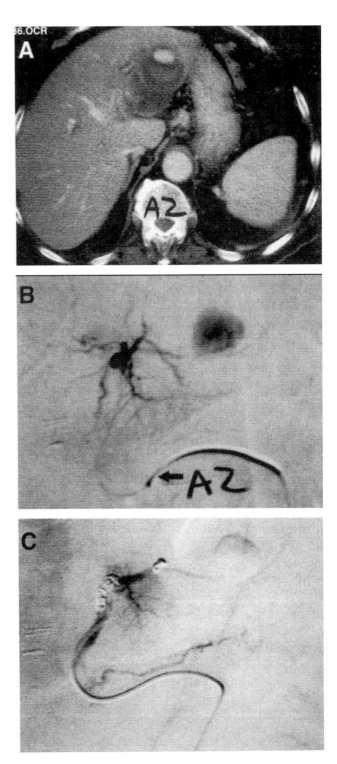

**Figure 8.2.** Hepatic artery pseudoaneurysm as demonstrated on computed tomography (CT) (A) and angiography after percutaneous radiofrequency ablation of a single colorectal metastasis. Angiograms demonstrate the pseudoaneurysm before (B) and after (C) embolization. Source: "Radiofrequency ablation of unresectable hepatic malignancies: lessons learned," by Bilchik AJ, Wood TF, Allegra DP, published in *The Oncologist* 2001;6:24–33 © AlphaMed Press 1083–7159. Reprinted with permission.

**Table 8.3 Recommended Prophylactic Measures for Use with Electrocautery in Patients with Implanted Cardiac Devices[16]**

| |
|---|
| Resolve electrical instability preoperatively |
|    Electrolyte imbalance |
|    Myocardial ischemia |
|    Hypoxemia |
| Check position and lead integrity |
| Evaluate device function |
| Determine patient dependence on device countershocks |
| Place grounding pad so current flows away from device |
| Do not arc current to another instrument en route to patient |
| Use alternate monitoring devices during current application |
| Keep the programming device in the operating room for emergent need |

© 1999 Lippincott Williams & Wilkins. Reprinted with permission. See reference 16.

febrile or has a leukocytosis, studies should be repeated to look for possible abscess formation. Drainage and antibiotics should be used liberally when indicated by imaging and clinical suspicion.

## Approach-Specific Complications

### Open RFA

The surgeon performing RFA at laparotomy is subject to the same precautions that apply to other abdominal procedures. Careful tissue handling, aseptic technique, and adequate exposure are of paramount importance. As outlined in Table 8.1, complications using this approach are varied, and with the exception of abscesses (particularly in larger lesions), seem sporadic.

### Laparoscopic RFA

The major issues that a surgeon must be aware of in laparoscopic RFA are those due to the laparoscopy itself. Even prior to beginning any laparoscopic procedure, setup and placement of trocars can involve complications. The most significant of these is vascular injury, which has a mortality rate of 15%.[17] Techniques involving blind trocar insertion and Veress needle placement are the most common complications related to laparoscopy,[18] with combined morbidity estimated at approximately 0.2%.[19] The "open" Hasson technique for trocar placement also is not without complications. Avulsion of adhesions, injuring or tearing the involved viscera, and periodic resultant bleeding or even perforation are possible. Major vascular injury can occur but is quite rare.[20] Nonetheless, despite a paucity of randomized data, the Hasson technique probably has a lower risk of complications.

Insufflation of the abdomen creates an environment that alters physiology predominantly by absorption of carbon dioxide. Barotrauma, hypothermia, and postoperative bleeding from insufflation-induced intraoperative venous tamponade have all been described. Should a gas embolism develop, a "mill wheel" heart murmur may be present.[21]

Electrosurgical injuries are not uncommon with laparoscopy because monopolar devices like cautery are commonly used. The estimated incidence of strictures, fistulae, and perforation is 0.1% to 0.5%.[22] Because cellular temperatures reach $\geq 200°C$ during fulguration,[22] any tissue in proximity is subject to the effects of this heat dispersion. Incomplete instrument insulation and unintentional application of cautery can also contribute to this class of injury.

Care also must be taken when dealing with laparoscopic equipment; suction injuries to the viscera can occur when handling a high-pressure suction irrigator. Grounding pads in incomplete contact can result in dispersive burns for cautery current. Additionally, caution must be exercised when handling an unattached light-source cord, because it generates a significant amount of heat.

### Percutaneous RFA

A percutaneous approach allows RFA to be undertaken in some patients who are not candidates for open or laparoscopic approaches. It has the distinct advantage of being the least invasive method of RFA and can be performed as an outpatient procedure. Unfortunately, however, it is responsible for the largest number of documented complications. Only an experienced interventional radiologist, in conjunction with a multidisciplinary team, should decide what tumors are safe and appropriate to ablate via this route.

Percutaneous ablation can damage structures unrelated to the ablation target. There was one postablation pneumothorax in the John Wayne Cancer Institute series,[8A] likely from penetration of the pleura and possible laceration of the lung. Percutaneous procedures lack the advantage of direct diaphragmatic visualization. Transdiaphragmatic probe insertion can thus occur, even in CT-guided attempts to place the probe into high hepatic lesions. Curley et al[12] also noted one instance of a hydropneumothorax.

Misidentification and nonidentification of structures can also cause visceral injuries, such as bowel and ureteral complications. All three of our documented fistulae were noted after percutaneous procedures.[8A] Additionally, a ureteral injury was noted in one patient, accounting for 0.7% incidence in our series.

One unique complication of percutaneous RFA is pain severe enough to require aborting the procedure. Jiao et al[8] reported three such cases, and we have noted one similar case. As with the vast majority of percutaneous procedures, these were performed under local anesthetic with sedation. While the need to repeat an ablation is not without cost and risk, performance of general anesthesia on every patient to avoid this rare complication does not seem warranted at this time.

## Prophylactic Measures

Tumor location is one of the most important considerations during ablation, as shown by many of the complications outlined. While many injuries are unforeseeable, damage to the biliary system is often predictable based on tumor location. Because of the high frequency of peribiliary tumors, however, it would be unfortunate to exclude all of these malignancies. To reduce the chance of a bile duct injury, we stent the biliary system via endoscopic retrograde cholangiopancreatography (ERCP) before performing the RFA. To date this has been performed in 10 patients with no biliary injury after RFA (Fig. 8.3). The stents are then removed 4 to 6 weeks after the procedure.

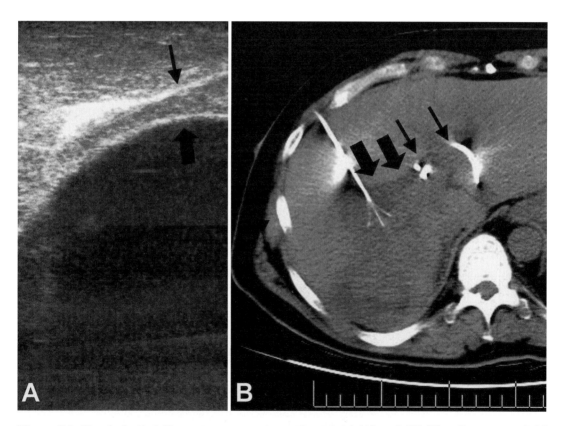

**Figure 8.3.** Prophylactic biliary stents as seen on ultrasound (A) and CT (B), adjacent to a field of ablation. Thick arrows highlight the edge of the ablated lesion, and thin arrows point to the stent.

As mentioned, preoperative assessment includes determination of the relative volume of tumor to normal liver. If tumor burden is close to the maximum volume permissible for ablation, portal vein embolization to hypertrophy the liver parenchyma can confer a margin of safety during ablation.[23] Such a procedure requires the expertise of an interventional radiologist and the luxury of time to wait for the liver to hypertrophy, which occurs by approximately 2 months.[23] This delay often increases a patient's anxiety and in a few cases may allow the tumor to progress beyond the scope of RFA. However, the appearance of an extrahepatic tumor usually indicates that those sites were already seeded and would have grown despite RFA. Therefore, this would not change the patient's management.

## Conclusion

Radiofrequency ablation is a technology that has demonstrated promise for cytoreduction of many primary and metastatic hepatic malignancies that cannot be resected. This new technology can be applied at laparotomy, laparoscopy, or via a percutaneous approach. Because the largest laparoscopic series does not report complications,[24] documented complications of laparoscopic RFA are few. While the benefits of RFA are great, complications have been noted to occur, and perioperative measures in addition to intraoperative vigilance may help minimize risk.

Knowledge of potential pitfalls is required to perform the procedure in a safe and effective manner. It is thus crucial that institutions utilizing RFA continually monitor their outcomes. Complications, attempts to minimize risk, long-term results, and mortalities are all end points that must be monitored to ensure safe application of this technology.

### References

1. Huang SK, Graham AR, Wharton K. Radiofrequency catheter ablation of the left and right ventricles: anatomic and electrophysiologic observations. Pacing Clin Electrophysiol 1988; 11:449–459.
2. Manolis AS, Wang PJ, Estes NA III. Radiofrequency catheter ablation for cardiac tachyarrhythmias. Ann Intern Med 1994; 121:452–461.
3. Bilchik A, Rose DM, Allegra DP. Radiofrequency ablation: a minimally invasive technique with multiple applications. Cancer J Sci Am 1999; 5:356–361.
4. Jarnagin WR, Bodniewicz J, Dougherty E, Conlon K, Blumgart LH, Fong Y. A prospective analysis of staging laparoscopy in patients with primary and secondary hepatobiliary malignancies. J Gastrointest Surg 2000; 4:34–43.

5. Rose DM, Allegra DP, Bostick PJ, Foshag LJ, Bilchik AJ. Radiofrequency ablation: a novel primary and adjunctive ablative technique for hepatic malignancies. Am Surg 1999; 65:1009–1014.

6. Yamasaki T, Kurokawa F, Shirahashi H, Kusano N, Hironaka K, Okita K. Percutaneous radiofrequency ablation therapy with combined angiography and computed tomography assistance for patients with hepatocellular carcinoma. Cancer 2001; 91:1342–1348.

7. Bowles BJ, Machi J, Limm WML, et al. Safety and efficacy of radiofrequency thermal ablation in advanced liver tumors. Arch Surg 2001; 136:864–869.

8. Jiao LR, Hansen PD, Havlik R, Mitry RR, Pignatelli M, Habib N. Clinical short-term results of radiofrequency ablation in primary and secondary liver tumors. Am J Surg 1999; 177:303–306.

8A. Bleicher RJ, Allegra DP, Nora DT, Wood TF, Foshag LJ, Bilchik AJ. Radiofrequency ablation in 447 unresectable liver tumors: lessons learned. Ann Surg Oncol 2003;10:52–58.

9. Meyers WC, Callery MP, Schaffer BK, Shah SA. Staging, resection, and ablation of liver tumors. In: Townsend CM, Beauchamp DR, Evers MB, Mattox KL, Sabiston DC, eds. Sabiston Textbook of Surgery: The Biological Basis of Modern Surgical Practice. Philadelphia: WB Saunders, 2001:1035–1043.

10. Curley SA, Izzo F, Delrio P, et al. Radiofrequency ablation of unresectable primary and metastatic hepatic malignancies: results in 123 patients. Ann Surg 1999; 230:1–8.

11. Wood TF, Rose DM, Chung M, Allegra DP, Foshag LJ, Bilchik AJ. Radiofrequency ablation of 231 unresectable hepatic tumors: indications, limitations, and complications. Ann Surg Oncol 2000; 7:593–600.

12. Curley SA, Izzo F, Ellis LM, Vauthey JN, Vallone P. Radiofrequency ablation of hepatocellular cancer in 110 patients with cirrhosis. Ann Surg 2000; 232:381–391.

13. de Baere T, Elias D, Dromain C, et al. Radiofrequency ablation of 100 hepatic metastases with a mean follow-up of more than 1 year. AJR 2000; 175:1619–1625.

14. Izzo F, Thomas R, Delrio P, et al. Radiofrequency ablation in patients with primary breast carcinoma: a pilot study in 26 patients. Cancer 2001; 92:2036–2044.

15. Bilchik AJ, Wood TF, Allegra DP. Radiofrequency ablation of unresectable hepatic malignancies: lessons learned. Oncologist 2001; 6:24–33.

16. Madigan JD, Choudhri AF, Chen J, Spotnitz HM, Oz MC, Edwards N. Surgical management of the patient with an implanted cardiac device. Ann Surg 1999; 230:639–647.

17. Nordestgaard AG, Bodily KC, Osborne RW, Buttorff JD. Major vascular injuries during laparoscopic procedures. Am J Surg 1995; 169:543–545.

18. Hashizume M, Sugimachi K. Needle and trocar injury during laparoscopic surgery in Japan. Surg Endosc 1997; 11:1198–1201.

19. Schafer M, Lauper M, Krahenbuhl L. Trocar and Veress needle injuries during laparoscopy. Surg Endosc 2001; 15:275–280.

20. Hanney RM, Carmalt HL, Merrett N, Tait N. Vascular injuries during laparoscopy associated with the Hasson technique. J Am Coll Surg 1999; 188:337–338.
21. Kashuk JL, Penn I. Air embolism after central venous catheterization. Surg Gynecol Obstet 1984; 159:249–252.
22. Wu MP, Ou CS, Chen SL, Yen EYT, Rowbotham R. Complications and recommended practices for electrosurgery in laparoscopy. Am J Surg 2000; 179:67–73.
23. Azoulay D, Castaing D, Smail A, et al. Resection of nonresectable liver metastases from colorectal cancer after percutaneous portal vein embolization. Ann Surg 2000; 231:480–486.
24. Siperstein A, Garland A, Engle K, et al. Laparoscopic radiofrequency ablation of primary and metastatic liver tumors: technical considerations. Surg Endosc 2000; 14:400–405.

# Radiofrequency Ablation of Solid Tumors at Various Sites

# Radiofrequency Ablation of Early-Stage Breast Cancer

Merrick I. Ross and Bruno D. Fornage

The surgical management of breast cancer has gradually evolved over the past century from the exclusive use of radical mastectomy to the present-day prevalence of segmental mastectomy and radiation therapy. This evolution to a breast-conserving surgical approach that is less mutilating and more self-image preserving has occurred for the following reasons: (1) patients are presenting with smaller tumor size as a result of earlier diagnosis facilitated by public education and screening mammography programs, (2) a better understanding of the natural history of breast cancer and the biologic events predicting distant dissemination, (3) prospective randomized trials demonstrating survival equivalence between radical and conservative surgical approaches,[1,2] (4) more frequent use of preoperative chemotherapy regimens that can significantly downstage large tumors, (5) the universal desire for less overall surgical morbidity, and (6) a heightened sensitivity to women's health issues.

This movement to less aggressive surgical approaches in the management of breast cancer has been expanded to the surgical treatment of the axilla and has led to the recent introduction and subsequent acceptance of lymphatic mapping and sentinel node biopsy as an alternative to the routine use of formal level I and II axillary dissections in clinically node-negative patients. This innovative technology is rapidly becoming universally commonplace and offers not only the promise of reduced surgical morbidity but also the potential for improved axillary staging.

As an extension of the mindset to embrace less invasive and less extensive surgical approaches, interest has emerged in evaluating nonsurgical ablative modalities in treating the primary tumor in patients with breast cancer. Further motivating the investigation of nonsurgical modalities is the recognition that the current surgical standards of care have limitations: (1) the cosmetic results may not be acceptable with surgical approaches, particularly in those patients with relatively small breasts or centrally located tumors (Fig. 9.1); and (2) in-breast recurrence rates approach 10% in the selected "ideal" candidate group and are greater in other higher risk groups.[3] In addition, increasing percentages of breast cancer patients are diagnosed with core as opposed to excisional biopsies, which not only further indicates a commitment to minimally invasive procedures but also expands the patient population that can be treated with nonsurgical ablative techniques, since the index primary tumor is still for the most part intact.

Nonsurgical ablative techniques are available that may either cool or heat tumors sufficiently to cause complete cell death. Cryotherapy, in the context of treating metastatic tumors to the liver,[4–6] has demonstrated success, but with a relatively high complication rate.[7] Heat has been used for medical purposes since neolithic times to control bleeding, promote wound healing, and treat ulcers and tumors.[8] The introduction of electromagnetic energy sources to produce heat has facilitated the application of thermal treatments in medicine. A variety of technologies are currently available to administer heat as local therapy including laser, microwave, focused ultrasound, and radiofrequency. Radiofrequency is the most promising nonsurgical ablative modality that is currently under active investigation in the treatment of primary breast cancer.

### Why Radiofrequency Ablation (RFA)?

An extensive discussion of the thermal properties of radiofrequency (RF) is presented in Chapter 1. In short, local heat is generated through the friction that is created between tissue ions that are forced to rapidly change direction by administering a high-frequency alternating current. This current, which is generated ex vivo, is passed between a small electrode positioned in the target tissue and discharge electrode pads placed on the surface of the skin (Fig. 9.2). RFA has been demonstrated to be effective in the treatment of unresectable metastatic disease in the liver as well as primary hepatocellular carcinoma, and promising results have been achieved in the treatment of tumors in lung, bone, brain, kidney, and prostate with minimal morbidity.[9–12] This encouraging clinical experience, combined with the fact that RFA

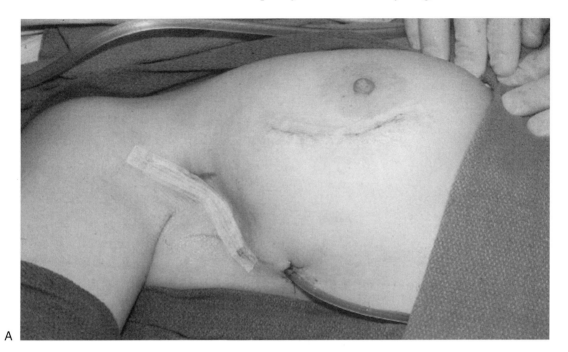

A

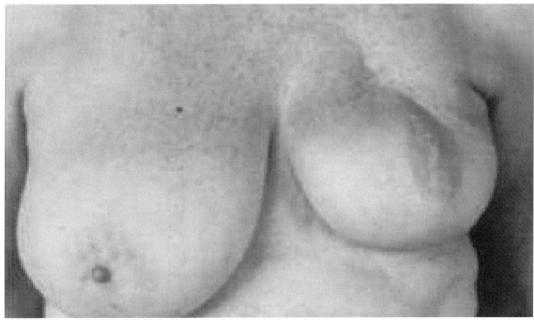

B

**Figure 9.1.** Examples of excellent (A) and poor (B) cosmetic results following breast conservation surgery.

can be administered without significant complications, has provided ample motivation to investigate the effectiveness of this modality in treating primary breast cancer. Furthermore, precise percutaneous placement of the electrode in the epicenter of the tumor can be accomplished in real time with ultrasound guid-

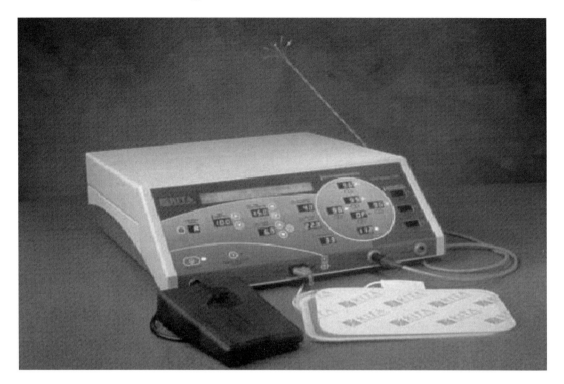

**Figure 9.2.** Basic equipment needed for radiofrequency ablation (RFA) of small breast cancers. Pictured are the radiofrequency generator (A), the electrosurgical probe with arrays deployed (B), skin electrode pads (C), and foot pedal (D).

ance. The widespread use of ultrasound as an excellent imaging modality for the visualization of both nonpalpable and palpable tumors in the breast has facilitated the natural extension of the RF technology to breast cancer.

Other features specifically related to the breast promote a favorable environment in which to apply this technology. Because there are no large blood vessels in the parenchyma of the breast, convectional heat loss, which can occur during ablation when tumors are located in proximity to major blood vessels, is unlikely to occur. Furthermore, thermal injury to surrounding normal tissue such as the overlying skin and underlying pectoralis muscle can be easily avoided by excluding the treatment of tumors that are determined by ultrasound to be too close to these structures.

## Initial Feasibility Studies

Initial feasibility studies evaluating RFA have been limited both in number and size but have provided valuable information concerning efficacy as well as insights into the design of future studies of RFA in primary breast cancer. The first published experience from Jeffrey et al[13] summarized the collaborative efforts of the Stanford University School of Medicine and the University of California–Davis School of Veterinary Medicine. The study comprised five patients with locally advanced invasive breast cancer whose tumors were ablated intraoperatively just prior to resection by either total or partial mastectomy. The ablation was carried out under ultrasound guidance via a 15-gauge multiple needle electrode to a maximum of 60 W in two 15-minute time periods. The tumor sizes ranged from 4 to 7 cm, and by design only a portion of the tumor was treated to facilitate the pathologic assessment of the extent of ablated tissue in distinction from the surrounding nonablated tumor. Routine hematoxylin and eosin (H&E) and reduced nicotinamide adenine dinucleotide-diaphorase (NADH-diaphorase) viability stains were employed to correlate the extent of cell kill with the gross descriptions of the extent of coagulation necrosis. Complete cell death was achieved within ablation zones ranging from 0.8 to 1.8 cm in diameter in four patients, and in the fifth patient a small area of viable cells persisted in lining a cyst. However, accurate pathologic assessment as to the ablative effect may be questioned in part because four of the five patients had received preoperative chemotherapy either with or without preoperative radiation therapy. Despite these limitations in assessing efficacy of the ablation, it was important to demonstrate that no treatment-related complications were encountered in any patient. The authors of the study concluded that RFA could be effectively accomplished in primary breast cancers and would be applicable for primary tumors <3 cm.

## Italian Experience

A relatively large single-institution study was recently reported by Izzo et al.[14] Ultrasound-guided RFA was performed in 26 patients with T1 and T2 breast cancers followed by immediate surgical resection. Complete coagulation necrosis of the tumor was achieved in 25 (96%) of 26 patients. The remaining patient was found to have a small focus of viable tumor adjacent to the electrode shaft. One patient experienced a full-thickness burn of the skin overlying the tumor as the sole complication in this study.

These two aforementioned experiences not only demonstrated the potential efficacy of RFA in the treatment of primary breast cancer but also helped to establish guidelines and parameters to be used in subsequent pilot studies. A complete cell kill could be achieved in a relatively short treatment period (15 minutes), at which time impedance increased exponentially. Because of this rise in impedance, additional treatment time not only may be ineffective but also may lead to increased complications. While the denaturation[8,15,16] of cellular proteins and subsequent cell death can occur at temperatures ranging from 45° to 50°C, this particular temperature range delivered by the electrode may not be sufficient to treat the entire target tissue volume. Since heat is transported in gradients, resulting in lower temperatures achieved with increasing distances from the heat source, tissues at greater distance from the electrode may receive insufficient thermal energy for cell kill.[17] Therefore, higher temperatures in the range of 90° to 95°C are desired to deliver a lethal hit to the entire target tissue volume. The temperature should be gradually increased to this level over 5 to 7 minutes to avoid charring around the electrode and the associated increase in tissue impedance that could hinder the adequate transport of thermal energy.[15,18] It is also important to make sure that the temperature does not reach the boiling point of 100°C to avoid burning of the skin that may result from liquefied material moving along the shaft of the electrode onto the skin.

### Multicenter Feasibility Study

Similar to the aforementioned study by Izzo et al, the M.D. Anderson Cancer Center embarked upon a pilot feasibility study of ultrasound-guided RFA treating primary breast cancers ≤2 cm in diameter. The study began in 1999 and was initially a single-institution program that was subsequently amended to include two additional institutions: John Wayne Cancer Institute and the New York–Weill Cornell Medical Center.

The ultimate goal of using RFA to treat primary breast tumors is to produce a lethal damage volume that encompasses the tumor and a rim of surrounding normal tissue to destroy peripheral extensions of microscopic disease that mimics what can be achieved with surgery. The specific goal of this particular pilot study was to determine the completeness of thermal ablation assessed by pathologic evaluation of specimens obtained by standard surgical procedures employed immediately following intraoperative tumor ablation. This is an ongoing clinical trial that will accrue 50 patients meeting the following eligibility criteria: (1) documented invasive cancer by core needle biopsy, (2) tumor clearly identifiable and measurable by ultrasound, (3) standard prognostic information inclusive of estrogen and progesterone receptor status obtained with core biopsy prior to treatment of the tumor, and (4) tumor location not less than 1 cm from the overlying skin or underlying pectoralis muscle. This last point warrants some discussion as initial ultrasound evaluation may demonstrate that the tumor lies in very close proximity to deep structures but can be mobilized further away with a simple lateral compression maneuver of the breast.

This maneuver must be applied and then maintained during the ablation to ensure that the appropriate distance is preserved (Fig. 9.3).

The RF equipment being utilized includes an electrosurgical RF energy generator, and a 15-gauge multiarray electrosurgical probe with five thermocouples distributed throughout the tips of the array for on-line monitoring of target tissue temperatures (Fig. 9.4) The ablation takes place in the operating room with the electrosurgical probe placed under ultrasound guidance. If the patient requires axillary staging with sentinel node biopsy, the sentinel node procedure, which includes the injection of radiolabeled colloid prior to surgery and the injection of Lymphazurin intraoperatively, is performed prior to RFA. The sequencing of the sentinel node procedure before or after the ablation was an important issue to resolve as two concerns were raised as we designed this protocol to make sure that the appropriate standards of breast cancer care were preserved and that the ablative effect would not be compromised. One concern was that the injection

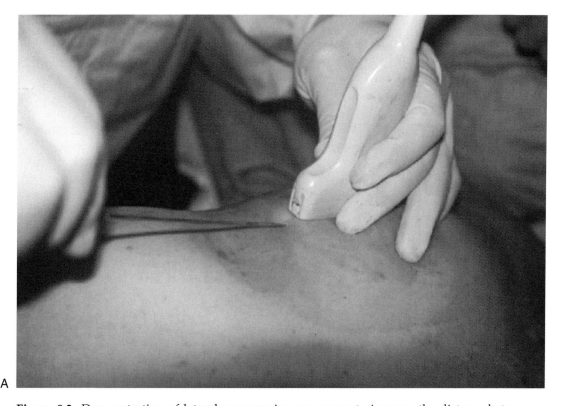

A

**Figure 9.3.** Demonstration of lateral compression maneuver to increase the distance between a deep-seated tumor and the underlying pectoralis musculature. (A) The electrosurgical probe is inserted in real time under ultrasound guidance.

(*continued*)

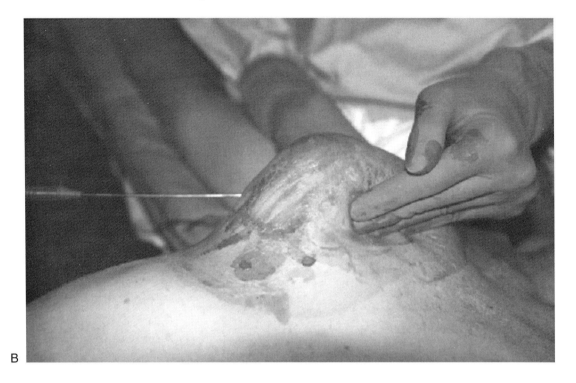

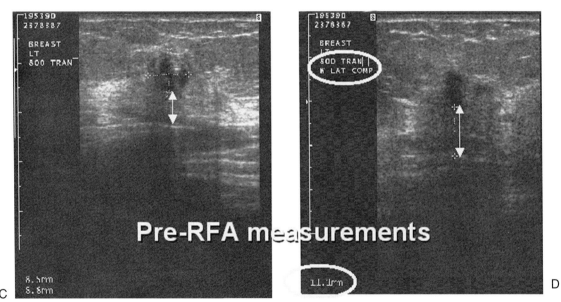

**Figure 9.3.** (B) The lateral compression maneuver is applied. Ultrasound evaluation confirms that the distance from the lesion to the chest wall increased from 8 mm (C) to 11 mm (D).

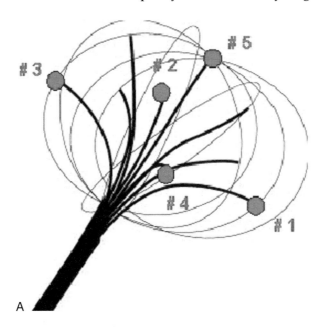

A

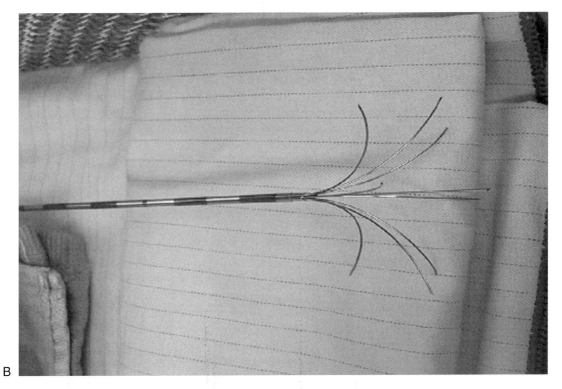

B

**Figure 9.4.** (A) Schematic of the five temperature sensors distributed throughout the nine arrays of the electrosurgical probe. (B) A photograph of the StarBurst™ probe with arrays deployed.

of the radiolabeled colloid and/or Lymphazurin around the tumor could affect the transport of thermal energy into the desired target tissue and in turn limit the effectiveness of the ablation. The second concern was that if the sentinel node biopsy was performed after the ablation, the thermal injury delivered to the surrounding tissue could result in thrombosis or sclerosis of the lymphatics and impede or alter the migration of the injected mapping agents. Such an event could negatively affect both the ability to identify the sentinel node and/or the accuracy of the sentinel node procedure. Since the RFA is the experimental component of the study, the accuracy of the standard axillary staging procedure had to take precedence; therefore, the sentinel node biopsy was performed prior to the ablation.

Subsequent to the completion of the sentinel node biopsy the electrosurgical probe is placed under ultrasound guidance and then deployed over a 3-cm area (Fig. 9.5). The ablations are carried out over a 15-minute period at 95°C followed by a 30- to 60-second cool down and then removal of the electrosurgical probe. During the ablation, on-line monitoring of temperature, impedance, and power is done (Fig. 9.6). Formal segmental mastectomy or total mastectomy is carried out to complete the standard surgical treatment.

Both gross and histologic assessment of the effectiveness of ablation is then carried out for each surgical specimen. The gross examination looks for the presence of the white central coagulum, which represents the ablated zone of tumor and the surrounding margin of normal breast tissue, as well as for the presence and extent of the "red zone" that develops directly adjacent to ablated tissue. A typical example of these gross finding is illustrated in Fig. 9.7. The red zone is an interesting physiologic response to thermal injury that is a result of damage to the blood vessels and normal breast tissue surrounding the ablation zone, followed by a complex series of vasoactive events that include hemostasis, hemorrhage, and then hyperemia.[19,20] Hemostasis is caused by direct thermal coagulation of small blood vessels, hemorrhage is a result of an intact live organ providing continued inflow of blood with a pressure gradient forcing red blood cells out of thermally damaged blood vessels, and hyperemia is a result of the vasoactive substances that are produced by thermal injury to the vascular endothelium and normal tissue breast parenchyma.[20,21] This red zone as well as the white zone coagulation that extends beyond the tumor may effectively treat microscopic extensions of carcinoma beyond the clinical extent of disease and therefore provide an additional treatment margin that is functionally similar to the removal of a 0.5- to 1-cm rim of normal breast tissue during a standard lumpectomy procedure.

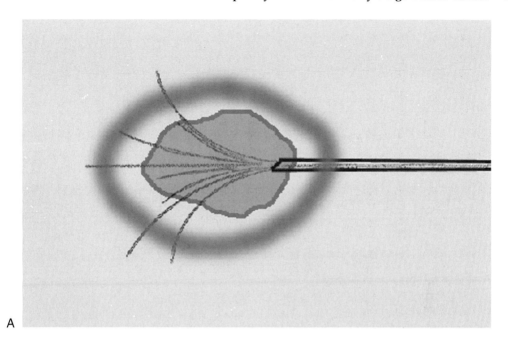

A

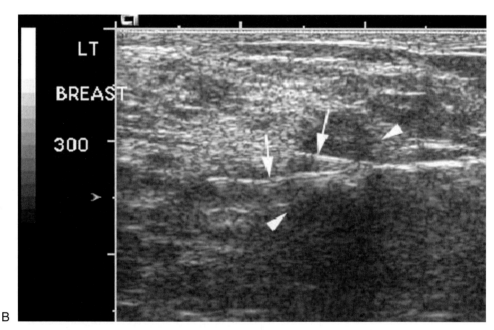

B

**Figure 9.5.** (A) A schematic representation of an electrosurgical probe deployed in the tumor and the volume to the ablated. (B) An ultrasound verification of intratumoral deployment of the arrays. Arrows designate ultrasound visualization of arrays.

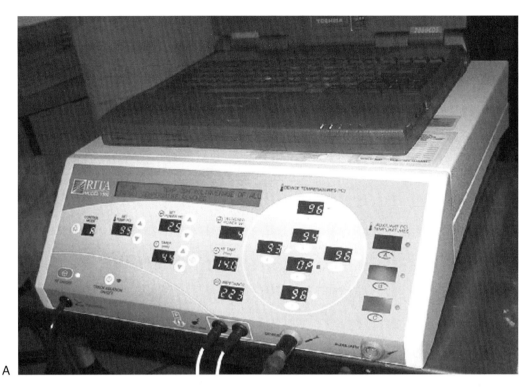

A

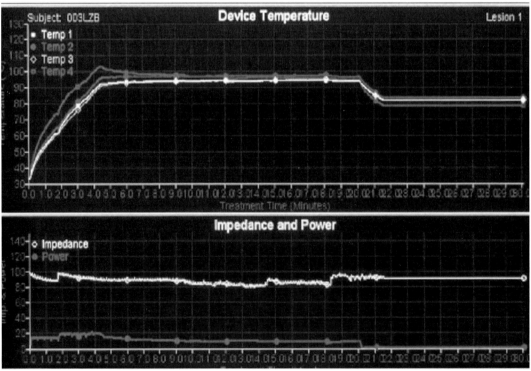

B

**Figure 9.6.** (A) Laptop computer connected to the RF generator for on-line monitoring of temperature during the ablation. (B) An example of on-line computer read-out of impedance and power.

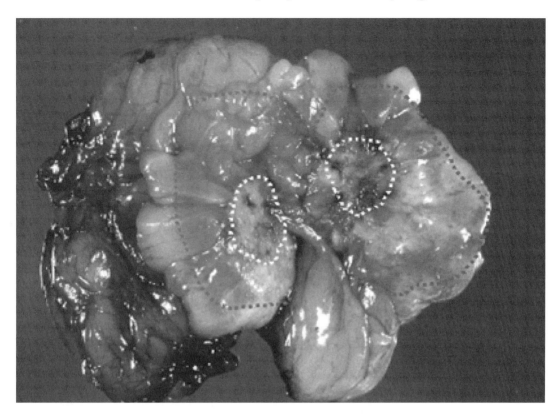

**Figure 9.7.** A bivalved segmental mastectomy specimen. The gross pathologic appearance of the central white coagulum representing the extent of ablation encompassing the tumor is delineated by broken white lines and surrounding reactive "dark zone" indicated by broken dark lines.

Microscopic examination includes routine H&E as well as NADH staining to assess cell viability. Since the surgery takes place immediately following the ablation, not enough time has elapsed for the development of the pathologic hallmarks of co-agulative necrosis. After this short time period the H&E stain still demonstrates an intact tumor architecture, but the tumor cells exhibit thermal injury; it is the NADH stain that confirms the presence of cell death (Fig. 9.8). Thus far a total of 26 lesions in 25 patients have been treated at the three centers in this multi-center pilot study. The results from each center are described below and are summarized in Table 9.1.

### M.D. Anderson Cancer Center

Seventeen patients have been entered in the pilot study, with 18 lesions being treated. Overall, median tumor size was 1.2 cm, and 88% of the lesions were invasive ductal carcinoma with or without associated ductal carcinoma in situ. Within the area of ablation 100% cell kill was accomplished as determined by the NADH stain, and the zone of nonviability coincided directly with the

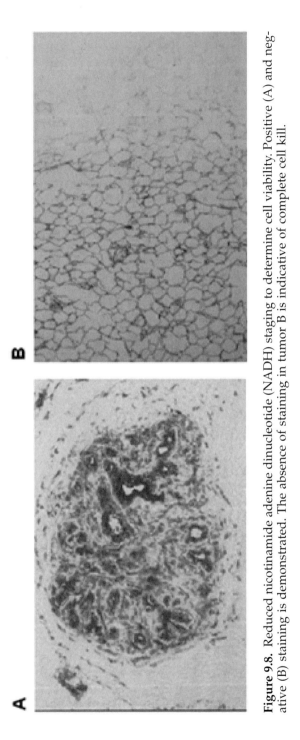

**Figure 9.8.** Reduced nicotinamide adenine dinucleotide (NADH) staging to determine cell viability. Positive (A) and negative (B) staining is demonstrated. The absence of staining in tumor B is indicative of complete cell kill.

**Table 9.1  Ultrasound (US)-Guided Radiofrequency Ablation (RFA) of Small Breast Cancer: Results of Multicenter Pilot Study**

M.D. Anderson Cancer Center, $n = 17$ patients (18 lesions)
  Median size, 1.2 cm
  88% invasive duct with or without ductal carcinoma in situ
  100% response in treated volume
  95% complete tumor ablation
  In two patients ultrasound underestimated extent of disease; one of
    the two received preoperative chemotherapy
  No complications

New York–Weill Cornell Medical Center, $n = 5$
  Three of five patients had complete tumor ablation
  One patient was not well visualized with ultrasound
  One minor skin burn

John Wayne Cancer Institute, $n = 3$
  Two of three patients had 100% ablation
  Ultrasound underestimation in the one patient without complete
    ablation

gross assessment of thermal injury. These results alleviated our concern that the injection of the sentinel node localizing agents prior to the RFA procedure would reduce the effectiveness of the ablation. However, in one patient, occult invasive carcinoma was found microscopically beyond the ablated volume. Retrospective assessment determined that the microscopic extent of tumor was underestimated by the sonographic descriptions and measurements. This occurred in one of the two patients who had received preoperative chemotherapy prior to the ablative procedure. No detectable adverse affect on the overlying skin or the underlying chest wall was documented in any of the patients.

*John Wayne Cancer Institute*
Three patients have been treated at this center, and in two of these patients 100% of the tumor was successfully ablated by the RF procedure. In the remaining patient, 75% tumor kill was accomplished and, similarly to the M.D. Anderson Cancer Center experience, the tumor size was underestimated by ultrasound imaging.

*New York–Weill Cornell Medical Center*
To date five patients have been treated, and in three patients 100% of the tumor was successfully ablated. In the remaining two patients residual tumor was identified outside the ablated area. Consistent with the failures from the other two centers, the true extent of the tumor was not well delineated by the ultrasound examination. At this center one minor skin burn represented the sole adverse event in the study thus far.

### Results

Overall, a total of 26 lesions have been treated, of which 22 revealed complete ablation. In the remaining four patients, ultrasound examination underestimated the true extent of the tumor. There was one minor skin burn. The data suggest that in the ablated area as targeted by ultrasound, at least according to NADH staining, the RF procedure was completely successful; therefore, failures have been related to the imaging rather than to the treatment of the tumor.

### Limitations

While the aforementioned pilot data are very encouraging and support the conclusion that ultrasound-guided percutaneous ablation of small invasive breast cancers is achievable and safe using commercially available RF equipment, this experience also raises a number of issues:

1. The most significant concern, as illustrated in the pilot experience, is the underestimation of the true microscopic extent of the tumor using ultrasound. If these microscopic extensions are limited and distributed circumferentially in a symmetric fashion, then the ablated zone, which may include at least 0.5 to 1 cm of normal breast tissue around the grossly detectable lesion, as is accomplished with standard surgical resection, would be adequate, assuming that the electrode is placed consistently in the epicenter of the tumor and deployed accurately. However, in some situations the microscopic extent can be very large and at times asymmetric. Without surgical resection coupled to frozen section or final pathologic evaluation, as would be the case in future trials that were designed to use RFA alone, unablated and therefore untreated tumor would go undetected. This could lead to a higher risk of local recurrences. How often this is truly a clinical problem when using current standards of surgical care is unclear, but when it is encountered it can be adequately addressed by additional surgery either to obtain more margins or to perform a complete mastectomy if necessary. Some of these events can be predicted prior to treatment by the percentage of extensive ductal carcinoma in situ (DCIS) in the diagnostic core biopsy. Patients with extensive DCIS associated with invasive cancer may then be excluded from RFA trials.
2. Many patients have tumors that cannot be imaged with ultrasound and are appreciated only as calcifications on mammograms. Such patients are currently not included in these ongoing ablation studies. Since patients with microcalcifications represent a significant percentage of patients diagnosed with early-stage invasive cancer, the exclusive use of ultra-

sound guidance for ablation could limit the utilization of this approach. The potential treatment of these patients will require stereotactic placement of the electrosurgical probes. However, precise placement of probes in the epicenter of the tumor would be difficult since stereotactic procedures are not performed in real time. Despite these theoretical/technical concerns, a small series has been reported in which ablation electrodes were placed under stereotactic guidance.[22]

3. Widespread availability of interventional ultrasound expertise ultimately limits the overall infiltration of this approach into the general treating community. Many courses are now available to instruct and familiarize surgeons with ultrasound technology and ultrasound guided biopsies. It is unclear that the expertise required for this procedure in terms of exact localization and determination of extent of the target lesion is exportable to the general surgical community. If it is not, the acceptance of this technology as a potential alternative to surgery may be limited by the availability of expert sonographers.

4. Ultrasound monitoring during ablation is difficult as the margins of the tumor become relatively indistinct and therefore the area of ablation is difficult to measure. This is an important issue as it relates to the ability to accurately assess the ablated zone in future trials in which the treated tumor is left in situ rather than excised. Accurate posttreatment assessment for the completeness of ablation as determined by the presence of either tissue necrosis or residual viable tumor via ultrasound-guided biopsy may be compromised.

5. Individual variation in breast tissue compositions in terms of percent fatty tissue versus percent glandular tissue may affect results. The transport of heat and therefore the potential effectiveness of the ablation may be affected by breast tissue composition; for example, fatty tissue does not conduct thermal energy very efficiently.

6. In patients who may undergo ablation as a potential alternative to surgical excision, appropriate prognostic factor analysis will have to be accomplished solely with core needle biopsies. While the technology for acquiring this information with a core needle biopsy is widely available, the amount of tissue removed may be small and limit the ability to perform retrospective analyses of paraffin-embedded tissue to determine the presence of critical novel prognostic factors that may become established in the future.

## Questions

As investigators have planned to move forward rationally and logically in the evaluation of this modality as a potential replacement for surgical resection in selected patients, a number of questions need to be answered:

1. Will all ablated tumors go on to complete necrosis? To date we have information related only to the effectiveness of the ablation based on immediate evaluation of the target tissue through NADH viability stains. Whether or not these findings are predictive of eventual complete necrosis over time after ablation is of paramount importance. Two issues must be considered: First, it must be cautioned that pathologic evaluation of surgically removed specimens could be inaccurate in some cases as a result of sampling errors. Isolated areas of viable tumor may be present that are missed depending on how carefully the specimen is sectioned. Second, a variety of pathologic markers of thermal damage develop that are time dependent. These markers include the peripheral red zone surrounding the central white coagulation zone, both of which are established in minutes, as opposed to tissue necrosis and the subsequent removal of necrotic cellular debris, which occurs in living tissue in anywhere from 1 to 3 days and then finally is followed by the reparative healing process.[8,20,21] These time-dependent events need to be considered when designing future trials that would include RF as the sole ablative modality followed by planned core biopsies of the ablated area.

2. Is there an accurate way to access in situ the completeness of tumor kill sometime after the ablative procedure? This question is related to the first question but focuses more on the pathologic assessment of the ablated target tissues. Since core biopsies are effective in the diagnosis of primary tumors such as these, they may also be accurate in assessing the treated area for the presence or absence of residual viable tumor cells. Of concern is that ultrasound evaluation of the ablated area immediately after the procedure is performed is somewhat difficult. On physical examination after the ablation, a clear area of induration remains, which is easily palpable. It is likely that this palpable marker of thermal injury will resolve over time and therefore cannot be used to help in the targeting of postablation core biopsies. How useful ultrasound will be in the accurate visualization of the ablated tissue and therefore subsequent targeting for postablation biopsies is presently unknown and may ultimately call into question the reliability of these biopsies.

3. What are the long-term local control rates with ablation alone followed by x-ray therapy (XRT)? This is clearly the most important end point for future RFA trials that will be designed to use RFA as an alternative procedure to surgical ablation. Incidences of ipsilateral breast failures after present-day stan-

dards of local therapy approaches are well established and are secondary to residual, untreated multifocal disease, occult extension of disease not encompassed by lumpectomy, or the development of second primary carcinomas. Whether or not targeted RFA that results in coagulative necrosis of the tumor with a surrounding rim of cell destruction adequately mimics a surgical procedure and results in a similar long-term local control should be the major end point of any future study.

4. What is the long-term cosmetic results after ablation? While it may be predicted that the cosmetic results would be excellent because a surgical resection and its resultant scar, retraction, and/or deformity is avoided, the natural history of the repair process, extent of tissue retraction and tissue fibrosis, and the ultimate impact of radiation therapy in a thermally treated area is not only underdetermined but may vary from patient to patient.

5. How difficult will it be to follow patients after ablation with standard imaging modalities and physical examinations? One of the most important issues in the overall management of patients undergoing breast conservation therapy is careful follow-up and expeditious identification of local failures. While there is some experience in the follow-up of patients who undergo RFA of hepatic tumors with computed tomography (CT) imaging, no data are available in the imaging of the breast with ultrasound or mammograms after ablative procedures. Given the aforementioned concern about standard imaging modalities of ablated tissue, we should take the opportunity to assess other imaging approaches that may be useful in these patients, such as magnetic resonance imaging (MRI) or positron emission tomography (PET) before and after ablation.

## Future Studies

The results of the pilot studies suggest that RFA may represent a viable alternative to surgical resection as a breast-conserving modality. In these studies the small tumors were ablated with a high success rate and minor adverse events were observed in only one patient. Further studies are clearly warranted and must be designed in a way that incorporates what was learned in the pilot studies and addresses the questions posed. To this end our group at M.D. Anderson Cancer Center is embarking on a phase II nonrandomized prospective evaluation of RFA alone as primary local therapy in patients who are breast conservation candidates without immediate surgical resection. Those patients with tumors ≤1.5 cm, identifiable with ultrasound, and at least 1 cm removed from the chest wall and overlying skin are eligi-

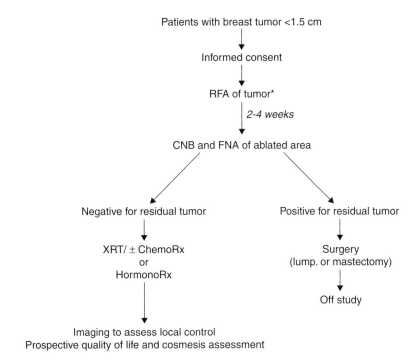

**Figure 9.9.** Algorithm for planned phase II prospective study of ablation followed by in vivo assessment of the ablation areas by core biopsy. *Axillary sentinel node staging performed at this point prior to radiofrequency ablation (RFA). CNB, core needle biopsy; FNA, fine needle aspiration.

ble. Core biopsies will be obtained pretreatment for the determination of invasive disease as well as prognostic factors. The following exclusion criteria have been established: (1) invasive lobular histology, (2) presence of ductal carcinoma in situ of greater than 25%, and (3) preoperative chemotherapy. The purpose of these exclusion criteria is to minimize the underestimation of tumor size by ultrasound, an issue that led to some failures in the pilot studies. The algorithm for this trial is described below and displayed in Fig. 9.9.

In the operating room patients will first undergo a sentinel node biopsy if appropriate, followed by ultrasound-guided RFA for 15 minutes at 95°C. At the completion of the ablation an ultrasonographically identifiable clip will be placed under ultrasound guidance in the epicenter of the ablated tissue. The marker will be used to accurately target multiple core needle biopsies to be obtained at 2 to 4 weeks after the ablative procedure. This should allow ample time for the complete ablative process and subsequent removal of necrotic tissue to transpire and the refractive process to begin. Patients who are found to have evidence of residual carcinoma in any of the biopsies will then undergo a formal surgical segmental mastectomy alone or at the same time as an axillary dissection if the sentinel node was positive on permanent sections. Patients without identifiable residual disease will then undergo XRT. These patients will also be imaged with ultrasound and mammogram at the time of post-treatment biopsy and at the 6-month interval. A separate correlative imaging study with MRI and PET is planned as well to determine the value of these studies. A prospective quality of life protocol to assess cosmesis and patients acceptance of the procedure is also planned.

## Conclusion

Based on the evolving trends to embrace minimally invasive treatments in cancer, it is not surprising that interest has emerged in evaluating nonsurgical ablative approaches in the treatment of primary breast cancer as an alternative to the current standard. Initial results with RFA have been encouraging, and planned phase II studies of ablation and XRT in a breast-conserving setting will be of great interest and provide valuable insights into the potential utility of this modality. Ultimately, a large-scale phase III randomized trial of ablation and XRT versus surgery and XRT may be performed with survival, local control, and quality of life as the primary end points.

### References

1. Fisher V, Redmond C, Poisson R, et al. Eight-year results of a randomized clinical trial comparing total mastectomy and lumpectomy with or without irradiation in the treatment of breast cancer. N Engl J Med 1989; 320:822–828.
2. Veronesi U, Salvadini B, Luini A, et al. Conservation treatment of early breast cancer: long-term results of 1,232 cases treated with quadrantectomy, axillary dissection, and radiotherapy. Ann Surg 1990; 211:250–259.
3. Early Breast Cancer Trialists Collaborative Group. Effects of radiotherapy and surgery in early breast cancer. N Engl J Med 1995; 333:1444–1455.
4. Quebbeman EJ, Wallace JR. Cryosurgery for hepatic metastases. In: Condon RE, ed. Current Techniques in General Surgery. New York: CV Mosby, 1997:1–75.
5. Gagne DJ, Roh MS. Cryosurgery for hepatic malignancies. In: Curley SA, ed. Liver Cancer. New York: Springer-Verlag, 1998:173–200.
6. Stewart GJ, Proketes A, Horton KM, et al. Hepatic cryotherapy: double-freeze cycles achieve greater hepatocellular injury in man. Cryobiology 1995; 32(3):215–219.
7. Sarantou T, Bilchik A, Ramming KP. Complications of hepatic cryosurgery. Semin Surg Oncol 1998; 14(2):156–162.

8. Thomsen S. Qualitative and quantitative pathology of clinically relevant thermal lesions. In Matching the Energy Source to the Clinical Need. Proceedings of a conference held January 23–24, 2000, San Jose, California, vol CR75, page 425.

9. Mirza AN, Fornage BC, Sneige N, et al. Radiofrequency ablation of solid tumors. Cancer J 2001; 7(2):95–102.

10. Hamazoe R, Maeta M, Murakami A, Yamashiro H, Kaibara N. Heating efficiency of radiofrequency capacitive hyperthermia for treatment of deep-seated tumors in the peritoneal cavity. J Surg Oncol 1991; 48(3):176–179.

11. Miao Y, Ni Y, Mulier S, et al. Ex vivo experiment on radiofrequency liver ablation with saline infusion through a screw-tip cannulated electrode. J Surg Res 1997; 71(1):19–24.

12. Leveillee RJ, Hoey MF, Hulbert JC, Mulier P, Lee D, Jesserun J. Enhanced radiofrequency ablation of canine prostate utilizing a liquid conductor: the virtual electrode. J Endourol 1996; 10(1):5–11.

13. Jeffrey SS, Birdwell RI, Ikeda DM, et al. Radiofrequency ablation of breast cancer: first report of an emerging technology. Arch Surg 1999; 134(10):1064–1068.

14. Izzo F, Thomas R, Delrio P, et al. Radiofrequency ablation in patients with primary breast carcinoma: a pilot study in 26 patients. Cancer 2001; 92(8):2036–2044.

15. Organ LW. Electrophysiologic principles of radiofrequency lesion making. Appl Neurophysiol 1976; 39(2):69–76.

16. Nath S, Haines DE. Biophysics and pathology of catheter energy delivery systems. Prog Cardiovasc Dis 1995; 37(4):185–204.

17. Henriques FC, Mortiz AR. Studies of thermal injury in the conduction of heat to and through skin and the temperatures attained therein: a theoretical and experimental investigation. Am J Pathol 1947; 23:531–549.

18. Haines DE, Verow AF. Observations on electrode-tissue interface temperature and effect on electrical impedance during radiofrequency ablation of ventricular myocardium. Circulation 1990; 82(3):1034–1038.

19. Mortiz AR. Studies of thermal injury II. The pathology and pathogenesis of cutaneous burns: an experimental study. Am J Pathol 1947; 23:695–720.

20. Henriques FC. Studies of thermal injury. V. The predictability and significance of thermally-induced rate processes leading to irreversible epidermal injury. Arch Pathol 1947; 43:489–502.

21. Thomsen S. Identification of lethal thermal injury at the time of photothermal treatment. In: Muller G, Rogan A, eds. Laser-Induced Interstitial Thermotherapy. Bellingham, WA: SPIE PM 25, 1995:459–467.

22. Elliott RL, Rice PB, Suits JA, Ostrowe AJ, Head JF. Radiofrequency ablation of a stereotactically localized non-palpable breast carcinoma. Am Surg 2002; 68:1–5.

# 10

# Radiofrequency Ablation of Osteoid Osteoma

Martin Torriani and Daniel I. Rosenthal

Osteoid osteoma is a painful bone tumor that is usually found in the lower extremities of children and young adults. The tumors rarely exceed 1.5 cm in diameter. They are benign and have little or no growth potential, even when followed for long periods of time. Very rarely, there may be adverse affects on the adjacent tissues (joints, growth plates). However, in the great majority of patients, treatment is undertaken only for pain control.

Because of these features and the belief that given adequate periods of time many lesions may regress spontaneously, some authorities advocate medical management.[1] In our experience, most patients prefer tumor removal to medical management, particularly when given the option of minimally invasive percutaneous treatment.

Surgical treatment is generally thought to require complete removal of the tumor. Failure to do so can lead to local recurrence. The tumor can be difficult to identify at surgery because it is small, and because of the surrounding bone formation, edema, and joint effusion. Generous surgical margins increase the probability of cure, but resection of weight-bearing bone requires a long recovery period, and may necessitate internal fixation and/or bone grafting.[2] Even conservative surgical techniques require a hospital stay and a rehabilitation period that can last for several months.[3]

Many attempts have been made to match the extent of operative intervention to the size of the tumor. Improved imaging has helped to limit the extent of bone removal. Radioisotope scanning is highly sensitive to the presence of these lesions, and can be used intraoperatively to localize the lesion[4,5] and to ensure removal of the tumor.[6] Computed tomography (CT) scanning is also extremely effective at finding the tumor nidus and can be used to guide placement of needles, Kirschner (K) wires,[7,8] or methylene blue[7,9,10] to assist with surgical identification. Arthroscopic removal of osteoid osteomas has been reported.[11]

In recent years, percutaneous excision using relatively large-caliber hollow needles and drills has been performed under CT guidance, especially in Europe.[12,13] Although it is less invasive than open surgery, complications such as fractures and osteomyelitis have been reported.[12] In addition, hospitalization[12,13] and a period of limited weight bearing[12] may be required.

Most recently, CT-guided ablative methods have been introduced in which the tumor is destroyed in situ. These methods include drilling of the nidus followed by ethanol injection[14,15]; magnetic resonance imaging (MRI)-guided cryo-treatment[16]; interstitial laser photocoagulation through an optical fiber[17–19]; and percutaneous radiofrequency (RF) thermocoagulation.

Since our initial description of the technique,[20] we have performed almost 300 RF treatments for osteoid osteoma. We believe that RF ablation is a robust technique, suitable for most patients, and feasible in most centers, and that it has significant advantages when compared with other available minimally invasive methods.

## Imaging

Successful treatment depends on precise identification of the tumor. Osteoid osteomas may arise in cortical bone, on the periosteal surface of bone, or less often in the bone marrow. The lesion may contain a variable amount of internal ossification, but in most cases at least part of the tumor is lucent. The lesion is usually either spherical, or elongated in the direction of the long axis of the bone. In our experience, 90% of tumors are between 3 and 10 mm in diameter. In some instances, elongation of the tumor can be striking, giving the appearance of a "string of beads" (Fig. 10.1). Rarely, multiple distinctly separate tumors may be seen adjacent to each other in the same bone. Multiple tumors in different bones have been reported, but are extremely rare.[21]

Tumors may be difficult to identify on plain films if they are surrounded by very dense sclerosis or not demarcated by any sclerosis at all. Radioisotope bone scans consistently demonstrate

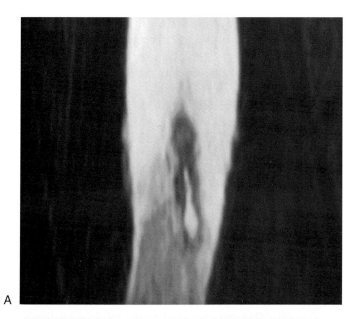

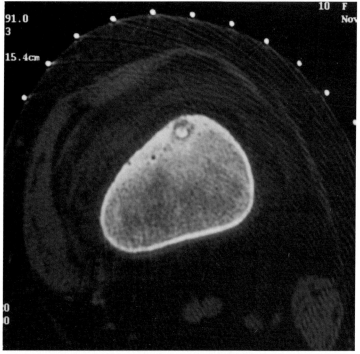

**Figure 10.1.** (A) Sagittal reformation of computed tomography (CT) images demonstrates an elongated lytic lesion measuring almost 3 cm in craniocaudal extent. The lesion exhibits distinctly widened areas, separated by a slender isthmus. (B) Axial images from the same CT scan show typical rounded focus of tumor containing central ossification. The tumor measures approximately 5 mm in cross section.

the lesions. Although the literature indicates that osteoid osteoma may occasionally fail to show uptake, we have not seen such an example. Thin-section CT (<2.0 mm thick) is the preferred method for diagnosis of osteoid osteoma. Although MRI reveals the marrow and soft tissue edema that surrounds the lesions, the reactive tissues can occasionally obscure the tumor itself.[22,23]

## Differential Diagnosis

Some believe that the diagnostic accuracy of clinical and imaging features makes biopsy unnecessary.[3] We agree that diagnosis based on imaging and clinical features is highly accurate for patients with typical features. However, several different entities can be mistaken for osteoid osteoma.

*Chondroblastoma* is often larger than osteoid osteoma, and has a predilection for the upper extremity and epiphysis. Like osteoid osteomas, these lesions are often surrounded by edema. *Eosinophilic granuloma* is also often larger and has a more irregular shape than osteoid osteoma. It is also surrounded by edema, and sometimes by a sclerotic reaction in the healing state. *Osteoblastoma* presents histologic findings identical to those of osteoid osteoma, and therefore biopsy is not helpful in distinguishing them. The important distinction is that osteoid osteoma is a growth-limited lesion, something that can only be determined in retrospect. *Stress fractures* can have a variety of different shapes and may be surrounded by edematous and sclerotic tissue. In most instances the clinical distinction is clear, as these lesions tend to be symptomatic with activity and to heal with rest. However, the pain of osteoid osteoma is frequently exacerbated by activity, and sometimes the distinction is difficult. *Herniation pits* on the anterior surface of the femur may be confused with an osteoid osteoma (Fig. 10.2). However, herniation pits are asymptomatic, may be bilateral, and occur in older patients. An *abscess* also could potentially mimic osteoid osteoma. Both entities are surrounded by edematous and sclerotic tissue. However, the lytic center of an abscess generally does not have the simple spherical or oval shape of an osteoid osteoma. Interestingly, we have not encountered a single abscess in the course of treating osteoid osteoma, perhaps due to the perceptiveness of referring clinicians.

## Patients

We usually do not treat lesions of the spine or the hand. Although needle placement is not difficult, most spinal tumors involve the posterior elements, and thus are in close proximity to nerves

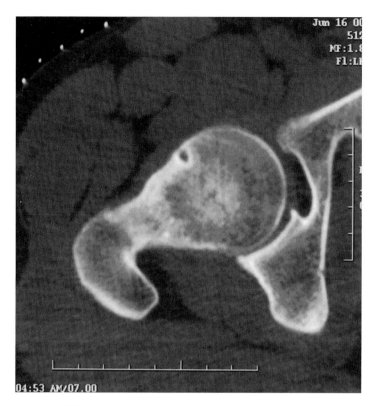

**Figure 10.2.** CT scan reveals a rounded lytic lesion on the anterior surface of the femoral neck, surrounded by a limited amount of sclerosis in a 38-year-old man. This lesion proved to be an osteoid osteoma.

within the spinal canal, the lateral recesses, or the neural foramina. Although cortical bone may be a relative barrier to heat transmission,[24] our own laboratory experiments and clinical experience indicate that it is not a reliable insulator, and we consider the risks to nerves due to heat conduction to be unacceptable. Similar considerations apply in the hand. In addition, convalescence following operative treatment of these tumors is shorter than that which follows lower extremity lesions. Therefore, compared with long bone lesions, the risks are greater and the benefits less.

Tumors on, or immediately beneath, joint surfaces can be safely treated in many instances. Although the articular cartilage is at risk for a focal injury, this appears to be well tolerated by the patient, as we have yet to encounter a patient with significant symptoms following the procedure. Perhaps very long-term follow-up will reveal premature degenerative changes; however, the subarticular location of the tumor and the resultant synovitis may itself produce this result.

Bleeding has not been a problem, despite the fact that most patients take significant amounts of nonsteroidal antiinflammatory medications and presumably have prolonged bleeding times.

Patients often are referred after a long period of diagnostic uncertainty. In many instances the symptoms have been blamed on stress fractures, tendinitis, or "growing pains." There is no reason to second-guess the clinical process, and patients should be reassured that delayed diagnosis is common. In other cases, an initial diagnosis of malignant bone tumor may have been made, and the patients may still harbor such concerns. It is important to address these fears directly and to allay them specifically.

We advise our patients that the probability of complete and permanent success from a single procedure (no symptoms and no medications 2 years later) is about 85%. About 7% to 8% of patients undergo a second procedure because of recurrence, and another 7% to 8% describe some continuing symptoms, but not enough to merit intervention.

The probability of a definitive diagnosis from the biopsy taken at the time of the procedure is about 70%. If the biopsy is nondiagnostic and the patient is free of symptoms, we advise the patient that it is of no clinical significance. A change in approach may be warranted in the rare event that the pathologist returns another diagnosis.

## Anesthesia

We have performed this procedure using conscious sedation and spinal anesthesia; however, we prefer general anesthesia. Children and teenagers find it frightening to be awake for the procedure, and the paralysis induced by the spinal anesthesia is alarming. Pain control provided by local anesthesia with or without conscious sedation is adequate for most bone biopsies. However, needle puncture of an osteoid osteoma is more painful than biopsy of other lesions. When the biopsy needle enters the tumor, patients often exhibit sudden, marked tachycardia and tachypnea, even under general anesthesia. It is important that the anesthetist be aware of this phenomenon to prevent patient movement. An intravenous nonsteroidal antiinflammatory drug such as ketorolac given approximately 20 minutes before completion helps with postprocedure pain.

This is an outpatient procedure in our institution. The patient must be fasting for 8 hours before anesthesia. The preanesthesia interview is done when the patient arrives at the CT suite, and the average procedure requires between 1.5 and 2 hours of CT time.

## Technique

### Approaching the Tumor

Once the patient is anesthetized, a grounding plate is attached to the skin opposite to the site of entry. The patient is positioned on the CT table for preprocedural localization of the nidus. We believe that any CT scanner capable of obtaining contiguous 3-mm-thick sections is suitable for guidance. Helical acquisitions, although useful, are not essential.

A Fast Find Grid (EZ Grid, E-Z EM, Inc., Westbury, NY) is applied to the skin overlying the tumor and contiguous 3-mm-thick sections are acquired to determine the easiest and safest path for the needle. Once the lesion has been adequately demonstrated, the radiation exposure can be minimized by decreasing milliamperage (mA) to the lowest level of which the equipment is capable. Although this results in artifacts and decreased spatial resolution, it is usually adequate for assessment of the needle tip. If it is not, we increase the mA in a stepwise fashion until it is minimally adequate.

In general, we recommend choosing the level that demonstrates the tumor in its largest diameter. If the lesion is large or elongated, it may exceed the treatment radius of the probe (5–6 mm). In such cases, it may be necessary to treat the lesion at two adjacent levels to ensure complete ablation of the tumor.

After skin preparation, a 22-gauge needle is introduced in the direction to be followed for the biopsy. An image is obtained to confirm the puncture site and to estimate angulation, following which a stab incision is made with a number 11 scalpel.

When it is necessary to penetrate dense cortical bone we use a hand-operated drill, which appears safer and more versatile than power drills. We generally use the Bonopty Penetration Set (RADI Medical System AB, Uppsala, Sweden), which produces a hole large enough to admit a 16-gauge (1.6-mm) biopsy needle. It is also possible to use a trephine needle alone or in conjunction with a hand drill.[25] Whether a drill or a trephine is used, it is necessary to pause at frequent intervals to clear the trephine or the threads of the drill. If this is not done, it becomes increasingly difficult to continue advancing, and indeed the biopsy device may become wedged in the bone, making it very difficult to withdraw. The best method to prevent this frustrating and alarming situation is to advance by small steps with frequent clearing when drilling through hard bone.

To minimize the risk of slipping, the needle should be as perpendicular to the surface of the bone as possible. For the relatively common lesions of the medial and even posterior upper femur, the patient can be placed in the "frog-lateral" position once anesthetized (Fig. 10.3). This position usually rotates the femur sufficiently to allow an anterior approach. Sometimes even with this positioning it is necessary to approach from a very medial direction, through the adductors. Finally, when there is no safe direct access to the lesion, a transosseous approach can be used, drilling through the entire thickness of the bone from the contralateral side (Fig. 10.4).

Additional CT images are obtained as the instrument is advanced through bone. When the drill comes into close proximity with the tumor (1 mm) but has not entered it, it is exchanged for the biopsy needle.

### Biopsy

We perform a biopsy in every case, even when the diagnosis is apparent from the clinical features and imaging studies. It does not add to the difficulty or duration of the procedure, and can provide significant reassurance to the patient. When the tumor arises on the surface of the bone, and is not surrounded by dense sclerosis, almost any biopsy needle can be used. We prefer the Ostycut Bone Biopsy Needle (C. R. Bard Inc., Covington, GA) because the sharp stylet exhibits little tendency to slip on the surface of the bone, the external screw threads are helpful in advancing through the lesion, and it yields a biopsy sample of good quality. A 1.6-mm (16-gauge) needle is appropriate for the 1-mm outer diameter of the electrode.

The biopsy needle is advanced through the full width of the tumor. As mentioned earlier, a marked physiologic response should be expected when penetrating the tumor. The biopsy sample is taken and immersed in 0.9% sodium chloride. We generally do not request frozen-section analysis because tissue preservation is not optimal by this method, and the histologic diagnosis will rarely alter the treatment. The one exception is when infection is a serious diagnostic possibility, as thermocoagulation could potentially worsen the condition by producing a sequestrum.

### Treatment

The biopsy needle is exchanged for the radiofrequency electrode and CT imaging is done to confirm the placement of the tip within the nidus. We use electrodes with either 5 or 8 mm of exposed tip, depending on the diameter of the lesion. Once the CT scan has demonstrated adequate position of the electrode, it is connected to the RF generator (RFG-3C, Radionics, Burlington, MA), and the tip temperature is slowly raised to 90°C (one degree every 1 to 2 seconds).

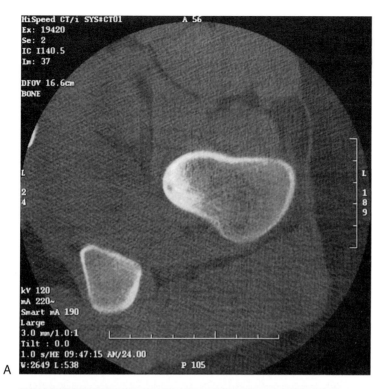

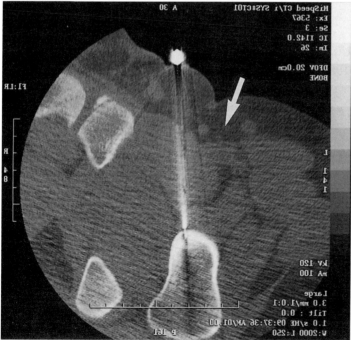

**Figure 10.3.** (A) CT scan of the left hip shows an osteoid osteoma in the posteromedial cortex of the proximal femur. (B) Images obtained with the patient in the "frog-lateral" position. This rotates the lesion anteriorly, allowing it to be safely approached medial to the femoral triangle (arrow).

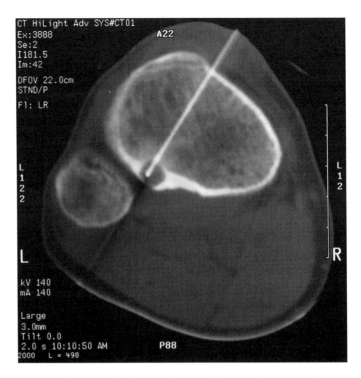

**Figure 10.4.** CT scan of the proximal tibia reveals an osteoid osteoma of the posterior cortex. Because of the proximity of the neurovascular structures, it was elected to approach this lesion from the front, by drilling through the tibia. Although technically demanding, this approach is quite safe.

Except for the exposed tip, the remainder of the electrode is insulated and does not cause heating of adjacent structures. We maintain the tip temperature for 6 minutes, after which the generator is turned off, and the procedure is complete. The electrode and sleeve through which it was inserted (drill or biopsy needle sleeve) are removed, and the small skin wound is closed with a Steri-Strip.

These parameters (90°C, 6 minutes) consistently result in a spherical (5-mm electrode) or cylindrical (8-mm electrode) lesion with a radius of 5 to 6 mm. With a 6-minute duration, a steady state is reached, resulting in the maximum extent of thermal damage that is possible at that temperature. Slightly higher or lower temperatures can increase or decrease the radius by a small amount, but the effect is minor.[26] Therefore, the electrode placement must be such that no portion of the tumor is more than 5 to 6 mm away from its exposed tip. If the tumor is large, or if electrode placement is off-center, it will be necessary to perform more than one puncture and treatment with overlapping fields to ensure that the entire tumor is covered.

It is apparent from the foregoing that a 6-mm minimum separation between the electrode and any vital structures is required do avoid tissue damage. We generally do not perform this procedure when the distance is less than 1 cm.

In our experience, no intralesional administration of anesthetics or postprocedure imaging is required or helpful.

## After the Procedure

Pain in the recovery room is very variable. In those individuals who have pain, it is most severe almost immediately upon awakening. It may require narcotics for control, but once brought under control, it improves steadily and rapidly. Patients are discharged with a prescription for enough oral narcotics to last 24 hours, but they seldom need more than one or two doses. Occasionally a patient complains of moderate to severe pain lasting several days after the procedure.

It should very rarely be necessary for a patient to stay in the hospital overnight.[27–32] The patient should be able to walk out of the hospital without the use of casts, braces, or crutches, and resume all daily activities within 24 hours. During the first few years of our experience we recommended avoiding sports for 3 months due to the theoretical weakening of bone during the resorptive phase of healing. However, no fractures have occurred, and we have loosened our recommendations to avoid only those activities involving prolonged running and/or jumping.

On the day following the procedure we communicate by telephone to assess the appearance of the treatment site. There should be no evidence of bleeding, swelling, or inflammation. Most patients feel markedly better; about half state with confidence that the tumor is gone. The remainder improve over the next several days, so that the symptoms are almost always gone within a week. Approximately 1 week after the procedure we again speak with the patient to discuss the histopathologic findings.

The radiographic appearance of the tumor changes very slowly after treatment. We obtain an x-ray examination approximately 3 to 4 weeks after treatment. The tumor does not change in appearance during this interval. The film serves as a baseline in the event of future complications. If the patient is asymptomatic, we obtain a further follow-up at 1 year, by which time there should be clear evidence of healing. Younger children heal more rapidly, with the x-ray examination becoming normal after a few months.

We have occasionally obtained interval films at 6 weeks to 3 months following treatment. These films can sometimes show a faint, lucent line demarcating a spherical region of 1 cm diameter at a distance of 5 mm from the electrode site. This presumably represents the margin of the thermal necrosis.

## Outcomes

In our experience, most recurrences are seen between 3 and 6 months following treatment. Recurrences after a year without symptoms are rare, and after 2 years exceedingly rare. We therefore believe that a follow-up of 2 years is adequate to confirm a successful treatment.

Several studies of osteoid osteoma treatment by RF ablation have shown cure rates from 75% to 95% with mean follow-up periods ranging between 3 and 23 months.[20,27–31] Recurrence rates are similar to those observed following operative treatment.[32] In all cases a second RF treatment cured the recurrence.[27–29,32]

## Complications

A few patients have had somewhat prolonged postprocedural pain of unknown significance that resolved spontaneously after approximately 1 week. In one case, an apparent cellulitis was treated with oral antibiotics and resolved. In another case, an unusual skin discoloration probably of vascular origin resolved spontaneously. Neither fractures nor major or delayed complications have been reported.[27–29,32]

## Summary

Percutaneous CT-guided radiofrequency treatment of osteoid osteoma is a minimally invasive alternative to the surgical and medical management of osteoid osteoma. Experience with a large number of patients has shown that it can be performed safely and effectively in the great majority of patients with this condition. With success rates similar to those for operative treatment, minimal complications, and rapid recovery, it has largely eliminated surgical treatment and long-term medical management in our institution.

### References

1. Kneisl JS, Simon MA. Medical management compared with operative treatment for osteoid-osteoma. J Bone Joint Surg 1992; 74A: 179–185.
2. Rosenthal DI, Hornicek FJ, Wolfe MW, Jennings LC, Gebhardt MC, Mankin HJ. Decreasing length of hospital stay in treatment of osteoid osteoma. Clin Orthop 1999 (361):186–191.

3. Campanacci M, Ruggieri P, Gasbarrini A, Ferraro A, Campanacci L. Osteoid osteoma. Direct visual identification and intralesional excision of the nidus with minimal removal of bone. J Bone Joint Surg 1999; 81B:814–820.

4. Kirchner B, Hillmann A, Lottes G, et al. Intraoperative, probe-guided curettage of osteoid osteoma. Eur J Nucl Med 1993; 20: 609–613.

5. Lee DH, Malawer MM. Staging and treatment of primary and persistent (recurrent) osteoid osteoma. Evaluation of intraoperative nuclear scanning, tetracycline fluorescence, and tomography. Clin Orthop 1992 (281):229–238.

6. Roger B, Bellin MF, Wioland M, Grenier P. Osteoid osteoma: CT-guided percutaneous excision confirmed with immediate follow-up scintigraphy in 16 outpatients. Radiology 1996; 201:239–242.

7. Magre GR, Menendez LR. Preoperative CT localization and marking of osteoid osteoma: description of a new technique. J Comput Assist Tomogr 1996; 20:526–529.

8. Steinberg GG, Coumas JM, Breen T. Preoperative localization of osteoid osteoma: a new technique that uses CT. AJR 1990; 155:883–885.

9. Logan PM, Janzen DL, Munk PL, Connell DG. A technique for preoperative localization of osteoid osteoma. Can Assoc Radiol J 1995; 46:471–474.

10. Ziegler DN, Scheid DK. A method for location of an osteoid-osteoma of the femur at operation. A case report. J Bone Joint Surg 1992; 74A:1549–1552.

11. Resnick RB, Jarolem KL, Sheskier SC, Desai P, Cisa J. Arthroscopic removal of an osteoid osteoma of the talus: a case report. Foot Ankle Int 1995; 16:212–215.

12. Sans N, Galy-Fourcade D, Assoun J, et al. Osteoid osteoma: CT-guided percutaneous resection and follow-up in 38 patients. Radiology 1999; 212:687–692.

13. Parlier-Cuau C, Champsaur P, Nizard R, Hamze B, Laredo JD. Percutaneous removal of osteoid osteoma. Radiol Clin North Am 1998; 36:559–566.

14. Adam G, Neuerburg J, Vorwerk D, Forst J, Gunther RW. Percutaneous treatment of osteoid osteomas: combination of drill biopsy and subsequent ethanol injection. Semin Musculoskelet Radiol 1997; 1:281–284.

15. Sanhaji L, Gharbaoui IS, Hassani RE, Chakir N, Jiddane M, Boukhrissi N. [A new treatment of osteoid osteoma: percutaneous sclerosis with ethanol under scanner guidance]. J Radiol 1996; 77:37–40.

16. Skjeldal S, Lilleas F, Folleras G, et al. Real time MRI-guided excision and cryo-treatment of osteoid osteoma in os ischii—a case report. Acta Orthop Scand 2000; 71:637–638.

17. Gangi A, Dietemann JL, Gasser B, et al. Interstitial laser photocoagulation of osteoid osteomas with use of CT guidance. Radiology 1997; 203:843–848.

18. Gangi A, Dietemann JL, Guth S, et al. Percutaneous laser photocoagulation of spinal osteoid osteomas under CT guidance. AJNR 1998; 19:1955–1958.

19. Gangi A, Dietemann JL, Gasser B, et al. Interventional radiology with laser in bone and joint. Radiol Clin North Am 1998; 36:547–557.
20. Rosenthal DI, Alexander A, Rosenberg AE, Springfield D. Ablation of osteoid osteomas with a percutaneously placed electrode: a new procedure. Radiology 1992; 183:29–33.
21. Kenan S, Abdelwahab IF, Klein MJ, Hermann G, Lewis MM. Case report 864. Elliptical, multicentric periosteal osteoid osteoma. Skeletal Radiol 1994; 23:565–568.
22. Kribbs S, Munk PL, Vellet AD, Levin MF. Diagnosis of osteoid osteoma using STIR magnetic resonance imaging. Australas Radiol 1993; 37:292–296.
23. Hayes CW, Conway WF, Sundaram M. Misleading aggressive MR imaging appearance of some benign musculoskeletal lesions. Radiographics 1992; 12:1119–1136.
24. Dupuy DE, Hong R, Oliver B, Goldberg SN. Radiofrequency ablation of spinal tumors: temperature distribution in the spinal canal. AJR 2000; 175:1263–1266.
25. Kattapuram SV, Rosenthal DI, Phillips WC. Trephine biopsy of the skeleton with the aid of a hand drill. Radiology 1984; 152:231.
26. Goldberg SN, Gazelle GS, Halpern EF, Rittman WJ, Mueller PR, Rosenthal DI. Radiofrequency tissue ablation: importance of local temperature along the electrode tip exposure in determining lesion shape and size. Acad Radiol 1996; 3:212–218.
27. de Berg JC, Pattynama PM, Obermann WR, Bode PJ, Vielvoye GJ, Taminiau AH. Percutaneous computed-tomography-guided thermocoagulation for osteoid osteomas. Lancet 1995; 346:350–351.
28. Lindner NJ, Ozaki T, Roedl R, Gosheger G, Winkelmann W, Wortler K. Percutaneous radiofrequency ablation in osteoid osteoma. J Bone Joint Surg 2001; 83B:391–396.
29. Woertler K, Vestring T, Boettner F, Winkelmann W, Heindel W, Lindner N. Osteoid osteoma: CT-guided percutaneous radiofrequency ablation and follow-up in 47 patients. J Vasc Intervent Radiol 2001; 12:717–722.
30. Barei DP, Moreau G, Scarborough MT, Neel MD. Percutaneous radiofrequency ablation of osteoid osteoma. Clin Orthop 2000 (373):115–124.
31. Rosenthal DI, Springfield DS, Gebhardt MC, Rosenberg AE, Mankin HJ. Osteoid osteoma: percutaneous radio-frequency ablation. Radiology 1995; 197:451–454.
32. Rosenthal DI, Hornicek FJ, Wolfe MW, Jennings LC, Gebhardt MC, Mankin HJ. Percutaneous radiofrequency coagulation of osteoid osteoma compared with operative treatment. J Bone Joint Surg 1998; 80A:815–821.

# 11

# Percutaneous Radiofrequency Ablation of Osseous Metastases

Damian E. Dupuy

Osseous metastatic disease is by far the most common cause of cancer pain. Conventional treatment relies primarily on external beam radiation and chemotherapy, although these treatments are not completely effective and many patients live with inadequate analgesia. Radiofrequency ablation (RFA) is an image-guided minimally invasive treatment for solid tumors. Patients who have not responded to conventional treatment for osseous metastases and have limited disease may benefit from palliation with RFA. RFA has been used for patients who have persistent pain from a solitary focus of metastatic disease that has been previously treated or in localized disease where a more local ablative therapy can be performed as an alternative to external beam radiotherapy. In addition, RFA can be used in combination with conventional therapy such as external beam radiotherapy or with some of the newer therapies such as vertebroplasty. This chapter briefly discusses the clinical problem of osseous metastatic disease and presents recent results from early RFA treatment. Clinical examples are provided.

## Background

Metastatic cancer is the most common neoplasm involving the skeletal system.[1] Of approximately 965,000 new cancer cases each year in the United States, approximately 30% to 70% will develop skeletal metastases. Given the high prevalence of carcinomas of the breast, lung, and prostate, these cancers account for more than 80% of the cases of metastatic bone disease. Bone metastases lead to significant morbidity due to pain, pathologic fracture, and neural compression.

Pain from bone metastases can be related to mechanical or chemical factors. Mass effect and elevated intraosseous pressure cause local or radiating pain. Bleeding from local bone osteolysis from osteoclastic activity causes a local release of bradykinin, prostaglandins, histamine, and substance P that can irritate the nerves in the area.[2] Primary treatment has relied on radiation therapy[3] with or without systemic chemotherapy or hormonal therapy. Systemic therapy with radionuclides[4,5] and bisphosphonates[6,7] has also shown some success. Radiotherapy is successful because it destroys the local tumor and inflammatory cells that are responsible for the pain. Several clinical trials have been performed analyzing external beam radiation therapy's ability to palliate pain or control progression of osseous metastatic disease.[8–15] The Radiation Therapy Oncology Group study by Tong et al[8] measured the patient's response to radiation therapy with a pain scale and narcotic requirement scale of 1 to 4. The study showed a complete response rate of 54% and a partial response rate of 90% within the first 4 weeks. Ninety-six percent of the patients had at least minimal relief, but only 50% had complete relief in 4 weeks. Interestingly, there was a significant relapse rate of 30% in the patients who survived at least 12 weeks. Another interesting point from this study is that lung cancer patients or patients with severe constant pain at the outset tended not to improve after radiation. A study by Madsen[9] reported a response rate of only 48% when measuring a patient's pain using a visual analogue scale. Overall response rates vary according to the length of follow-up, type of radiation treatment, and the measurement of patient response. As pointed out in a review by Ratanatharathorn et al[16] of all published reports, the relapse after initial response is frequent, the pain relief in all studies is poor, and the practices of radiation therapy need to be improved. This point, although not uniformly accepted in the field of radiation oncology, supports the addition of new therapy to help this group of patients. A more effective modality of local treatment for bone metastases could substantially improve quality of life. The life expectancy of patients with osseous metastatic disease is limited, with an average median survival of between 3 and 6 months. Therefore, finding an effective local therapy that can be done at a single outpatient sitting would be beneficial.

Recently percutaneous procedures for providing local tumor ablative therapy such as ethanol injection,[17] vertebroplasty,[18] and RFA[19,20] have shown some promise in palliation of metastatic bone lesions. Percutaneous RFA is a technique that was originally pioneered decades ago for the treatment of trigeminal neuralgia.[21] For the treatment of bone lesions the technique involves placing an electrode under computed tomography (CT) guidance directly into the metastasis. The electrode is coupled to a radiofrequency (RF) generator and causes tissue necrosis by heating of adjacent tissues. The potential advantages of RFA versus other destructive methods are multifold: cell death is immediate, lesion size can be accurately controlled, lesion temperature can be monitored, electrode placement can be achieved with a percutaneous image-guided procedure, and RFA can be performed under local anesthesia and conscious sedation. Currently, RFA is commonly used in the musculoskeletal system for treatment of intractable back pain due to failed back syndrome,[22] and chronic back pain due to facet joint osteoarthritis.[23] CT-guided RFA has been shown to be a cost-effective surgical alternative in the treatment of osteoid osteomas.[20] A preliminary study investigated RFA for patients with metastatic bone tumors that remain painful after radiation therapy or are solitary and can be treated without subjecting the bone marrow to immunosuppressive doses of external beam radiation therapy.[24]

## Technique

At our institution RFA is performed under intravenous conscious sedation with midazolam and fentanyl. Patients are monitored with continuous pulse oximetry, and electrocardiogram (ECG) with blood pressure performed every 5 minutes. We feel this is preferable over general anesthesia for two reasons: patients can have sensorimotor testing when an ablation is performed near a neurovascular bundle, and the procedure time and expense are reduced, making it more applicable to the outpatient arena. Computed tomography is used to localize the metastasis. Standard surgical prepping and draping is done, and local anesthesia with 1% lidocaine both intradermally and around the periosteum is administered. A 14-gauge coaxial bone biopsy needle is placed into the lesion if the cortical bone is intact. After the core is removed by the trephine needle, the RF electrode is placed through the outer cannula into the metastasis. It is important to withdraw the outer cannula prior to the application of RF energy so the current doesn't conduct into the metal cannula, thus causing thermal injury along the needle track. In cases with larger tumors that have destroyed the bone cortex, the RF electrode is placed directly into the metastasis. Tumors over 4 cm in size are treated with a cluster RF electrode consisting of three 17-gauge needles spaced 5 mm apart. Tumors smaller than 4 cm are treated with a single RF electrode. The tip of the RF electrode is posi-

tioned against the deepest margin of the tumor. Axial and cra-
niocaudad placement of the RF electrode is confirmed with CT.

The RF electrode contains an internal thermocouple for temperature measurement. The electrode is coupled to a Radionics
CC-1 radiofrequency generator and perfusion pump (Radionics
Inc., Burlington, MA). Internal cooling of the electrode (tip temperature 10°–20°C) is performed with continuous infusion of ice
water at 80 mL/min with the accompanying perfusion pump. At
the end of each treatment the perfusion is stopped and the maximum temperature recorded. At least one RF treatment is created
with the maximal allowable current given the impedance of the
system (typical current range 1100–1600 mA) for a time of no
greater than 4 minutes. The maximal intratumoral temperature
is recorded. An intratumoral temperature greater than 60°C is obtained to ensure adequate thermocoagulation. If the temperature
exceeds 60°C at the end of the treatment, then the RF electrode
is withdrawn in increments of 1 cm up to the length of the active tip (e.g., three 1-cm increments for a 3-cm active tip single
electrode or 3 cm for a 2.5-cm active tip cluster electrode) while
measuring the intratumoral temperature. If the temperature falls
below 60°C and the RF electrode is still within the tumor mass
as determined by imaging, then another 4-minute treatment is
performed at the new position. If after the first 4-minute treatment the maximum intratumoral temperature does not exceed
60°C, then an additional 4-minute treatment is performed at the
same position. This is repeated for a maximum time of 12 minutes (i.e., three treatments) at any given electrode position. Rarely,
a hypervascular metastasis such as from renal cell carcinoma may
require embolization prior to RFA due to the heat sink effect from
the tumor blood flow. After the entire longitudinal dimension of
the tumor is treated with a series of overlapping temperature-
based treatments, the RF electrode is positioned into a new portion of tumor so that the electrode shaft is 1.5 to 2 cm away from
the longitudinal axis of the previous series of treatments. This is
repeated until these elliptical-shaped treatment regions encompass the volume of the tumor mass. This temperature-dependent
treatment attempts to standardize the RF therapy for any given
tumor despite differences in the tumor size, local blood flow, and
histology. The current is grounded by the application of four
grounding pads (in the horizontal configuration) (1800 cm$^3$/
each) to the anterior and posterior aspect of the patient's thighs.

## Results

The largest clinical application for RFA and bone metastases is
pain palliation. Our early results from a pilot study that were

presented recently at the American Society of Clinical Oncology, in which we treated 18 metastatic bone tumors in 16 patients, indicated that RFA reduced pain in a heterogeneous group of patients, some of whom could not have additional radiation therapy.[25] By the visual analogue pain scale of 0 (no pain) to 10 (worst), the mean of average pain intensity was 6.5 prior to RFA and 4.62 at 1 week ($p = .039$) and 4.64 at 1 month ($p = .036$) after the procedure. Similarly the mean of the worst pain described by the patients was 8.5 before the procedure, and 6.93 ($p = .005$) and 5.64 ($p = .003$) at 1 week and 1 month, respectively. No incidences of bleeding or infection at the site of procedure were identified, and the only side effects were swelling, local pain, and postablation syndrome whereby flu-like symptoms occur for several days after the treatment. Patients with larger tumors involving the pelvis and sacroiliac joints did not have significant pain relief. However, patients with smaller tumors and tumors involving the chest wall had significant pain relief (Figs. 11.1 and 11.2). Our study also showed that RFA has very low morbidity and is well tolerated in the outpatient arena. Additional benefits in adding RFA to the palliation of patients with osseous metastases are the ability to perform concomitant chemotherapy and the avoidance of marrow suppresion in more localized disease. A larger multiinstitution trial has just begun through the Amercian College of Radiology Imaging Network (Web site: www.acrin.org) to further study the potential beneficial effects of RFA in the treatment of painful osseous metastatic disease.

Radiofrequency ablation may be used as an alternative to radiation therapy. In patients with very localized disease that can be safely treated with RFA, tumor control can be achieved. In addition, in larger tumors when radiation therapy alone is less effective, a combination approach could be used (Fig. 11.3). In any event, RFA should always be considered a less invasive and probably less costly alternative when tumor burden is small and well confined. In addition, RFA may be an effective up-front cytoreduction treatment prior to conventional external beam radiotherapy and/or systemic chemotherapy.

Radiofrequency ablation can also be applied to malignancies in the spinal axis, a common location for painful bone metastases. Spinal RFA can be performed safely in the vertebral body without cytotoxic temperature elevations observed within the spinal canal if the vertebral body cortex is intact and a cerebrospinal fluid (CSF) space exists between the mass and spinal canal.[25] Despite the use of internally cooled electrodes at maximum output, significant elevation of temperatures in the epidural space did not occur in this experimental study. Ex vivo studies confirmed decreased heat transmission in cancellous bone and an insulative effect of cortical bone. An additional

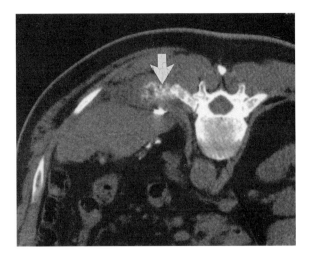

A

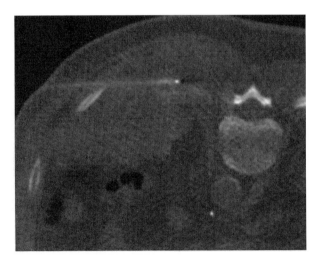

B

**Figure 11.1.** A 62-year-old man with metastatic renal cell carcinoma and a painful destructive metastasis involving the right posterior tenth rib and adjacent transverse process. (A) Prone computed tomography (CT) image shows the destructive bone and associated soft tissue mass (arrow). Due to the localized extent of the disease, radiofrequency ablation (RFA) was employed as the treatment method of choice. (B) Prone CT fluoroscopy image shows a single radiofrequency (RF) electrode within the mass. Four overlapping treatments were performed. The patient remains asymptomatic 6 months after the therapy.

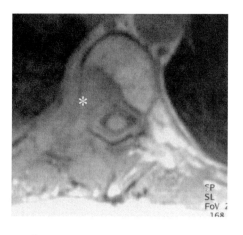
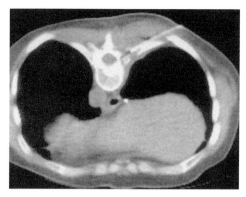

A                                              B

**Figure 11.2.** A 48-year-old woman with metastatic non–small cell lung cancer to the spine and chest wall with persistent pain despite external beam radiotherapy. (A) Axial T1-weighted magnetic resonance imaging (MRI) shows the tumor involvement in the vertebral body, right transverse process, rib, and adjacent soft tissues (*). (B) Prone CT-fluoroscopy image shows the RF electrode within the mass. The patient had significant pain relief after the procedure that lasted 3 months.

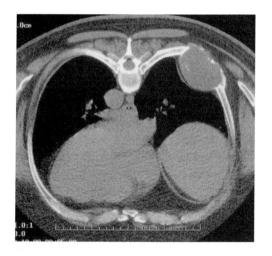
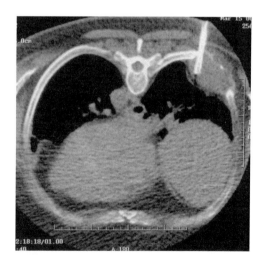

A                                              B

**Figure 11.3.** A 58-year-old man with metastatic thyroid cancer and a painful expansile posterior rib metastasis shown on this prone CT image (A). The patient had had a prior sternectomy for metastatic disease and did not want repeat surgery or radiation; therefore, the patient elected RFA. (B) Under CT-fluoroscopic guidance a cluster electrode was placed, and nine overlapping ablation spheres were created. The patient's pain resolved and a repeat biopsy 5 months later showed 95% necrosis.

factor that more than likely accounts for the differences in heat distribution observed are local heat sinks from the rich epidural venous plexus and CSF pulsations. Perfusion-mediated tissue cooling has been demonstrated as negatively influencing the extent of coagulation that can be produced in in-vivo liver, and decrease of blood flow by mechanical or pharmacologic means can increase the diameter of coagulation necrosis. The clinical application of RFA to the vertebral body may be important in the future. Osseous metastatic disease commonly involves the spine and often leads to debilitating pain, surgical decompression, and paraplegia. If a less invasive means of treating local tumor burden were available, then surgical decompression may be avoided in some cases. In cases where there is preserved cancellous or better yet cortical bone between the lesion and the spine, a margin of safety may be provided. In patients with extensive osteolysis with no intact cortex between tumor and spinal cord or nerve roots, RFA may not be an option due to potential thermal injury to adjacent neural tissue. Theoretically, if a CSF space were present between the tumor and neural tissue, RFA could be applied without unwanted neurotoxicity. The use of a remote temperature sensor (Fig. 11.4) may offer a prudent margin of safety as the procedure could be terminated if deleterious temperature

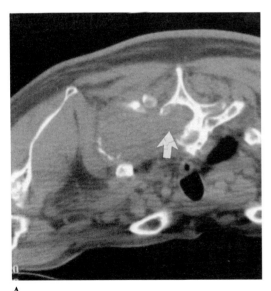
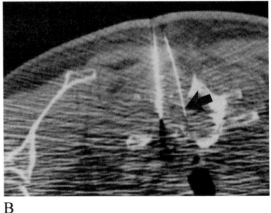

A                          B

**Figure 11.4.** A 65-year-old man with metastatic renal cell carcinoma to the left first rib and vertebral body status post–external beam radiotherapy and systemic immunotherapy. (A) Prone CT image shows the mass with extensive bone destruction adjacent to the spinal canal (arrow). Therefore, remote thermometry was performed to prevent thermal cord injury. (B) Prone CT-fluoroscopy image shows the medially placed thermocouple (arrow) between the RF electrode and the spinal cord. RFA was performed safely without any thermal untoward side effects to the spinal cord.

increases are observed adjacent to nervous tissue (i.e., greater than 45°C). In addition to destroying local tumor with heat, combination strengthening procedures such as vertebroplasty can be done at the same sitting (Fig. 11.5). Anecdotally, we have per-

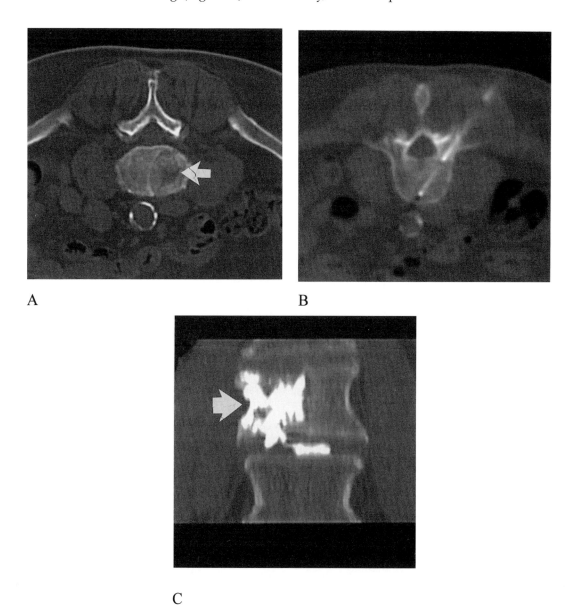

A                                             B

C

**Figure 11.5.** A 78-year-old man with metastatic prostate cancer to L4 status post–external beam radiotherapy with persistent pain. (A) Prone axial CT image shows a mixed lytic and blastic lesion within the right side of the L4 vertebral body with an associated pathologic fracture of the endplate (arrow). (B) CT-guided transpedicular RFA was performed prior to the injection of methylmethacrylate. (C) Coronal reconstructed CT image after the injection of methylmethacrylate shows the cement distribution throughout the area of metastasis (arrow). The patient's pain resolved immediately after the procedure.

formed RFA and vertebroplasty in several patients, and the results have been clinically beneficial. Up-front RFA may contract the tumor enabling improved distribution of cement.

In summary, RFA is an exciting new treatment modality that can be safely applied to metastatic bone disease. Its synergy with other therapies and its outpatient nature make it an attractive treatment option for this fragile group of patients. The precise role of RFA in this group of patients is not clearly defined, and continued work is underway in the hope that it will benefit those patients who currently have no treatment options and succumb to their disease without adequate therapy.

## References

1. Stoll BA, Parbhoo S, eds. Bone Metastasis: Monitoring and Treatment. New York: Raven Press, 1983.
2. Twycross RG. Management of pain in skeletal metastases. Clin Orthop 1995; 312:187–196.
3. Janjan NA. Radiation for bone metastases: conventional techniques and the role of systemic pharmaceuticals. Cancer 1997; 80:1628–1645.
4. Quilty PM, Kirk D, Bolger JJ, et al. A comparison of the palliative effects of strontium-89 and external beam radiotherapy in metastatic prostate cancer. Radiother Oncol 1994; 31:33–40.
5. Serafini AN, et al. Palliation of pain associated with metastatic bone cancer using samarium-153 lexidronam: a double blind placebo-controlled trial. J Clin Oncol 1998; 16:1574–1581.
6. Hortobagyi GB, et al. Efficacy of pamidronate in reducing skeletal complications in patients with breast cancer and lytic bone metastases. Protocol 19 Aredia Breast Cancer Study Group. N Engl J Med 1999; 12:1785–1791.
7. Conte PF, et al. Delay in progression of bone metastases in breast cancer patients treated with intravenous pamidronate: results from a multinational randomized controlled trial. The Aredia Multinational Cooperative Group. J Clin Oncol 1996; 14:2552–2559.
8. Tong D, Gillick L, Hendrickson FR. The palliation of symptomatic osseous metastases; final results of the study by the radiation therapy oncology group. Cancer 1982; 50:893–899.
9. Madsen EL. Painful bone metastasis: efficacy of radiotherapy assessed by the patients: a randomized trial comparing 4 Gy versus 10 Gy × 2. Int J Radiat Oncol Biol Phys 1983; 9:1775–1779.
10. Blitzer PH. Reanalysis of the RTOG study of the palliation of symptomatic osseous metastasis. Cancer 1984; 55:1468–1472.
11. Price P, et al. Prospective randomized trial of single and multifraction radiotherapy schedules in the treatment of painful bony metastases. Radiother Oncol 1986; 6:247–255.
12. Arcangeli G, et al. The responsiveness of bone metastases to radiotherapy: the effect of site, histology and radiation dose on pain relief. Radiother Oncol 1989; 14:95–101.
13. Cole DJ. A randomized trial of a single treatment versus conven-

tional fractionation in the palliative radiotherapy of painful bone metastases. Clin Oncol 1989; 1:59–62.

14. Poulter CA, et al. A report of RTOG 8206: a phase III study of whether the addition of single dose hemibody irradiation to standard fractionated local field irradiation is more effective than local field irradiation alone in the treatment of symptomatic osseous metastases. Int J Radiat Oncol Biol Phys 1992; 23:207–214.

15. Arcangeli G, et al. Radiation therapy in the management of symptomatic bone metastases: the effect of total dose and histology on pain relief and response duration. Int J Radiat Oncol Biol Phys 1998; 42:1119–1126.

16. Ratanatharathorn V, Powers WE, Moss WT, Perez CA. Bone metastasis: review and critical analysis of random allocation trials of local field treatment. Int J Radiat Oncol Biol Phys 1999; 44:1–18.

17. Gangi A, Kastler BA, Klinkert A, Dietemann JL. Injection of alcohol into bone metastases under CT guidance. J Comput Assist Tomogr 1994; 18:932–935.

18. Levine SA, Perin LA, Hayes D, Hayes WS. An evidence-based evaluation of percutaneous vertebroplasty. Manag Care 2000; 9:56–60,63.

19. Dupuy DE, Hong RJ, Oliver B, Goldberg SN. Radiofrequency ablation of spinal tumors: temperature distrubution in the spinal canal. AJR 2000; 175:1263–1266.

20. Rosenthal DI, Hornicek FJ, Wolf MW, Jennings LC, Gebhardt MC, Mankin HJ. Percutaneous radiofrequency coagulation of osteoid osteoma compared with operative treatment. J Bone Joint Surg 1998; 80A:815–821.

21. Sweet WH, Wepsic JG. Controlled thermocoagulation of trigeminal ganglion and rootlets for differential destruction of pain fibers. J Neurosurg 1974; 40:10–17, 143–156.

22. Sluijter ME. The use of radiofrequency lesions for pain relief in failed back patients. Int Disabil Stud 1988; 10:10–17.

23. Ogsbury JS, Simons H, Lehman RAW. Facet denervation in treatment of low back syndrome. Pain 1977; 2:257–263.

24. Dupuy DE, Safran H, Mayo-Smith WW, Goldberg SN. Radiofrequency ablation of painful osseous metastatic disease. Radiology 1998; 209(P);389.

25. Dupuy DE, Ahmed M, Rodrigues B, Safran H. Percutaneous radiofrequency ablation of painful osseous metastases: a phase II trial. Proceedings of the American Society of Clinical Oncology 2001; 20:1537 (abstract).

# Radiofrequency Ablation of Solid Renal Tumors

Raymond A. Costabile and Jack R. Walter

The majority of solid renal masses are malignant, principally renal cell adenocarcinoma (Fig. 12.1). Renal cell carcinoma is the third most common genitourinary malignancy, with over 26,000 cases diagnosed annually in the United States. Presently the only effective treatment for renal cell carcinoma is surgical extirpation. Renal cell carcinoma is not responsive to ionizing radiation or conventional chemotherapy. In 1965, Robson established radical nephrectomy, surgical removal of the kidney and all contents with Gerota's fascia, as the standard surgical treatment for renal cell carcinoma. Radical nephrectomy proved to offer significant survival advantages over simple nephrectomy and was the treatment of choice until the mid-1980s. With the increased use of abdominal imaging techniques [computed tomography (CT) and ultrasound], the mean size and stage of renal tumors became significantly smaller and of lower stage. These smaller tumors were amenable to local resection, and numerous centers demonstrated that partial nephrectomy, or renal sparing surgery consisting of removal of the tumor and a clear margin of normal renal tissue, was effective at preventing tumor recurrence and metastasis. Renal sparing surgery was also effective at preserving renal function. Long-term studies have further demonstrated the safety and efficacy of partial nephrectomy for the treatment of renal cell carcinoma.

As patient access and provider utilization of abdominal imaging techniques have become more widespread, there has been a

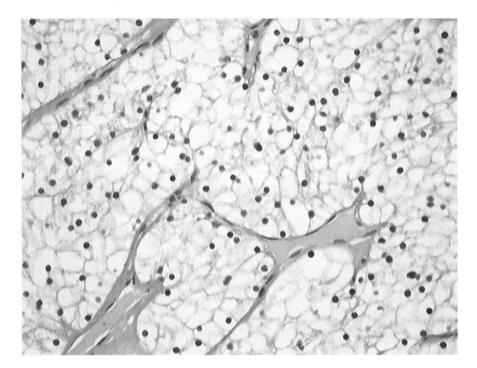

**Figure 12.1.** Renal cell carcinoma.

significant increase in the so-called incidentally discovered solid renal mass. Over 85% of renal cell carcinomas are now diagnosed exclusively by imaging methods without presenting symptoms. Most of these tumors are less than 4.0 cm in greatest dimension and are amenable to local excision.

The movement toward minimally invasive surgical treatment of renal cell carcinoma has led to new procedures including laparoscopic radical nephrectomy and laparoscopic partial nephrectomy. Laparoscopic procedures have significantly improved postoperative pain and reduced recovery time. Despite this improvement in recovery, laparoscopic procedures have significant perioperative risk. Many patients with renal cell carcinoma are in the sixth and seventh decade of life and have significant comorbidities limiting surgical options. Observation of the renal masses over time has been recommended for patients deemed too great an operative risk for radical extirpative surgery. Unfortunately, observation increases the likelihood that the renal cell carcinoma will metastasize and become untreatable. In an effort to develop a surgical treatment option for these patients, new ablative techniques are being studied. Cryoablation under laparoscopic and percutaneous guidance has been demonstrated to ablate renal tumors in several studies.[1] This chapter discusses the present status of radiofrequency ablation (RFA) of solid renal tumors as a minimally invasive treatment option for the treatment of renal cell carcinoma.

## Animal Studies of Radiofrequency Ablation in the Kidney

Animal studies of the feasibility and efficacy of RFA began in earnest in the early 1990s using both "wet" and "dry" radiofrequency electrodes. Initial studies looking at the effects of radiofrequency energy on the kidneys of rabbits demonstrated the ability to induce reproducible thermal injury on normal renal tissue. Pathologic evaluation demonstrated coagulation necrosis in the treated areas of the kidney. To increase lesion size, Patel et al[2] utilized an electrolyte coupler ("wet" electrode) during radiofrequency application. They studied the wet electrode in 33 New Zealand rabbits and were able to produce predictable zones of tissue necrosis in vivo. The electrodes were placed under laparoscopic guidance to ensure correct placement and depth in the kidney. All animals survived treatment, and no urinomas or pyelocutaneous fistulae were found in any animal. Porcine models were later used to demonstrate the feasibility of RFA in the kidneys in a large animal.[1,3–6] Porcine kidneys are very similar to human kidneys in terms of size, anatomy, and renal blood flow. As in the rabbit model, reproducible lesions were found in all animals using commercially available "dry" radiofrequency arrays. Animals tolerated the procedure well under general anesthesia. Complications noted after RFA include ablation of portions of the psoas muscle and damage to the bladder. Rupture of the kidney was seen in one animal with subsequent hemorrhage and death.

A variety of operative techniques have been studied in animal models to ensure correct electrode placement. Direct operative placement, laparoscopic guidance as well as ultrasound-, CT-, and magnetic resonance imaging (MRI)-guided percutaneous placement have been used for these animal studies.

Attempts have been made in animal models to increase the size of the zone of necrosis induced by RFA by manipulating tissue characteristics and characteristics of the radiofrequency delivery system. As previously mentioned, an ionic coupler was used in rabbit models to further dissipate radiofrequency energy. Other methods include altering the time, application, tissue resistance, and temperature to compensate for the high renal blood flow acting as an efficient heat sink to reduce the effects of radiofrequency energy. Altering these parameters met with variable success in the majority of these studies.

Several researchers attempted to alter tissue characteristics of the kidney that may limit the efficacy of RFA (high renal blood flow, adjacent vessels and organs, dense perinephric fat pad, etc.). Balloon tamponade of the main renal artery prior to application of radiofrequency energy significantly increased the zone of coagulation necrosis in the treated kidney,[6] as did temporary clamping of the renal artery prior to ablation in porcine models.[7] Hydrodissection and $CO_2$ gas dissection of the surrounding perinephric fat pad were also used to increase the zone of necrosis and decrease potential damage to surrounding organs. No difference was noted between the use of saline or gas dissection.[4]

Follow-up radiographic studies were performed to evaluate lesion size after RFA. Ultrasound, CT, and MRI follow-up demonstrated the ability to noninvasively evaluate the effects of RFA on the treated kidneys.

These and other animal studies paved the way for evaluating the use of RFA on solid renal tumors. Certainly the tissue characteristics of renal cell carcinoma (diffuse intralesional hemorrhage, necrotic tumor, altered blood vessels and flow, etc.) differ significantly from normal renal tissue. Few animal studies are available to evaluate this difference.

## Radiofrequency Ablation of Human Renal Tumors

Case reports utilizing radiofrequency energy to treat small solid renal masses were first published in 1998.[8] These case reports demonstrated the use of percutaneous RFA on small renal masses in patients whose comorbidity prevented the performance of radical nephrectomy or nephron sparing energy. All of these lesions were <4 cm in diameter and had increased in size on serial radiographic studies prior to considering treatment. Percutaneous RFA was performed under conscious sedation without significant side effects. Radiographic follow-up with CT scan or MRI demonstrated a persistent nonenhancing lesion in the treated area. Short-term follow-up (2–24 months) showed no evidence of tumor growth or the development of metastatic disease.

Patients with von Hippel–Lindau (VHL) disease are one cohort in which RFA may be particularly useful. These patients frequently develop multiple bilateral renal cell carcinomas. Current treatment for VHL is by bilateral radical nephrectomy with subsequent renal transplant or serial partial nephrectomies. Unfortunately, partial nephrectomy is a difficult procedure to perform in a previously operated kidney. Radiographic (MRI)-guided RFA of small renal masses in VHL patients has been used with low morbidity.[5,9] Follow-up resection of 11 tumors treated with RFA in patients with VHL demonstrated loss of nuclear detail and nonvisualization of nucleoli. These pathologic changes were not noted in lesions not exposed to radiofrequency energy.[10]

We have had an ongoing study over the past 2 years looking at radiofrequency energy to ablate solid renal masses. Presently our protocol has two treatment arms: an ablate and resect group, and an ablation-only group. Patients in the ablation-only protocol have small solid renal masses consistent with renal cell carcinoma but are not considered surgical candidates due to significant comorbidity. Patients in this arm can opt for observation only (considered present standard of care) or be treated with percutaneous RFA under conscious sedation. Six patients have been treated in the ablation-only arm using the LeVeen (Radiotherapeutics, Mountain View, CA) array at standard application settings for hepatic masses (Fig. 12.2). Patients are followed up every 3 months for the first year after treatment with serial laboratory (CBC, BUN/creatinine), CT/MRI studies, and examination, and every 6 months thereafter. All patients have tolerated the procedure very well, with slight discomfort during application of radiofrequency energy and no other side effects. Hematuria, post-

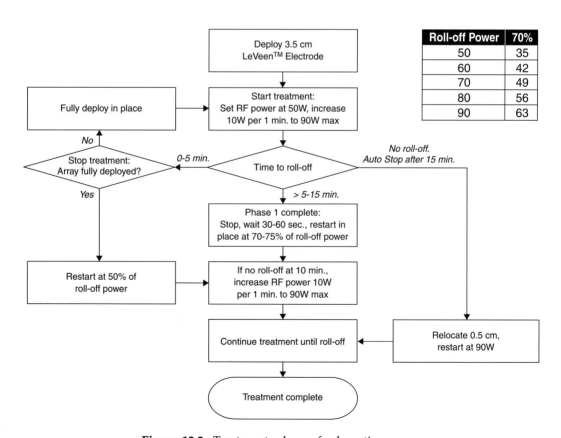

Figure 12.2. Treatment schema for hepatic masses.

procedure pain, or changes in serum creatinine have not been seen in any patient after treatment.

The longest follow-up in the ablation-only population (24 months) has demonstrated no evidence of metastatic disease. Two patients had significant progression of disease detected at 9 and 11 months. These patients subsequently underwent open radical nephrectomy. One mortality occurred in our series secondary to progression of disease.

The limited experience with the use of radiofrequency energy has demonstrated the feasibility of using percutaneous RFA in the treatment of solid renal masses in patients for whom surgery is not an option. It is a significant leap to suggest that RFA could supplant traditional surgical therapy. To further study the effects of radiofrequency energy on solid renal masses, we evaluated a series of patients undergoing extirpative renal surgery for renal cell carcinoma. Prior to ligating the renal artery and vein, a 2.5-cm LeVeen radiofrequency array was placed under direct vision into the renal mass. Again using the standardized treatment schema for ablation of hepatic lesions, an area of the renal mass was treated and marked with a silk suture. Pathologic evaluation was performed with hematoxylin and eosin staining as well as reduced nicotinamide adenine dinucleotide phosphate (NADPH) diaphorase stains to assess cell viability. A predictable zone of coagulation necrosis was seen on over 86% of renal masses treated in the ablate and resect arm. Tumor necrosis in the primary tumor prevented staining and evaluation in 14% of treated lesions. One treated region was not evaluable due to inadequate tissue preservation and staining techniques. The ablate and resect arm has demonstrated the ability of radiofrequency energy to create coagulation necrosis in renal cell carcinoma.

Other investigators have also demonstrated coagulation necrosis in renal masses treated with RFA. Areas of viable tumor have been seen to remain at the rim of the treated area in several cases. The presence of viable tumor suggests that either the array size or the treatment schema used for hepatic lesions may not be applicable for renal masses. Complete tumor destruction must be obtained to consider RFA curative in the treatment of renal cell carcinoma.

Radiofrequency ablation offers several logistic advantages for the treatment of small renal masses. Radiofrequency energy may be applied during open or laparoscopic surgery or with percutaneous technique. CT guidance is preferable for percutaneous placement, as it offers superior visualization of electrode placement as well as real-time monitoring of tissue ablation. Ultrasound guidance has also been used for percutaneous guidance. We have found that it is difficult to visualize a small renal mass and the array with ultrasound guidance. The large volume of perinephric fat decreases the ability of ultrasound to visualize small renal masses. Bubbles produced by the vaporization of renal tissue can further obscure ultrasonic visualization.

## Conclusions

Animal and human studies have demonstrated that radiofrequency energy can be applied safely as a minimally invasive treatment modality for small solid renal masses. Percutaneous placement under conscious sedation is presently recommended only in an investigational setting in patients for whom traditional radical nephrectomy or nephron sparing surgery is not possible. Numerous questions remain about the efficacy and reproducibility of radiofrequency energy to completely ablate renal cell carcinoma. Several studies have demonstrated viable tumor after RFA. Unfortunately, clinical studies to date have principally utilized existing treatment schema for hepatic lesions on renal masses. New treatment protocols need to be developed that are specific for the tissue characteristics of renal cell carcinoma. New techniques, perhaps using previously studied tissue-altering characteristics in animal models, may increase treatment area and reduce tumor viability. Radiofrequency ablation is an exciting new treatment modality that may significantly decrease the morbidity of the surgical treatment of small incidentally discovered renal masses.

## References

1. Shingleton WB, Farabaugh P, Hughson M, Sewell PE. Percutaneous cryoablation of porcine kidneys with magnetic resonance image monitoring. J Urol 2001; 166:289–291.
2. Patel VR, Leveilee RJ, Hoey MF, Burich JA, Hulbert JC. Radiofrequency ablation of the rabbit kidney using the liquid electrode: subacute observations. J Urol 1999; 163(4)(suppl).
3. Crowley JD, Shelton JB, Burton MP, Daltymple N, Bishoff JT. Laparoscopic radiofrequency ablation: acute and long-term clinical, radiographic and pathologic effects in an animal model. Kimbrough Urological Seminar, San Antonio, TX, 2000.
4. Rendon RA, Gertner MR, Sherar MD, et al. Development of a radiofrequency based thermal therapy technique in an in vivo porcine model for the treatment of small renal masses. J Urol 2000; 166:292–298.
5. Sulman A, Resnick MI, Oefelin MG, Lewin JS. MRI-guided radiofrequency interstitial thermal ablation of renal tumors: a minimally invasive alternative to traditional surgical approaches. J Urol 2000; 163(4)(abst).
6. Sulman A, Aschoff AJ, Martinez M, Resnick MI. Perfusion modulated MRI guided radiofrequency (RF) interstitial thermal ablation of the kidney in a porcine model. J Urol 2000; 163(4)(abst).

7. Corwin TS, Lindberg G, Traxier O, et al. Laparoscopic radiofrequency thermal ablation of renal tissue with and without hilar occlusion. J Urol 2001; 166:281–284.

8. McGovern FJ, Wood BJ, Goldberg SN, Mueller PR. Radio frequency ablation of renal cell carcinoma via image guided needle electrodes. J Urol 1998; 161:599–600.

9. Pavlovich CP, Wood BJ, Choyke PL, Linehan WM, Walther MM. Radiofrequency interstitial thermal ablation (RITA) of small tumors in von Hippel-Lindau disease. J Urol 2000; 163(4)(suppl).

10. Walther MW, Shawker TH, Libutti SK, et al. A phase 2 study of radiofrequency interstitial tissue ablation of localized renal tumors. J Urol 2000;163:1424–1427.

# 13

# Radiofrequency Ablation of Pulmonary Malignancies

Luis J. Herrera, Hiran C. Fernando, and James D. Luketich

Lung cancer is currently the most common cause of cancer-related death in the United States and represents the second most common malignancy in both men and women, with 171,400 new cases in the year 1999.[1,2] The current standard of care consists of surgical resection with or without multimodality therapy for patients with stage I to II disease, who have an acceptable operative risk and pulmonary reserve. Although patients who have stage IIIa lung cancer are not treated by resection alone, many of these patients participate in protocols that include neoadjuvant therapy followed by operation. The treatment options are limited for patients with significant comorbid disease or with poor pulmonary function who are not candidates for surgery.

This chapter presents alternative therapies for patients with primary lung cancer or limited pulmonary metastases who are not candidates for surgery. We have included a brief overview of lung cancer treatment and the management of pulmonary metastasis. We discuss the alternatives to resection of lung tumors, focusing on radiofrequency ablation (RFA). The current literature on RFA of lung tumors is scant, consisting mostly of animal studies and small case series in humans. We focus on the specific aspects of performing this procedure on the lung, its technical challenges, its applicability, and our experience with RFA at the University of Pittsburgh.

**Table 13.1** Non–Small Cell Lung Cancer (NSCLC) 5-Year
Survival Postresection per Pathologic Stage

| Stage | pTNM | 5-year Survival (%) |
|-------|------|---------------------|
| IA | T1N0M0 | 67 |
| IB | T2N0M0 | 57 |
| IIA | T1N1M0 | 55 |
| IIB | T2N1M0 | 39 |
| IIIA | T3N0M0 | 38 |
|  | T1–2N2M0 | 23 |
|  | T3N1M0 | 25 |
|  | T3N2M0 | 23 |

© 1989 American College of Chest Physicians. Reprinted with permission. See
reference 4.

## Lung Cancer Overview

The majority of lung cancer patients present with advanced disease.[3] Despite advances in the management of this disease, the best 5-year survival for stage I remains around 70% for patients who have undergone surgical resection.[4,5] Complete resection provides the best chance for cure and remains the gold standard of therapy for patients with acceptable surgical risk. The current tumor, node, metastasis (TNM) staging system adopted by the American Joint Committee on Cancer (AJCC) and the International Union Against Cancer (UICC) was revised in 1997[4] and is shown in Table 13.1. In stages I to III, lymph node involvement is the most important prognostic factor.

## Surgical Therapy for Early-Stage Non–Small Cell Lung Cancer (NSCLC)

Therapy for lung cancer patients is determined according to the stage of disease, taking into account the patient's comorbidities and pulmonary function, and the feasibility of completely resecting the disease. A multidisciplinary assessment is essential for determining the optimal therapeutic option for the patient. The main treatment for early-stage disease is complete surgical resection, providing the best overall survival and the best chance for cure. Only patients with the potential for complete resection with negative margins should be considered for surgery. T4 lesions with either direct invasion to mediastinal structures, malignant pleural effusions, or intraparenchymal metastasis have a poor prognosis and are generally not benefited by surgical treatment.

In general, patients with metastatic primary lung cancer are not considered for surgical therapy, but there have been highly selected patients with improved survival after resection of the primary tumor, together with ablation or resection of solitary metastases in the brain or adrenal glands.[6,7]

## Surgical Therapy for Management of Pulmonary Metastasis

The role of surgical resection of pulmonary metastasis in selected patients has become more widely accepted, and a survival advantage of agressive surgical therapy has been demonstrated. In particular, the early experience with metastasectomy of pulmonary sarcoma revealed an improvement in 5-year survival (from 17% to 32%).[8,9] Since then, a wide variety of metastatic lung tumors have been treated surgically, with improvement in survival for adequately selected patients. Selection criteria for pulmonary metastasectomy can vary, but essentially suitable patients are those whose disease is localized to the chest, and in whom control of the primary site and complete resection of metastases are possible[10,11] (Table 13.2). Adequate pulmonary reserve and reasonable operative risk are essential to establish.

Other criteria that are considered to determine the risk of local recurrence and survival benefit for resection include the disease-free interval from the time of resection of the primary tumor and the appearance of metastatic disease.[12,13] The number of pulmonary metastases and the tumor doubling time have also been used as prognostic factors.[14]

Surgical series have demonstrated 5-year survival rates of 25% to 42% in the surgical treatment of pulmonary metastasis from different primaries including colorectal cancer,[10,15] osteogenic sarcoma,[16] melanoma,[17] and others. In a prospective study of 5206 cases of lung metastasectomy, the International Registry of Lung Metastases reported an actuarial survival of 36% at 5 years and 26% at 10 years, which compares favorably with the survival of 13% at 5 years and 7% at 10 years in patients who had an incomplete resection. Factors that predicted longer survival after resection were long disease-free interval (>36 months), single lesions, and metastases from germ cell tumors.[18]

**Table 13.2  Criteria for Resection of Pulmonary Metastases**

| |
|---|
| Primary tumor controlled |
| All nodules potentially resectable with planned surgery |
| Adequate postoperative pulmonary reserve is expected |
| No extrathoracic metastasis |
| Systemic therapy options limited |

Patients with no surgical treatment have disease progression and worse prognosis. In the series from Memorial Sloan-Kettering Cancer Center, 144 patients with colorectal lung metastasis underwent resection, achieving a 5-year overall survival of 40%. However, 11 patients with colorectal metastasis who could not be completely resected due to poor pulmonary reserve died of progressive disease, with a median survival of 9 months.[19]

## Evaluation of Physiologic and Pulmonary Function

Assessment of pulmonary function is essential when planning therapy. A simple subjective determination can be made based on the patient's history of physical activity. We have also found that measurement of oxygen saturation before and after the patient walks up a flight of stairs is a useful test, particularly when contemplating pneumonectomy.[20] The risks of surgical therapy and resultant postresection pulmonary function must be acceptable to allow patients to return to normal activities.

In general, every patient being considered for resection should undergo pulmonary function testing of forced expiratory volume in 1 second (FEV$_1$), forced vital capacity (FVC), diffusing capacity of the lung for carbon monoxide (DLCO), and arterial blood gas (ABG). Several studies have measured different objective parameters such as ABG, pulmonary function tests, or diffusion capacity, but no single indicator is predictive of physiologic outcome. However, DLCO or the percent of predicted DLCO (ppDLCO) seems to correlate with postoperative pulmonary complications.[21,22] In addition, patients with poor pulmonary function can undergo exercise oxymetry and quantitative ventilation/perfusion (V/Q) scans in relation to the area to be resected, providing a more accurate estimate of postoperative spirometric

**Table 13.3 Preoperative Tests for Assessing Pulmonary Risk Prior to Major Lung Resection**

| Test | Values for Low-Risk Patients |
|---|---|
| FEV$_1$% | >60% |
| DLCO% | >60% |
| ppFEV$_1$ | >800 mL |
| ppFEV$_1$% | >40% |
| ppDLCO% | >40% |
| VO$_2$ max during exercise | >15 mL/kg/min |

DLCO, diffusing capacity of the lung for carbon monoxide; FEV$_1$, forced expiratory volume in 1 second; pp, percent of predicted.
© 1999 American College of Chest Physicians. Reprinted with permission. See reference 22.

function. Combining different parameters and calculating post-operative estimated pulmonary function in combination with clinical assessment by the surgeon seems to be the best indicator of the patient's capacity to tolerate a major lung resection (Table 13.3).

## Alternatives to Lung Resection in Patients with High Operative Risk

### Current Tumor Ablation or Minimal Resection Techniques

The standard resections for primary lung cancer include lobectomy or pneumonectomy depending on the size and location of the tumor. Limited resections, include segmentectomy or wedge resection of the lung, are the standard treatment for limited metastases and are good alternatives for patients with primary lung cancer and poor lung function who cannot tolerate a larger resection. The results of limited resection for primary lung cancer are best for patients with small (T1) tumors and no evidence of adenopathy. The only prospective randomized trial to address this issue was performed by the Lung Cancer Study Group in 276 patients with T1N0 NSCLC. Patients in the limited resection group suffered a 75% increase in the recurrence rate, and loco-regional recurrence was three times more common in the limited resection arm; no survival difference was seen between the two groups.[23] However, limited resection should continue to be viewed as a good option for metastasectomy but a compromise operation for primary lung cancer.

Some patients with metastases or early-stage lung cancer are not candidates for resection because of physiologic impairment or patient preference. These patients may benefit from RFA. However, the results of RFA will need to be compared to other non-resection modalities for this patient group, of which definitive radiotherapy is probably the most commonly employed alternative method of local cancer control.

Some investigators have advocated definitive radiation therapy for early-stage NSCLC patients who are not candidates for resection. In a meta-analysis of 149 stage I NSCLC patients who were considered inoperable based on operative risk, and who were treated with of 64.7 Gy of radiotherapy, a 5-year survival rate of 22% was achieved, and this improved to 31% with radiation of the mediastinal lymph node basin.[24] Another study evaluated the results of definitive radiotherapy with 62 Gy in 71 stage 1a or 1b NSCLC patients, and found a disease-specific 3-year survival of 49% for T1 lesions and a local control rate of 89%.[25]

Cryotherapy is another less invasive tissue ablation technique that has been used extensively for the treatment of hepatic malignancies. The extent of ablation is easier to follow intraoperatively using ultrasound, when compared to RFA. The technique may also be more effective than RFA for destruction of lesions larger than 5 cm. However, the major disadvantage of tissue cryoablation is the higher incidence of complications. In the treatment of liver lesions, a mortality rate of 4% has been reported, and complications include hemorrhage, abscess formation, and up to a 30% incidence of multisystem organ failure when large areas are treated.[26] To our knowledge, cryoablation has not been used to treat parenchymal lung lesions, but the higher complication rate reported makes it less attractive than RFA.

### Potential Role of RFA for Pulmonary Malignancies

After the widespread application of RFA for unresectable liver tumors, this technique has been considered as an alternative therapy for the destruction of other solid tumors. The experience in treating lung tumors is limited; however, the technique appears to be safe and feasible for ablation of peripheral lung nodules in the initial experience that has been reported. RFA also has the potential to provide local control of lung tumor for those patients who are either at high risk for resection or refuse operation. In cases of pulmonary metastases, high-risk patients would include those with impaired pulmonary function, sometimes after prior surgical resection, and those patients with other significant co-morbid disease. Situations may also occur where complete resection of pulmonary metastases is not possible, but RFA of remaining nodules may be an alternative. We have certainly found RFA to be of use in the situation where a wedge resection of a peripheral nodule was performed, and resection of a second centrally located nodule would have required a lobectomy but was treated instead with RFA. More central RFA treatments run the potential of damage to larger branches of the pulmonary artery with delayed hemorrhage, and should be considered only with extreme caution. If treatment of all disease is not possible by either operation or RFA, or if significant extrathoracic disease remains, RFA should not be used.

Animal models have been used to investigate the efficacy and feasibility of this technique in lung tissue. Goldberg et al[27] generated a model of lung tumors by infiltrating the pulmonary parenchyma of 11 rabbits with VX2 sarcoma cell suspensions. Seven lesions were treated with RFA for 6 minutes at 90°C, and the remaining four tumors were untreated to serve as controls. The authors noted computed tomography (CT) evidence of coagulation necrosis surrounding the tumor, manifested by increased opacity enveloping the lesion. This was followed by central tissue attenuation with peripheral hyperattenuation surrounding the treated site. Histologic analysis revealed that at least 95% of the tumor nodules were necrotic, although some rabbits (43%) had residual tumor nests at the periphery of the tumor. Pneumothorax was the only procedure-related complication, occurring in 29% of treated rabbits and in 25% of controls. In another study, Miao and colleagues[28] implanted VX2 tumor tissue in the lung of 18 rabbits (12 treated and 6 controls), and the lesions were then treated with RFA using a cooled-tip electrode for 60 seconds. Efficacy of therapy was assessed with magnetic resonance imaging (MRI), microangiography, and histopathology. Absolute tumor eradication was achieved with RFA in 33% and a partial response in 41.6% of rabbits that survived longer than 3 months. MRI evaluation of the lesion post-RFA demonstrated an early hyperintense peritumoral rim on T1- and T2-weighted MRI images, which subsequently turned into homogeneous signal and decreased lesion size with time. Microangiography revealed no perfusion to the ablated lesion. On histopathologic evaluation, the ablated lesion retained its tissue architecture, but with changes consistent with coagulation necrosis, surrounding edema, and inflammation of normal surrounding lung. After 1 to 3 months of treatment, the ablated tumor became an atrophied nodule of coagulation necrosis within a fibrotic capsule.

Putnam and colleagues[29] studied the effects of interstitial thermal energy on lung tumors 2 to 3.5 cm in size in a swine model. The authors used LeVeen electrodes to treat the lesions, and performed gross and histologic evaluations at different time points of 3, 7, and 28 days post-RFA. There were no complications from the procedure, and histologic evaluation demonstrated successful destruction of the lesion with preservation and minimal damage to the surrounding parenchyma. Characteristic changes in the lesion consisted of a central coagulum surrounded by a hyperemic rim early after therapy (Fig. 13.1). This was followed by organization of the lesion with surrounding inflammation and scar formation, with eventual decrease in size by 28 days (Fig. 13.2). The authors also noted some postprocedure pneumonitis and obstructive atelectasis adjacent to the treated lesion with some cases of limited intraparenchymal hemorrhage.

Given the experience with animal models suggesting feasibility and safety of pulmonary application, together with the success of RFA in the treatment of other solid tumors, interest has developed in the clinical application of this technique for the lung. The clinical experience of RFA in the treatment of pulmonary malignancies is limited and consists of pilot projects, but preliminary results suggest it can be applied successfully. Here

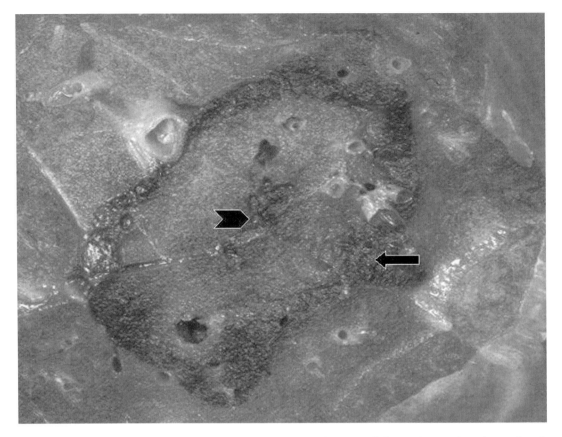

**Figure 13.1.** Ablated lung nodule in animal model. Note the central thermal coagulum (arrowhead) with surrounding hemorrhagic rim (arrow). (Courtesy of RadioTherapeutics, Mountain View, CA.)

we present an overview of the potential role of RFA to treat lung tumors, and the reported preliminary results.

## Indications and Contraindications for Using RFA in the Lung

Given the limited clinical experience of the application of RFA for treatment of lung tumors, there are no clear criteria to guide patient selection. However, Table 13.4 lists the selection criteria used by our group for RFA applications on lung tumors. As experience with this application broadens, these parameters are likely to evolve.

## Preoperative Evaluation and Considerations

As with any patient with a lung tumor, patients being considered for RFA must undergo a rigorous evaluation by a thoracic surgeon to determine if they would derive more benefit from standard surgical resection or another modality. Once a patient is identified as a candidate for lung RFA, particular attention

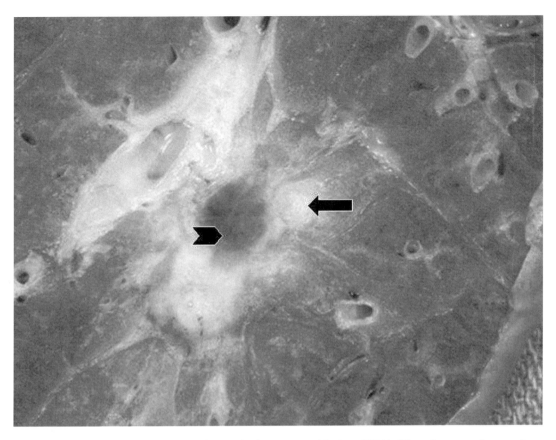

**Figure 13.2.** Lung lesion 28 days after radiofrequency ablation (RFA). Note the central coagulum (arrowhead), with surrounding scar formation (arrow) and decreased size of the lesion. (Courtesy of Radiotherapeutics, Mountain View, CA.)

should be focused on the technical feasibility of applying the technique, and of successfully ablating all the demonstrated lesions.

For each patient, the optimal approach to treat the disease needs to be determined. Many patients who are considered for lung RFA have undergone previous thoracotomies, particularly those with metastatic lung disease. Others will be considered for RFA due to prohibitive operative risk, including poor pulmonary reserve, or other risk factors that could increase the risk for general anesthesia. The following surgical options are possible:

1. Open thoracotomy: This approach provides the most controlled method for application of RFA, and can be used when a concomitant resection is planned, with ablation of a deep or unresectable lesion. Unfortunately, this is an invasive approach that can be of significant risk for patients with comorbidities or with poor pulmonary function.

2. Video-assisted thoracoscopy (VATS): Minimally invasive techniques have the benefit of reduced morbidity and pain and

**Table 13.4 Inclusion and Exclusion Criteria for Lung Radiofrequency Ablation (RFA)**

Inclusion criteria
  Patients with stage I–II non–small cell lung cancer (NSCLC) who are not candidates for resection based on comorbid disease or who refuse lung resection
  Patients with metastatic tumors to the lung who are not candidates for resection of all metastasis, but in which ablation can be applied without leaving residual disease
  Positive tissue diagnosis by recent resection (<6 months) or radiologic biopsy
  Patients with clinically suspicious disease defined as a new lesion on chest CT scan or a PET scan with a lesion demonstrating an SUV of 2.5 or greater
  RFA target lesions 4 cm or less
Exclusion criteria
  Central lesion <3 cm from hilum
  If metastatic tumor primary site is not controlled
  Patients with more than three tumors on one side
  Greater than six metastasis in total (bilateral)
  Pregnant or nursing mothers at time of procedure
  Malignant pleural effusion present

CT, computed tomography; PET, positron emission tomography; SUV, standard uptake value.

faster recovery, but at the expense of loss of tactile control of the ablated lesion. In addition, it is difficult to assess the position of the electrode within the lesion with the thoracoscope, and imaging modalities such as intraoperative ultrasonography are required.

3. Percutaneous CT-guided: This approach has the advantage of being minimally invasive, and has the potential of application of RFA under monitored controlled anesthesia. It provides an accurate imaging modality to guide placement of the electrode and has become the preferred approach by our surgical group. The main disadvantages are limited access to manipulating the lesion in case of inaccessibility, and the loss of tactile appreciation of the mass as well as other possible tumor deposits.

### Technique for Lung RFA

#### Equipment

In one early report of three patients, percutaneous treatment with RFA was performed in the radiology suite under CT guidance with local anesthesia.[30] We have performed the procedure under general anesthesia in an operating room suite with CT scan capabilities. This allows for complete anesthesia support, minimizing patient movement and discomfort, as well as rapid access to instruments and easy placement of pigtail or chest tubes for the commonly associated pneumothoraces that occur.

There are different radiofrequency (RF) current generators available, but we favor those with bipolar characteristics, with capabilities to adjust the power settings. In our current protocol, we use the Radio Therapeutics (Mountain View, CA) RF current generator (Fig. 13.3). Newer generation RF LeVeen multiarray needle electrodes, which vary in size from 2 to 4 cm in diameter, are preferred, achieving ablation of lesions up to 4 cm in diameter. After four grounding pads are placed on the patient's upper thighs, a LeVeen needle electrode size is selected according to the target lesion diameter. The generator is turned on and the power settings are adjusted according to probe size (Table 13.5). The lesion is treated until "roll off" is achieved, which means that a tissue impedance greater than 200 $\Omega$ or power less than 15 W is encountered. A second-phase treatment of the lesion is performed, with starting power that is 50% of the power at which

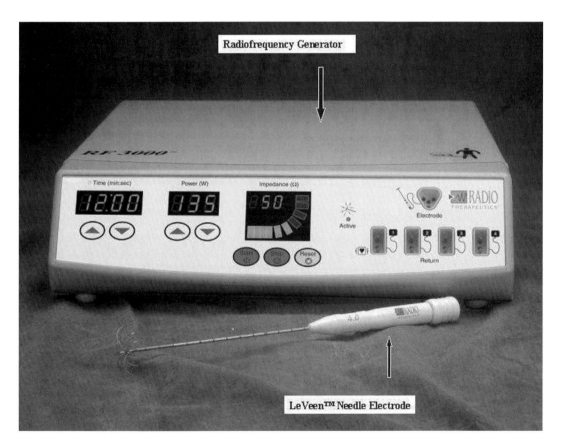

**Figure 13.3.** Radiofrequency current generator (RadioTherapeutics, Mountain View, CA), with 3.5-cm LeVeen needle electrode.

**Table 13.5  First-Phase Power Settings on RF Current Generator for First-Phase Treatment of Lung Lesions**

| Probe size (cm) | Start power (W) | 3 min | 6 min | 9 min | 12 min | 15 min | 18 min | 21 min | 24 min | 27 min | 30 min | 33 min | 36 min |
|---|---|---|---|---|---|---|---|---|---|---|---|---|---|
| 2.0 | 20 | 30 | 40 | 50 | 60* | | | | | | | | |
| 3.0 | 30 | 40 | 50 | 60 | 70 | 80* | | | | | | | |
| 3.5 | 40 | 50 | 60 | 70 | 80 | 90 | 100 | 110 | 120 | 130* | | | |
| 4.0 | 70 | 80 | 90 | 100 | 110 | 120 | 130 | 140 | 150 | 160 | 170 | 180 | 190* |

*Continue at max power until "roll off."

204

**Table 13.6  Second-Phase Power Settings**

| Probe size (cm) | Power (W) |
| --- | --- |
| 2.0 | 45 |
| 3.0 | 60 |
| 3.5 | 90 |
| 4.0 | 120 |

Second-phase treatment if "roll off" encountered after reaching maximum power. Do not increase power during second phase. If first phase roll off is detected before reaching maximum power, then set power at 50% of the power at which roll off occurred.

"roll off" was detected if this occurred before reaching maximum power (Table 13.6).

### RF Application

The goals of RFA of lung tumors are coagulation necrosis of the lesion of interest with a small rim extension into normal lung parenchyma. The technique uses RF energy to generate ionic vibration, which increases tissue temperature up to 100°C, causing protein denaturation, thermal coagulation, and tissue necrosis. To maximize the ablation diameter, tissue coagulation necrosis should be achieved without creating tissue boiling and cavitation, which results in increased tissue impedance.[31] For larger lesions (>3 cm), RFA results seem to be less consistent. It is important to maintain a systematic approach for the treatment of these lesions, in which six or more simultaneous ablations are applied in a cylindrical fashion starting from the most distal area and advancing to more superficial areas as described previously.[33]

### Results with Clinical Application of Lung RFA

In our initial experience at the University of Pittsburgh Medical Center, we treated 10 patients with RFA and included primary and metastatic lung tumors. Selected patients were not candidates for complete surgical resection based on surgical risk, multiple lesions, poor pulmonary reserve, or refusal of further surgery. Mean age was 57 years (range 27 to 95). A total of 17 nodules were treated with RFA in 10 patients (six males, four females) with metastatic carcinoma (four), sarcoma (three), or primary lung cancer (three), with a mean follow-up of 4.4 months (range 1 to 9). One patient with metastatic head and neck cancer who had undergone open resection combined with RFA received a second RFA treatment (percutaneously) 1 month after the initial procedure for two newly detected nodules bilaterally.

The technique is performed by thoracic surgeons in the operating room under general anesthesia, and the approach by either minithoracotomy (27.3%, $n = 3$) or CT-guided percutaneous route (72.7%, $n = 8$). In both approaches, the patient is placed in the lateral decubitus position. In the CT-guided procedures we employ the services of a CT technician, and the thoracic surgeon places a small finder needle into the center of the lung nodule. The surgeon confirms successful central placement of the finder needle during CT imaging, and the LeVeen needle electrode size is chosen according to the diameter of the target lesion. The needle electrode has a diameter of 14 gauge with a 15-cm shaft length, and it is introduced in the center of the lesion under CT guidance (Fig. 13.4). Several applications in different locations within the lesion may be required for larger masses, with the therapy beginning at the most distal area and progressing proximally. Chest tubes were placed in all open procedures and in 62.5% ($n = 8$) of percutaneous procedures for procedure-related pneumothoraces. This complication was treated with placement

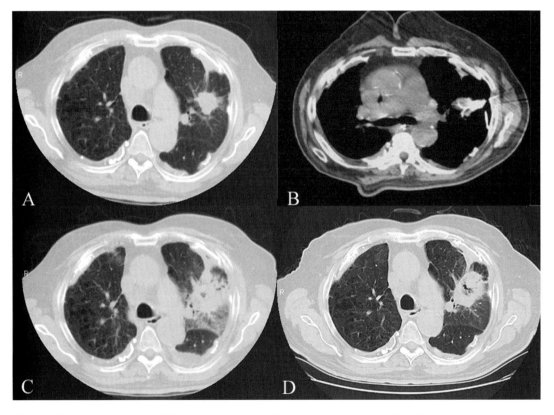

**Figure 13.4.** Percutaneous RFA treatment for 78-year-old patient with left lung non–small cell lung cancer (NSCLC) and severe cardiac risk factors. (A) Preprocedure computed tomography (CT) reveals 3 cm left upper lobe mass. (B) CT-guided percutaneous RFA treatment with 4-cm LeVeen probe. (C) CT scan on 2 days post-RFA showing inflammation and parenchymal bleeding. (D) CT scan 3 months post-RFA showing central cavity and decreased density of lesion.

of pleural pigtail catheters using Seldinger's technique. Evacuation of the pneumothoraces allowed for lung reexpansion and less lung motion for better access of the RFA electrode to the lesion. Mean length of stay was 3.6 days (range 2 to 7).

One patient with a central nodule died from massive hemoptysis 19 days post-RFA and 5 days after receiving brachytherapy for endobronchial disease. Two patients were readmitted with pneumonitis, one of whom later developed pneumonia and transient renal failure 20 days post-RFA. No other complications occurred. Preliminary radiographic assessment of response shows cavitation or liquefaction of treated sites smaller than 4 cm, with one lesion of 2 cm remaining unchanged. Positron emission tomography (PET) scan was used to further evaluate treated lesions when CT scan findings were indeterminate (Fig. 13.5). During this initial follow-up period, 50% of patients developed new metastasis, four of whom died of progressive disease. At this limited follow-up, the others remained free of disease and no patient developed a radiographic recurrence at the RFA-treated site. This pilot study demonstrates the feasibility of RFA for lung malignancies not amenable to resection. The rapid progression of

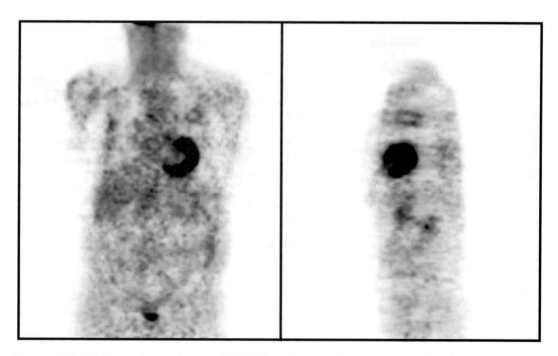

**Figure 13.5.** 18-Fluorodeoxyglucose (18-FDG) positron emission tomography (PET) scan of patient with left upper lobe (LUL) NSCLC treated percutaneously with RFA 5 months prior to this study. Note the tumor in the LUL with central photopenia on the anteroposterior (AP) (left) and lateral (right) views. A rim of peripheral 18-FDG uptake can be seen; however, the standard uptake value (SUV) is 1.5, compared to a pre-RFA SUV of 7.5.

disease of some of these patients reflects the advanced stage and large tumors that were treated in our initial experience. Better patient selection needs to be evaluated in future clinical trials.

The initial report of the Chinese experience with lung RFA was recently reported.[33] The authors treated eight patients with primary lung cancers, seven with metastatic breast cancers, and five with colorectal metastasis. Complications included five patients with pneumothorax and six with postprocedure fevers. Lesion assessment with PET scans demonstrated nonviability in lesions smaller than 3.5 cm. However, lesions larger than 3.5 cm had a partial response, with residual uptake in the tumor periphery.

Dupuy and colleagues[30] reported their initial experience with RFA of lung tumors in three patients with lung malignancies. All treatments were performed percutaneously under CT guidance with either sedation or general endotracheal anesthesia as an outpatient procedure. Only one pneumothorax developed, as shown on follow-up radiographs, which did not require intervention. All three patients developed pleural effusions and postprocedural fevers. Follow-up of the ablated nodules with CT scans at 6 weeks and 3 months postop in one patient revealed no residual disease, but a biopsy of the fibrotic nodule revealed atypical cells, prompting a second RFA treatment. The second patient died of unknown causes 5 weeks post-RFA and 3 weeks after external beam radiation. The third patient is alive, and PET scan at 3 months post-RFA revealed no residual disease. The authors concluded that RFA of lung malignancies is an alternative for patients who are not surgical candidates.

In a report of their initial experience, Sewell and colleagues[34] treated 10 patients with inoperable NSCLC using local anesthesia under CT guidance. Procedure-related complications included four pneumothoraces and pain at the treated site. Follow-up PET scans revealed nonviable cells at the treated site.

The early experience with RFA of lung tumors seems to be feasible and safe. This technique could have a potential role in the treatment of inoperable patients with lung tumors as a form of local control. Clinical trials are needed to assess the safety of the procedure and its impact on long-term survival.

### Follow-Up and Assessment of Response

There is no standard imaging modality for assessment of the response to therapy and for monitoring disease recurrence within an ablated nodule. The ideal follow-up would be histologic evaluation of the nodule, but this is impractical as it defeats the purpose of sparing these patients a resection, since needle biopsy has a large sampling error in a nonsolid ablated tissue. CT scan seems to be an adequate modality for these purposes. Initially, the ablated lesion becomes hyperattenuated, with an increased size, but with decreased density measured as a decrease in Hounsfield units. There can be areas of inflammation in surrounding normal lung parenchyma. With time, there can be formation of a central cavity with liquefaction of the nodule on CT imaging. Lesions that were treated successfully are expected to show a progressive decrease in size with time as the lesion scars and contracts. MRI can also be used to assess the ablated lesion, as it can provide a better definition of liquefaction, tissue densities, and margins. PET scan can be used as a primary or complementary modality for follow-up of these lesions.

## Summary

Radiofrequency ablation of lung tumors is a feasible alternative for the treatment of pulmonary malignancies in patients who cannot undergo surgical resection. It is essential that any patient considered for RFA of a lung nodule should first undergo evaluation by an experienced thoracic surgeon to exhaust any surgical resection options. This tool could also be complementary in the surgical treatment of lung tumors, and for the treatment of lesions that would otherwise require a pneumonectomy or other extensive resection. In the early experience with this technique applied to the lung, tumors can be successfully ablated with minimal complications. Larger studies need to be performed to evaluate the safety and benefits of this modality for treating lung tumors.

## References

1. Boring CC, Squires TS, Tong T, Montgomery S. Cancer statistics, 1994. CA Cancer J Clin 1994; 44:7–26.
2. Greenlee RT, Murray T, Bolden S, Wingo PA. Cancer statistics, 2000. CA Cancer J Clin 2000; 50:7–33.
3. Ries LA, Wingo PA, Miller DS, et al. The annual report to the nation on the status of cancer, 1973–1997, with a special section on colorectal cancer. Cancer 2000; 88:2398–2424.
4. Mountain CF. Value of the new TNM staging system for lung cancer. Chest 1989; 96:47S–49S.
5. Naruke T, Goya T, Tsuchiya R, Suemasu K. Prognosis and survival in resected lung carcinoma based on the new international staging system. J Thorac Cardiovasc Surg 1988; 96:440–447.
6. Luketich JD, Burt ME. Does resection of adrenal metastases from non-small cell lung cancer improve survival? Ann Thorac Surg 1996; 62:1614–1616.
7. Luketich JD, Martini N, Ginsberg RJ, Rigberg D, Burt ME. Successful treatment of solitary extracranial metastases from non-small cell lung cancer. Ann Thorac Surg 1995; 60:1609–1611.

8. Martini N, Bains MS, Huvos AG, Beattie EJ Jr. Surgical treatment of metastatic sarcoma to the lung. Surg Clin North Am 1974; 54:841–848.

9. Shah A, Exelby PR, Rao B, Marcove R, Rosen G, Beattie EJ Jr. Thoracotomy as adjuvant to chemotherapy in metastatic osteogenic sarcoma. J Pediatr Surg 1977; 12:983–990.

10. McCormack P. Surgical resection of pulmonary metastases. Semin Surg Oncol 1990; 6:297–302.

11. Mountain CF, McMurtrey MJ, Hermes KE. Surgery for pulmonary metastasis: a 20-year experience. Ann Thorac Surg 1984; 38:323–330.

12. Morrow CE, Vassilopoulos PP, Grage TB. Surgical resection for metastatic neoplasms of the lung: experience at the University of Minnesota Hospitals. Cancer 1980; 45:2981–2985.

13. Putnam JB Jr, Roth JA. Prognostic indicators in patients with pulmonary metastases. Semin Surg Oncol 1990; 6:291–296.

14. Rusch VW. Pulmonary metastasectomy. Current indications. Chest 1995; 107:322S–331S.

15. McAfee MK, Allen MS, Trastek VF, Ilstrup DM, Deschamps C, Pairolero PC. Colorectal lung metastases: results of surgical excision. Ann Thorac Surg 1992; 53:780–785.

16. Gadd MA, Casper ES, Woodruff JM, McCormack PM, Brennan MF. Development and treatment of pulmonary metastases in adult patients with extremity soft tissue sarcoma. Ann Surg 1993; 218:705–712.

17. Harpole DH Jr, Johnson CM, Wolfe WG, George SL, Seigler HF. Analysis of 945 cases of pulmonary metastatic melanoma. J Thorac Cardiovasc Surg 1992; 103:743–748.

18. Pastorino U, Buyse M, Friedel G, et al. Long-term results of lung metastasectomy: prognostic analyses based on 5206 cases. The International Registry of Lung Metastases. J Thorac Cardiovasc Surg 1997; 113:37–49.

19. McCormack PM, Burt ME, Bains MS, Martini N, Rusch VW, Ginsberg RJ. Lung resection for colorectal metastases. 10-year results. Arch Surg 1992; 127:1403–1406.

20. Ninan M, Sommers KE, Landreneau RJ, et al. Standardized exercise oximetry predicts postpneumonectomy outcome. Ann Thorac Surg 1997; 64:328–332.

21. Ferguson MK. Assessment of operative risk for pneumonectomy. Chest Surg Clin North Am 1999; 9:339–351.

22. Ferguson MK. Preoperative assessment of pulmonary risk. Chest 1999; 115:58S–63S.

23. Ginsberg RJ, Rubinstein LV. Randomized trial of lobectomy versus limited resection for T1 N0 non-small cell lung cancer. Lung Cancer Study Group. Ann Thorac Surg 1995; 60:615–622.

24. Morita K, Fuwa N, Suzuki Y, et al. Radical radiotherapy for medically inoperable non-small cell lung cancer in clinical stage I: a retrospective analysis of 149 patients. Radiother Oncol 1997; 42:31–36.

25. Kupelian PA, Komaki R, Allen P. Prognostic factors in the treatment of node-negative nonsmall cell lung carcinoma with radiotherapy alone. Int J Radiat Oncol Biol Phys 1996; 36:607–613.

26. Sarantou T, Bilchik A, Ramming KP. Complications of hepatic cryosurgery. Semin Surg Oncol 1998; 14:156–162.
27. Goldberg SN, Gazelle GS, Compton CC, Mueller PR, McLoud TC. Radio-frequency tissue ablation of VX2 tumor nodules in the rabbit lung. Acad Radiol 1996; 3:929–935.
28. Miao Y, Ni Y, Bosmans H, et al. Radiofrequency ablation for eradication of pulmonary tumor in rabbits. J Surg Res 2001; 99:265–271.
29. Putnam JB Jr, Thomsen SL, Siegenthale M. Therapeutic implications of heat-induced lung injury. Crit Rev Optical Sci Technol 2000; 75:139–160, 200.
30. Dupuy DE, Zagoria RJ, Akerley W, Mayo-Smith WW, Kavanagh PV, Safran H. Percutaneous radiofrequency ablation of malignancies in the lung. AJR 2000; 174:57–59.
31. Gazelle GS, Goldberg SN, Solbiati L, Livraghi T. Tumor ablation with radio-frequency energy. Radiology 2000; 217:633–646.
32. Rhim H, Dodd GD III. Radiofrequency thermal ablation of liver tumors. J Clin Ultrasound 1999; 27:221–229.
33. Kang S, Luo R, Liao W, Wang C, Luo Y. Effect of radiofrequency ablation on lung cancer. Proceedings of the 37th Annual Meeting of the American Society of Clinical Oncology, 2001 (abstract).
34. Sewell PE, Vance RB, Wang YD. Assessing radiofrequency ablation of non-small cell lung cancer with positron emission tomography (PET). Radiology 2000; 217(3 suppl):334.

# 14

# Radiofrequency Ablation of Recurrent Thyroid Cancer

Damian E. Dupuy and John M. Monchik

Papillary thyroid cancer is the most common type of thyroid cancer. It is generally associated with low morbidity and mortality rates, and a reported 10-year survival rate of 90%.[1] When the disease recurs it generally spreads to the level IV lymph nodes of the neck. Local spread is also seen to the level III (mid–jugular chain) and level VI (anterior space) lymph nodes. Factors associated with recurrence include young age at diagnosis, large size of the primary tumor, extracapsular spread, and a known distant metastasis.[2–5] Controversy exists regarding the effect of lymph node metastasis on survival.[1,6–10] Noguchi et al[1,11,12] reported lymph node metastasis to be a significant prognostic risk factor in this group of patients, and improved survival was shown after a modified radical neck dissection. In the past it was perceived that this disease ran an indolent course over many years with a variable prognosis, irrespective of the presence of cervical lymph node metastasis.[6,13] Despite this perspective the standard surgical therapy in patients with documented lymph node metastases is a modified radical neck dissection. Often, despite this extensive surgery, patients experience recurrence in the surgical field. These recurrences are usually documented with surveillance ultrasound (US) and tend to be small in patients who have yearly careful follow-up. Extensive postoperative scar tissue in these patients who have had multiple surgeries makes further surgery problematic from a morbidity standpoint, particularly with respect to the recurrent laryngeal nerve. In addition, since many of these recurrences are under 1 cm in size, even an experienced surgeon may find it difficult to locate them during surgery without intraoperative US. As we encountered a significant number of this problematic group of patients, we believed that they would benefit from an image-guided ablative therapy if the morbidity was lower than that with surgery and the results were comparable.

Minimally invasive surgical alternatives are becoming more attractive for the treatment of malignancy due to improvements in technology, reduced morbidity and mortality, and the ability to treat patients in the outpatient setting. Radiofrequency ablation (RF) has become a desirable image-guided ablative method because of its relative low cost, its ability to provide large regions of coagulative necrosis in a controlled fashion, and its relatively low toxicity. Although RFA has been extensively investigated in the liver, there has been minimal experience with this technique in the head and neck region. Therefore, we applied RFA to patients with recurrent well-differentiated thyroid cancer. This chapter describes our technique, discusses the early results, and illustrates the imaging findings with several clinical examples.

## Technique

All patients are seen in consultation preprocedure to determine the suitability of lesion ablation, to obtain informed written consent, and to ensure cessation of anticoagulant/antiplatelet medications prior to the procedure. Recurrences in the central compartment must be at least 5 to 10 mm from the expected course of the recurrent laryngeal and vagus nerves and be visualized with US. All lymph node metastases are documented via US-guided fine-needle aspiration biopsy prior to the ablation. In highly suspicious cases the biopsy is usually performed the same day of the ablation with on-site cytopathology. All patients undergo the ablation with intravenous conscious sedation and are premedicated with 0.625 mg intravenous droperidol and receive intravenous fentanyl (100–400 $\mu$g) and medazolam (1–4 mg) that is titrated to their discomfort level during the procedure. Under US guidance with a high-frequency (7–12 MHz) linear transducer, a radiofrequency (RF) electrode (Fig. 14.1) (Radionics, Burlington, MA) with a 1- or 2-cm active tip is inserted into the mass. The perfused treatment electrodes have a diameter of 18-gauge, but a thin, electrically insulated material coating increases its effective diameter to approximately 17 gauge. Each needle contains an RF electrode with a thermocouple embedded at the tip to measure temperature. Circuitry incorporated within the generator

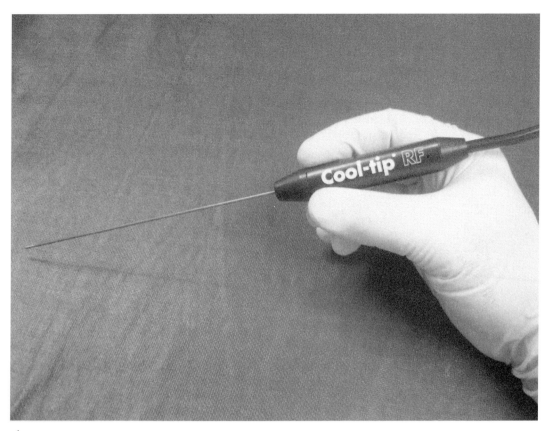

A.

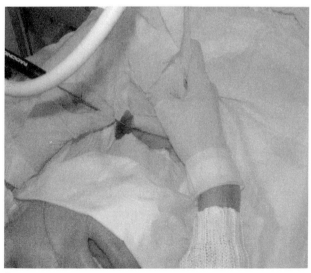

B.

**Figure 14.1.** (A) Radionics (Burlington, MA) 17-gauge Cool-tip radiofrequency electrode with a 1-cm uninsulated tip. The small tip exposure is optimal for treating small malignant lymph nodes from recurrent thyroid carcinoma. (B) Electrode insertion into lymph node with ultrasound guidance.

and needle permits continuous measurement of tissue impedance. Two internal lumina extend to each electrode tip. One is
used to deliver chilled perfusion fluid (sterile saline or water) to
the electrode tip, and the other returns the perfusion effluent to
a collection unit located external to the patient. A peristaltic pump
is used to infuse the perfusion fluid into the cooling lumen of the
electrode at 80 mL/min. Internal cooling is used only for masses
exceeding 1 cm in greatest dimension; otherwise, the electrode
tip temperature is maintained at 90°C for 2 minutes without internal cooling. Two 180-cm$^2$ grounding pads are placed horizontally on the patient's anterior or posterior chest wall and connected to the reference electrode port on the RF generator. The
pads must be placed horizontally to maximize the grounding effect and prevent thermal injury to the skin. The grounding pad(s)
and electrode are connected to the RF generator. When the RF
generator is activated, current flows between the conductive electrode tip and the grounding pad(s) or "dispersive electrode." The
increase in the tissue temperature is proportional to the current
density. Since the current density is highest near the conductive
electrode tip, coagulation is induced in the tissue surrounding
the treatment probe. When performing an RF treatment, the coagulation depth is controlled from the length of the uninsulatcd
"active" electrode tip. The diameter of coagulation necrosis produced around the tip of the treatment electrode depends on the
current, duration of treatment, and local tissue blood flow.

Continuous real-time US monitoring with gray scale and color
Doppler imaging is performed to identify proper electrode position and assess microbubble formation during the RF ablation.
Continuous impedance, current delivery, power output, and RF
electrode tip temperature is monitored with the RF generator. If
the impedance rises 20 Ω above the baseline three times within
1 minute during the internally perfused RF treatments, then the
treatment is stopped and the intratumoral temperature is
recorded. At the end of a given RF treatment, the RF electrode is
repositioned into the tumor mass to measure the intratumoral
temperatures adjacent to the previous treatment. If the temperature within the mass is below the cytotoxic threshold of 50°C,
then an additional RF treatment is performed at the new electrode position. Once the entire mass is treated to temperature levels above the cytotoxic threshold, the treatment is stopped. An
adhesive bandage is applied to the skin and the patients are followed in the radiology postprocedure recovery room for 2 to 4
hours with continuous vital sign monitoring. All patients are then
discharged on oral narcotics if necessary and nonsteroidal antiinflammatory medications. Clinical follow-up consists of a physical exam, thyroglobulin levels, and a follow-up high-resolution

neck ultrasound at 3-month intervals for the first year and then every 6 months thereafter.

## Outcomes

The procedure is well tolerated. Heating of the adjacent normal tissues is the most uncomfortable aspect of the procedure and is problematic only when larger masses are ablated. When smaller masses under 1.5 cm are treated, the procedure is relatively painless as internal perfusion of the electrode is unnecessary and the heat penetration does not extend very far into normal tissue. Careful consideration of which lymph nodes can be treated is important particularly in the central compartment. If a recurrence lies against the expected course of the recurrent laryngeal nerve, then hoarseness may result due to the thermal effects on the nerve. Therefore, we do not perform this procedure on recurrences abutting the recurrent laryngeal or vagus nerves. Self-limited neck swelling and regional discomfort last 1 to 2 weeks after the procedure and is easily controlled with either oral narcotics or nonsteroidal antiinflammatory medications.

The majority of the recurrences that we have treated have been under 1.5 cm in size, although we have treated tumor volumes as large as 3 to 4 cc$^3$. Most of our recurrences are detected when they are small since this group of patients has yearly high-resolution US exams, and generally these tumors are slow growing. After RF treatment, repeat thyroglobulin levels typically fall to normal levels if the ablated region is the only site of disease. We have treated patients with a solitary local recurrence in the neck and pulmonary metastases, and in these patients radioactive iodine is used in conjunction with the RF ablation.

Ultrasound evaluation at 3 months shows loss of the hypervascular color Doppler pattern that is usually seen prior to the treatment (Figs. 14.2, 14.3, and 14.4). The gray scale appearance of the lymph nodes also changes in that the lymph nodes that were initially hypoechoic are now echogenic with respect to muscle (Fig. 14.4). The size of the lymph nodes also decreases. At repeat, fine-needle aspiration biopsy necrosis with inflammatory cells is identified. In larger masses residual tumor may be identified on repeat biopsy or follow-up examination, and repeat RFA may need to be performed.

## Conclusions

Image-guide tumor ablation is an exciting new technique for treating solid tumors in patients who aren't good candidates for surgery.[14] The obvious advantage of ablative therapies when

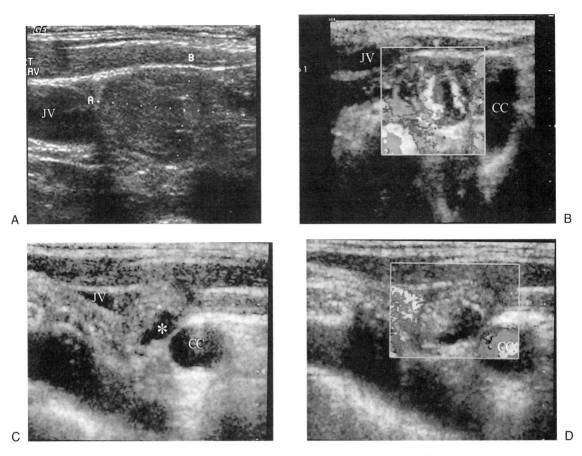

**Figure 14.2.** (A) A 34-year-old woman with a solitary recurrence of papillary carcinoma between the internal jugular vein (JV) and common carotid artery (CC) on the right. (B) Color Doppler interrogation shows extensive tumor vascularity. Three months after radiofrequency ablation (RFA) the area of tumor shows increased echogenicity and cystic changes (*) (C) as well as complete loss of internal color Doppler flow (D).

compared to surgical resection is the reduced morbidity and mortality, lower costs, and the ability to perform procedures in the outpatient setting. Radiofrequency-induced tissue coagulation has been used in early clinical trials for the treatment of liver tumors, both primary and metastatic.[15,16] Radiofrequency has also been successfully applied to osteoid osteomas.[17] Despite prom-

**Figure 14.3.** A 62-year-old woman with Hurthle cell variant of papillary carcinoma status post–total thyroidectomy and repeat surgery on the left presents with a new mass in the left supraclavicular fossa. (A) Color Doppler ultrasound image shows a hypervascular mass. (B) Thirty minutes post-RFA color Doppler image shows complete obliteration of the previously seen tumor hypervascularity.

*(continued)*

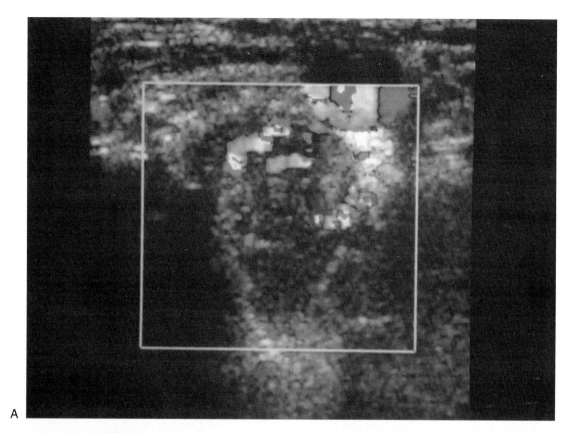

A

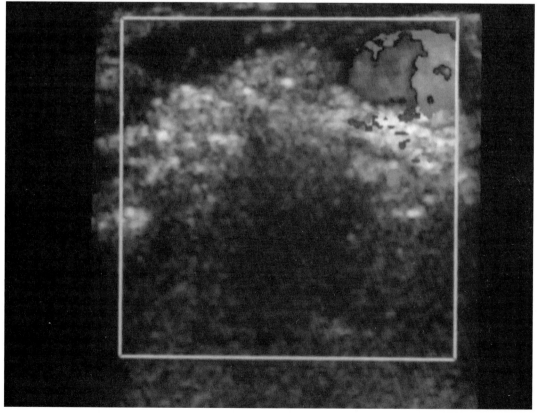

B

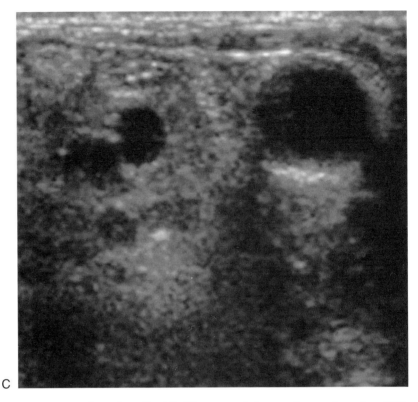

C

**Figure 14.3 (*continued*).** (C) Ultrasound image 3 months after RFA shows shrinkage of the lymph node with some internal cystic change and increased echogenicity.

ising early results in hepatic RFA, extrahepatic RFA has only just been investigated in several small studies involving the lung and kidney.[18,19] In the head and neck we reported success at local control of well-differentiated thyroid cancer.[20] Another recent report showed promise in the use of laser for thyroid masses in an ex vivo model.[21]

Patients with recurrent well-differentiated thyroid cancer can be problematic. They may have undergone total thyroidectomy or radioactive iodine ablation, and many have also had lymph node dissections. Radiofrequency ablation appears to be a particularly important means of therapy in patients who have recently undergone total thyroidectomy and modified neck dissection. A repeat operation in a neck that has been previously opened twice can be very difficult. The anatomic planes are distorted and small lymph node recurrences can be very difficult to find without US guidance. Since this group of patients has a good long-term prognosis and many of the local neck recurrences are identified with high-resolution US, it seems logical to apply a minimally invasive ablative procedure for local tumor eradica-

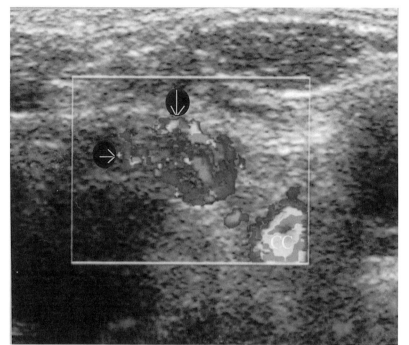

A.

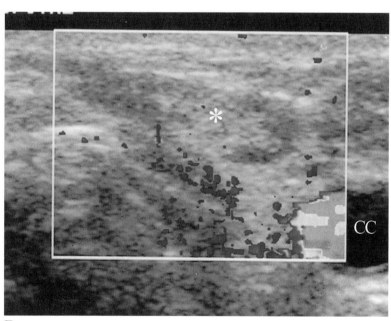

B.

**Figure 14.4.** A 41-year-old woman with a left-sided recurrence after total thyroidectomy 6 years previously and modified radical neck dissection 1 year previously. (A) Transverse ultrasound image of the recurrent mass with color Doppler shows hypervascular flow throughout the lymph node (arrows). (B) Follow-up ultrasound with color Doppler 3 months after RFA shows no hypervascularity and increased echogenicity of the treated lymph node (*). The patient remains disease free at 18 months after RFA.

tion. In our small experience we have shown that the lymph node masses are easily ablated with RFA in the outpatient setting, and that the ablated masses can be followed with US to document regression. Despite a single incidence of recurrent laryngeal nerve injury, the other patients have had no significant morbidity associated with the procedure. In the future, treatment near the recurrent laryngeal nerve probably should be avoided. Alternatively, a bolus of saline could be infused between the mass and the expected location of the nerve, thus providing a safe thermal barrier to the RF energy. Unlike radioactive iodine and surgery, RFA can be repeated on several occasions in areas of previous treatment. Our preliminary results are encouraging, and this new modality may prove useful in this group of patients, but further study in a larger group is warranted.

## References

1. Noguchi S, Murakami N, Yamashita H, Toda M, Kawamoto H. Papillary thyroid carcinoma: modified radical neck dissection improves prognosis. Arch Surg 1998; 133:276–280.
2. Noguchi S, Murakami N, Kawamoto H. Classification of papillary cancer of the thyroid based on prognosis. World J Surg 1994; 18:552–558.
3. Cady B, Rossi R. An expanded view of risk-group definition in differentiated thyroid carcinoma. Surgery 1988; 104:947–953.
4. Byar DP, Green SB, Dor P, et al. A prognostic index for thyroid carcinoma: a study of the EORTC Thyroid Cancer Cooperative Group. Eur J Cancer 1979; 15:1033–1041.
5. Hay ID, Grant CS, Taylor WF, et al. Ipsilateral lobectomy versus bilateral lobar resection in papillary thyroid carcinoma: a retrospective analysis of surgical outcome using a novel prognostic scoring system. Surgery 1987; 102:1088–1095.
6. Mazzaferri EL, Young RL. Papillary thyroid carcinoma: a 10-year follow-up report of the impact of therapy in 576 patients. Am J Med 1981; 70:511–518.
7. DeGroot LJ, Kaplan EL, McCormick M, et al. Natural history, treatment, and course of papillary thyroid carcinoma. J Clin Endocrinol Metab 1990; 71:414–424.
8. Hamming JF, van de Velde CJ, Goslings BM, et al. Preoperative diagnosis and treatment of metastases to the regional lymph nodes in papillary carcinoma of the thyroid gland. Surg Gynecol Obstet 1989; 169:107–114.
9. McHenry CR, Rosen IB, Walfish PG. Prospective management of nodal metastases in differentiated thyroid cancer. Am J Surg 1991; 162:353–356.
10. Yamashita H, Noguchi S, Murakami N, et al. Extracapsular invasion of lymph node metastasis is an indicator of distant metastasis and poor prognosis in patients with thyroid papillary carcinoma. Cancer 1997; 80:2268–2272.

11. Noguchi S, Noguchi A, Murakami N. Papillary carcinoma of the thyroid, II: value of prophylactic lymph node excision. Cancer 1970; 26:1061–1064.

12. Noguchi S, Murakami N. The value of lymph-node dissection in patients with differentiated thyroid cancer. Surg Clin North Am 1987; 67:251–261.

13. DeGroot LJ, Kaplan EL, McCormick M, Straus FH. Natural history, treatment, and course of papillary thyroid carcinoma. J Clin Endocrinol Metab 1990; 71:414–424.

14. Dupuy DE, Goldberg SN. Image-guided radiofrequency tumor ablation: challenges and opportunities; part II. J Vasc Intervent Radiol 2001; 12:1135–1148.

15. Livraghi T, Goldberg SN, Meloni F, Solbiati L, Gazelle GS. Hepatocellular carcinoma: comparison of efficacy between percutaneous ethanol instillation and radiofrequency. Radiology 1999; 210:655–661.

16. Curley SA, Izzo F, Delrio P, et al. Radiofrequency ablation of unresectable primary and metastatic hepatic malignancies. Ann Surg 1999; 230(1):1–8.

17. Rosenthal DI, Hornicek FJ, Wolfe MW, Jennings LC, Gephart MC, Mankin HJ. Changes in the management of osteoid osteoma. J Bone Joint Surg 1998; 80:815–821.

18. Dupuy DE, Zagoria RJ, Akerley W, Mayo-Smith WW, Kavanagh PV, Safran H. Percutaneous radiofrequency ablation of malignancies in the lung. AJR 2000; 174:57–59.

19. Gervais DA, McGovern FJ, Wood BJ, et al. Radio-frequency ablation of renal cell carcinoma: early clinical experience. Radiology 2000; 217:665–672.

20. Dupuy DE, Monchik JM, Decrea C, Pisharodi L. Radiofrequency ablation of regional recurrence from well-differentiated thyroid malignancy. Surgery 2001; 130:971–977.

21. Pacella CM, Bizzari G, Guglielmi R, et al. Thyroid tissue: US-guided percutaneous interstitial laser ablation—a feasibility study. Radiology 2000; 217:673–677.

# Imaging for Radiofrequency Ablation

# 15

# Sonographic Guidance for Radiofrequency Ablation of Liver Tumors

Bruno D. Fornage and Lee M. Ellis

Few patients with malignant liver tumors are candidates for surgical resection, which remains the gold standard for therapy. Patients with extrahepatic disease or multiple metastases in both lobes, those with metastases too close to major blood vessels or biliary structures, those with more than four or five lesions, and those without adequate hepatic reserve have traditionally been considered to have inoperable disease. These patients, however, may benefit from alternative therapies, including systemic or regional chemotherapy and local ablation. Techniques of local ablation aim at physically destroying the entire tumor(s), which in selected patients results in prolonged survival, improved quality of life, and possibly cure. Ablative techniques include cryoablation,[1] microwave coagulation therapy,[2] laser photocoagulation,[3] ethanol injection,[4] and radiofrequency (RF) ablation (RFA), which has become the most popular technique. This chapter describes our technique of ultrasound (US)-guided RFA of malignant liver tumors.

## Principles of Radiofrequency Ablation

The effect of RF current passing through living tissue and producing heat was first described by d'Arsonval in Paris more than a century ago. The best known application of this phenomenon is electrocautery. Modern RFA systems generate a high-frequency alternating electric current that passes from the uninsulated tip of the needle-electrode into the surrounding tissues in the direction of a dispersive electrode (grounding pad) placed on the skin of the back or the thigh. The alternating current causes ionic vibration as the ions attempt to follow the rapid changes in direction of the current. It is this ionic "friction" that heats up the tissues around the electrode. The tissue heats in the area that contacts the electrode tip, and heat is then transferred to more peripheral tissue.

The pathologic effects of RF-induced heat on malignant tumors have been well described. At 46°C, malignant cells die within 8 minutes, while at 51°C, 2 minutes is sufficient for cell death.[5,6] Above 60°C, intracellular proteins are denatured, the lipid bilayers melt, and cell death is inevitable. Thermal coagulation begins at 70°C. Higher temperatures (100°C and higher) cause tissue desiccation, vaporization, and charring.[7]

## RFA Equipment

Several types of RFA generators and needle-electrodes are commercially available. The first electrodes were straight monopolar needles, which create small, egg-shaped thermal lesions. To increase the ablated volume, bipolar devices were designed, but these had limited success.[8] Increasing the number of electrodes has been a more successful way to increase the size of the thermal lesion. This was achieved with a cluster of three parallel needles inserted 0.5 cm from each other.[9] Multiarray needles have allowed the generation of large, grossly rounded or spherical thermal lesions (RF 2000 generator system, RadioTherapeutics, Mountain View, CA; 1500 RF generator, RITA Medical Systems, Mountain View, CA). Multiarray RFA devices consist of a primary electrode—usually a stainless-steel cannula with a short portion exposed as an electrode—and a number (up to 12) of secondary electrodes, which are precurved, flexible metallic prongs deployed like an umbrella once they are pushed out of the cannula (Fig. 15.1). One manufacturer (RITA Medical Systems) has included temperature sensors at the tips of some of the prongs so that the temperature at these points can be monitored in real time during the procedure.

Another technique to increase the size of the RFA lesion is the injection of normal or hypertonic saline through the cannula directly into the lesion during the procedure[10] (Fig. 15.2). The infused saline solution acts as a liquid electrode and increases the volume of RF current conduction around the needle tips. However, the distribution of the fluid in three dimensions cannot be

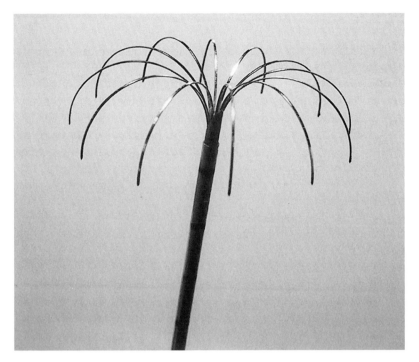

**Figure 15.1.** A multiarray radiofrequency ablation (RFA) device with its 12 prongs fully deployed (model 4.0, RadioTherapeutics, Mountain View, CA).

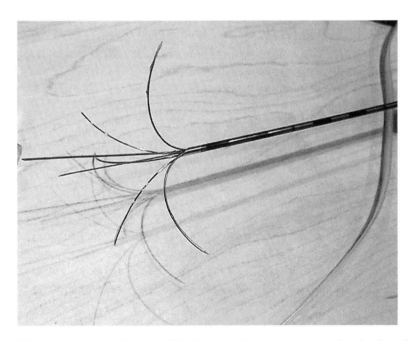

**Figure 15.2.** A multiarray RFA device whose prongs can be deployed over a distance of 7 cm with the theoretical capability of ablating lesions 7 cm in diameter. Ports allow fluid (saline) injection through five of the nine prongs for enhanced ablation (model Starburst™ XLI, RITA Medical Systems, Mountain View, CA).

controlled, and the shape of the thermal lesion may become irregular.

With every type of electrode, a limiting factor in the generation of the thermal lesion is the excessive temperature at the surface of the electrode; this may cause desiccation and char the tissues at the point of contact. The high impedance of the resulting charred tissue significantly reduces or even prevents the propagation of the RF current and therefore heating of the surrounding tissue. Solutions include the slow heating of the lesion with step-by-step increases in the generator's power output (incorporated into the operating software of the RFA units), progressive deployment of the prongs, and internal cooling of the electrode tip.[11]

## Ultrasound Equipment

At The University of Texas M. D. Anderson Cancer Center, RFA of liver tumors is performed under real-time US guidance. To obtain high-quality images for guidance, it is necessary to have a full line of dedicated intraoperative transducers of various frequencies, image geometries, shapes, and sizes, including a laparoscopic transducer if this approach is considered. For a percutaneous approach, a small-footprint phased-array transducer is usually the best option, especially for intercostal access. The transducers that we use most often for intraoperative US (IOUS) are I-shaped ("finger") and T-shaped probes (Figs. 15.3 and 15.4). To examine a large area of the liver and avoid the risk of scanning the liver incompletely, curved-array transducers (giving a sector image) are preferred to flat linear-array transducers, whose deep field of view remains too narrow.

Because it may be very difficult to gain US access to certain regions of the liver such as the posterior dome and because assessment of the proper positioning of the RFA device in three dimensions requires that the transducer be swiveled 90 degrees, the maneuverability of the transducer is of paramount importance. The smaller the transducer, the better. However, the maneuverability of the transducer involves other factors such as the rigidity of the cable and the design of the cable's attachment to the probe. Too stiff a cable may prevent adequate rotation of even a small transducer. When using an I-shaped probe, it is imperative to orient the probe so that the cable is not in the way of the operator or prevents the insertion of the RFA needle.

Color (power) Doppler US is used routinely during IOUS of the liver. This is particularly useful after RFA to confirm the complete "extinction" of any hypervascularity noted in the tumor,

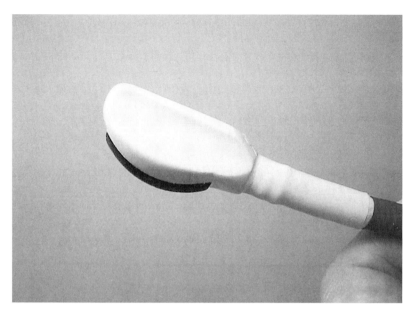

**Figure 15.3.** An l-shaped, 7.5-MHz convex-array intraoperative transducer (UST-995-7.5 Aloka, Wallingford, CT).

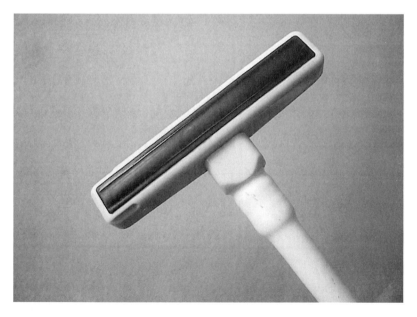

**Figure 15.4.** A T-shaped, 7.5-MHz side-firing flat linear-array intraoperative transducer (UST-5713T, Aloka).

thereby ruling out the presence of residual viable tumor. Color Doppler US can also be used to confirm the presence of an early local recurrence during the patient's follow-up.

The successful use of US contrast agents, initially with power Doppler US[12] and more recently with gray-scale harmonic imaging and pulse inversion,[13] has been reported to detect the presence of residual viable (nonablated) tumor immediately after the RFA procedure. Unfortunately, these contrast agents are only available in the United States for investigational use.

In the future, the use of three-dimensional (3D) US should eliminate the need for cumbersome rotation of the transducer to verify the location of the device in three dimensions. When they become available, small 3D transducers will greatly simplify the placement of the device and reduce—if not eliminate—the operator dependence of the procedure.

New small, portable US scanners have recently been commercialized; some of them incorporate features like color Doppler or harmonic imaging, which, until recently, were found only in high-end and mid-range machines. These scanners may represent an attractive option for IOUS if dedicated intraoperative transducers that can be attached to them become available.

The US scanner should be equipped with a high-capacity electronic storage device such as a magneto-optical (MO) drive or compact disk (CD) recorder to archive representative still frames or short digital videoclips of the critical phases of the procedure. Most nonportable US scanners are equipped with a VCR, and videotaping remains the most ubiquitous and cost-effective method to document the entire real-time procedure.

## Technique of US-Guided RFA

Although the diagnosis of malignancy is already established at the time of RFA, in certain cases, for example, a new small solid lesion detected solely by IOUS and indeterminate by US criteria, a needle biopsy may be indicated to obtain a tissue diagnosis prior to the RFA procedure. In case of intraoperative RFA, this can be done with US-guided FNA and/or core-needle biopsy (Fig. 15.5) with frozen-section examination; either can provide a diagnosis within 15 to 20 minutes.

### Percutaneous, Laparoscopic, or Open Surgical Approach?

In interventional radiology departments, RFA of liver tumors is often performed percutaneously with the patient under local anesthesia and conscious sedation.[11,14–17] In some cases, however, the percutaneous procedure has had to be aborted because of technical difficulties or intolerable pain.[18] Some authors have also

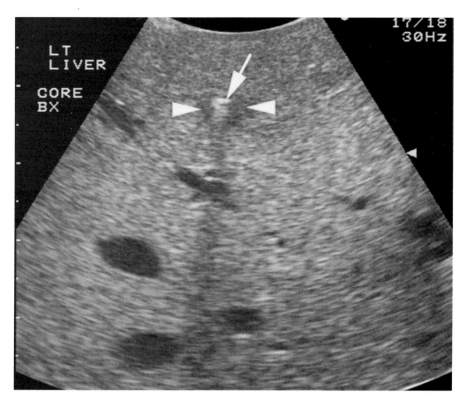

**Figure 15.5.** Intraoperative ultrasound (IOUS)-guided core-needle biopsy of a newly detected minute metastasis in the liver. Transverse intraoperative sonogram shows the echogenic cross section of the core biopsy needle (arrow) in the center of the 5-mm hypoechoic metastasis (arrowheads).

reported satisfactory results with laparoscopic guidance using dedicated laparoscopic US transducers.[19,20] With both the percutaneous and the laparoscopic approaches, the US examination of the liver may not be exhaustive, with the risk that a minute additional lesion that could be easily identified and destroyed with RFA during IOUS is not recognized. At M.D. Anderson, we have found that the most accurate placement of the RFA device—critical for the success of the procedure, especially for large tumors requiring multiple sessions—is best achieved during a laparotomy. Another advantage of IOUS-guided RFA is the possibility of performing the Pringle maneuver, clamping the main portal vein and hepatic artery to temporarily stop blood inflow to the liver and thereby minimize heat loss by convection through the blood vessels; this results in a larger RF lesion.[21] In our institution, percutaneous RFA is reserved for small, conspicuous, "easy-to-ablate" lesions located peripherally (Fig. 15.6). In such cases, the lesion must be easily identified on sonograms and located in a region of the liver that allows an easy and safe pathway for the

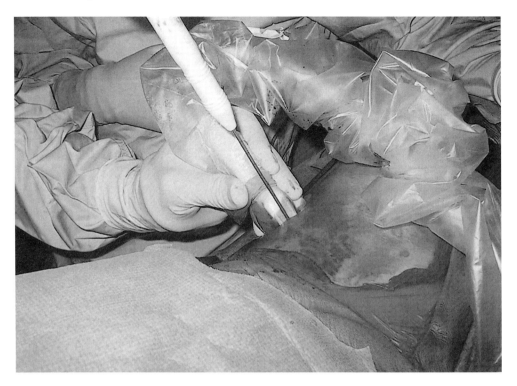

**Figure 15.6.** Percutaneous RFA. The RFA device is inserted from an intercostal approach. The needle-electrode is inserted parallel to the scan plane. The US probe has been gowned in a sterile sheath.

insertion of the needle-electrode (Fig. 15.7). Also, the lesion must be readily seen in two perpendicular planes for the 3D confirmation of the correct placement of the RFA device. This 3D confirmation is less critical for minute tumors, which will be destroyed by the oversized thermal lesion (Fig. 15.8) even if the needle is not perfectly centered, than it is for large tumors, for which a composite multisession thermal lesion is required.

*Review of Imaging*

The first step of IOUS-guided RFA of a liver tumor is to review meticulously the images from all modalities that have been utilized [e.g., computed tomography (CT), magnetic resonance imaging (MRI), US, positron emission tomography (PET), and angiography] and make sure that any lesion that needs to be ablated and that was demonstrated with other modalities will be unequivocally identified on US. Correlation must be perfect in terms of lesion size, shape, location, and surrounding anatomic landmarks. The golden rule for US-guided RFA is that the target must be clearly identified on US and lie in a location that permits satisfactory manipulation of both the transducer and the

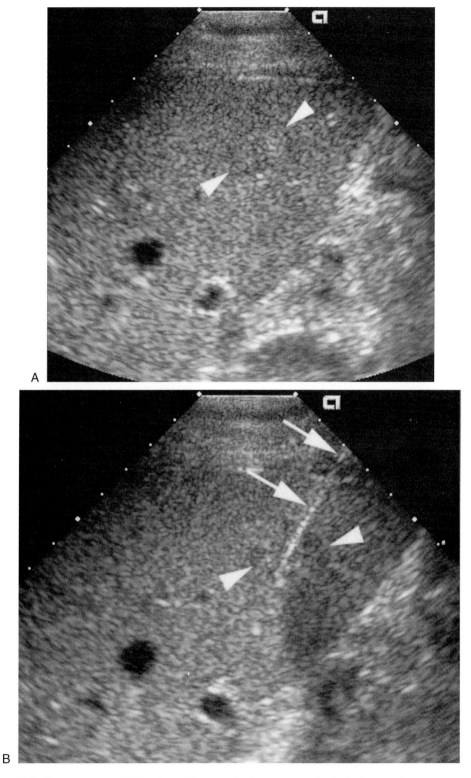

**Figure 15.7.** Percutaneous RFA of a solitary metachronous metastasis from colon cancer. (A) Pre-RFA transverse sonogram shows a well-defined 2-cm metastasis (arrowheads). (B) Sonogram obtained during needle insertion shows the needle (arrows) with its tip in the center of the lesion (arrowheads). *(continued)*

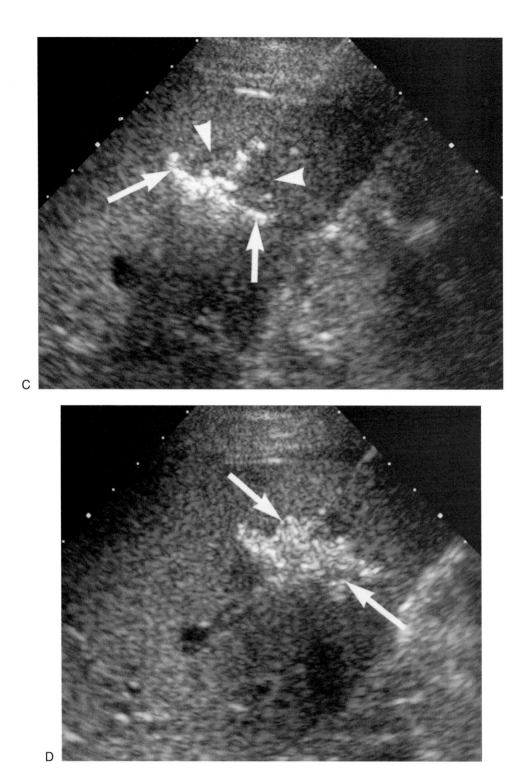

**Figure 15.7 (*continued*).** (C) Sonogram shows the echogenic prongs of the multiarray RFA device (RadioTherapeutics) (arrows) deployed at the posterior aspect of the lesion (arrowheads). (D) Sonogram obtained during the RFA shows a brightly echogenic area covering the tumor volume (arrows).

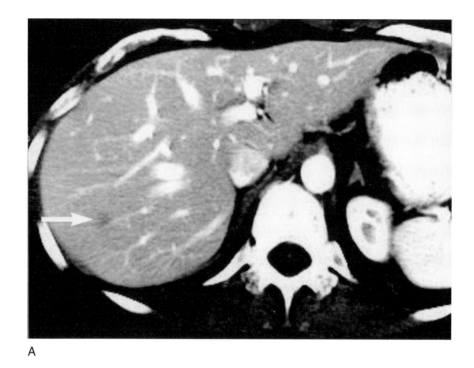

A

B                                    C

**Figure 15.8.** Percutaneous RFA of a solitary metachronous metastasis from colon cancer in segment 6 of the liver. (A) Contrast-enhanced computed tomography (CT) scan shows a new hypodense, nonenhancing lesion in segment 6 (arrow). (B) Pre-RFA longitudinal sonogram shows the small (less than 1 cm) echogenic metastasis. (C) Post-RFA longitudinal sonogram shows a large echogenic area (arrows), which includes the tumor.

RFA device. This usually is not a problem for IOUS-guided RFA, provided the liver can be easily mobilized. However, in the case of reoperation, mobilization of the liver may be very restricted, and the RFA may become technically challenging.

### IOUS

The second step of IOUS-guided RFA takes place in the operating room with the patient under general anesthesia and consists of a thorough IOUS study of the liver with a meticulous search for additional lesions that might have been missed with other modalities. This may lead to an IOUS-guided fine-needle aspiration (FNA) of a minute indeterminate solid mass. In addition to enabling the most complete examination of the liver at the highest resolution possible, the benefits of IOUS include the possibility of performing a dynamic examination of the liver with graded compression. This technique may in a few seconds differentiate an atypical (hypoechoic) hemangioma, which flattens under compression, from a metastasis, which does not. IOUS of the liver has been reported to change the surgical management of liver metastases from colorectal cancer in up to 44% of patients.[22]

### US Evaluation of the Target Lesion

The third step consists of the US evaluation of the target and determination of the optimal pathway for insertion of the RFA device. The shape of the tumor is carefully assessed, especially if instead of being spherical, it is ovoid, lobulated, or irregular. While a round mass can be approached from any direction, an oval mass will be most effectively treated if the RFA needle is inserted along the mass's longest diameter. The longest diameters of the target lesion are measured in three orthogonal dimensions with the built-in calipers. These measurements determine if the lesion can be ablated with a single or multiple RFA sessions and how the multiple sessions should be performed to ensure sufficient overlap of the ablated volumes.

The echotexture and echogenicity of the target lesion are evaluated. The presence of necrotic areas or large calcifications must be noted because they may interfere significantly with the deposition of RF energy or even the deployment of the prongs. Most liver metastases have a nonspecific hypoechoic appearance. However, hypervascular metastases, such as those from neuroendocrine tumors, tend to be isoechoic or hyperechoic, and their behavior during RFA is characterized by a very short ablation time.

It is important for the sonologist to evaluate carefully the relationship between the tumor and adjacent vessels that may act as heat sinks or may be in the pathway of the needle (Fig. 15.9).

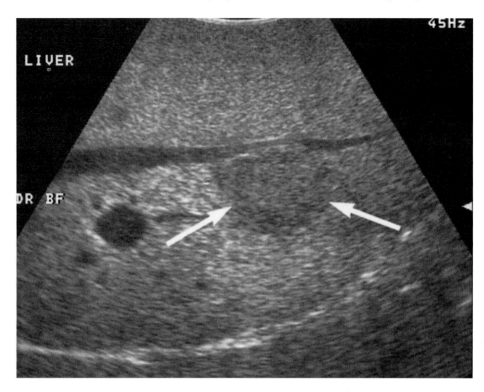

**Figure 15.9.** Intraoperative sonogram shows a liver metastasis (arrows) in close contact with the right hepatic vein. Complete ablation may be difficult to achieve because of the heat-sink effect of large adjacent vessels.

In addition, when instruments equipped with thermocouples at the tip of the prongs are used, the presence of a thermocouple in a vessel would result in a continuously low temperature reading that would interfere with the generator's software, which automatically adjusts the power output of the generator as a function of the temperature recorded at the tip of each prong.

### US-Guided Placement of the RFA Device

The standard technique of needle insertion is the oblique insertion technique, in which the cannula is inserted from the end of the transducer along the US scan plane with an obliquity that depends on the depth of the target. With this technique, the needle is visualized from the moment it enters the scan plane. The free-hand technique is preferred to the use of needle guides attached to the transducer because the former allows continuous adjustment of the needle's position in real time until the optimal position is obtained. The perfect alignment of the needle with the scan plane is verified through the display of the entire shaft of the needle as a brightly echogenic line.[23] The needle is then inserted halfway through the mass, and the transducer is swiveled 90 degrees to obtain a transverse sonogram confirming that the echogenic cross section of the needle is in the center of the target lesion. With the RadioTherapeutics device, the umbrella-shaped prongs are deployed at the very distal aspect of the tumor. With the RITA device, whose prongs are less curved, the needle is slightly withdrawn (but remains within the mass), and the prongs are deployed under real-time US through the mass so that they traverse the mass and protrude beyond it over a distance of about 1 cm (Fig. 15.10A). After the prongs are deployed, the position of the tip of the cannula, which also acts as an antenna and will be creating the most proximal "margin" of the ablated volume, may need to be adjusted to lie at the proximal edge of the tumor since it tends to be pushed back during the forward deployment of the prongs. Again, the transducer is swiveled 90 degrees to confirm that the cross sections of the prongs are distributed evenly throughout the tumor volume (Fig. 15.10B). The use of a small-footprint, easy-to-maneuver intraoperative transducer is critical to the 3D assessment of the correct positioning of the RFA device in lesions located at the dome and other hard-to-reach locations in the liver (Fig. 15.11).

It is important that the sonologist have a clear understanding of how the RFA device works and a clear 3D mental picture of the expected ablation volume based on the US display of the multiarray electrode's prongs. This is not always easy because the prongs are curved and thin and therefore not very reflective. Unless they are completely included in the scan plane (and usually only two prongs at a time are completely depicted), only very short segments may be visible. In addition, in firm or calcified tumors, the deployment of the prongs may be difficult because of their curvature and lack of stiffness. In that setting, the proper placement of a single straight needle-electrode is easier than the placement of a multiarray device. Other difficulties may arise when the target lesion abuts the surface of the liver. In such a case, direct insertion of the needle-electrode through the mass perpendicularly to the liver surface may be as efficacious as, and less cumbersome, than US-guided placement of the needle.

Because the success of the ablation is so dependent on the accurate placement of the RFA device in the very center of the target lesion, it is imperative that the device be inserted by an operator who is experienced in US and US-guided interventions and who has excellent eye-hand coordination and 3D "vision." The latter skills are indispensable when maneuvering in very tight spaces. The skill level required for US-guided RFA of solid tumors is greater than that required for US-guided needle biopsies. The major difference between the two procedures is the much greater needle placement accuracy required for US-guided

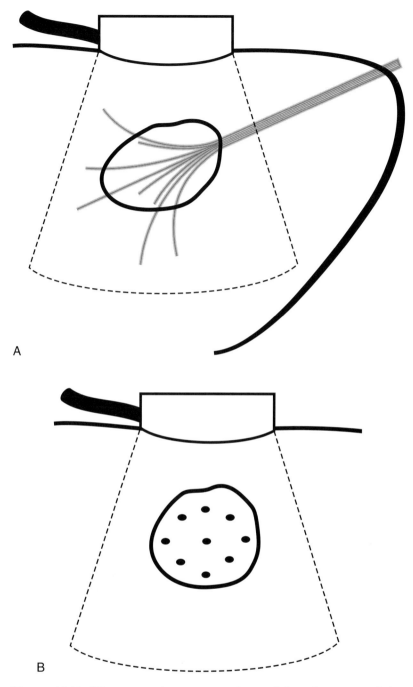

A

B

**Figure 15.10.** Diagrammatic representations of the placement of the multiarray RFA device under IOUS guidance show the relative positions of the deployed prongs and the tumor to be ablated. (A) Longitudinal view. (B) Transverse view shows the echogenic cross sections of the prongs inside the tumor.

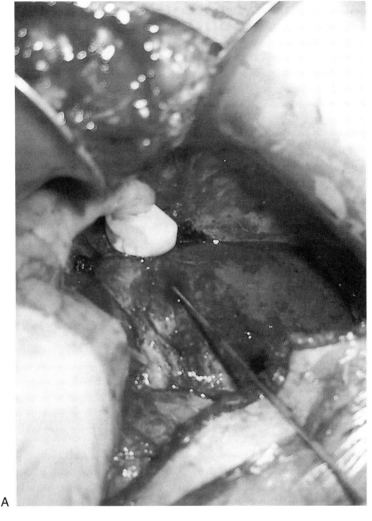

A

**Figure 15.11.** Intraoperative views of the US transducer's positions. (A) The needle is aligned with the small I-shaped convex-array transducer. Because of the location of the lesion at the dome of the liver and the limited space available, the transducer can be held by only one finger.

*(continued)*

RFA; a successful core-needle biopsy of a mass requires that the operator hit any part of the tumor only once (out of multiple passes), whereas a successful RFA requires that the operator not only hit the target but hit its precise center and make the tumor and the thermal lesion perfectly concentric.

### RFA Protocol

Once the placement of the needle and deployed prongs is deemed adequate, the generator is turned on and the RFA session begins. With the RadioTherapeutics RF 2000 generator, the initial power

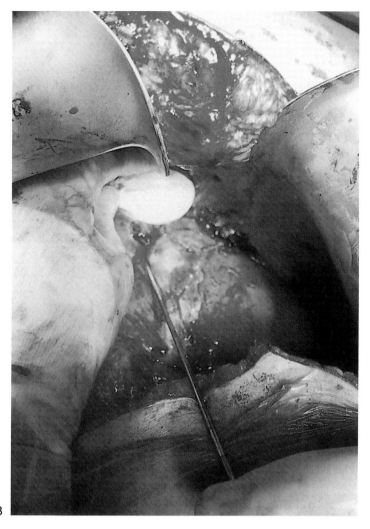

B

**Figure 15.11 (*continued*).** (B) The small-footprint transducer has been turned 90 degrees to display the cross section of the needle and verify its position.

is applied at 50 W and then increased in 10-W increments at 1, 2, 3, and 4 minutes to a maximum power of 90 W. The session continues until "power roll-off" occurs in response to a sudden rise in tissue impedance resulting from tissue boiling. After a 20-second pause, power is reapplied at 75% of the maximum power achieved until power roll-off again occurs. Thus, each tumor or area within a large tumor is treated with a two-phase application of RF power before the RFA device is removed or repositioned for another RFA session. With the RITA generator, the procedure is slightly different; the generator automatically adjusts its power output to raise and maintain the temperature at the tip of the active prongs throughout the session based on the continuous real-time reading of the temperatures recorded by the thermocouples at the tips of some prongs. (Editors' Note: These protocols are constantly being modified. Therefore, one should consult with the latest set of instructions provided by the manufacturer.)

### US Changes During RFA

As the temperature slowly rises, no US changes are noticed. Only late in the session, as the power roll-off is imminent, are changes noted in the US appearance of the tumor. The echogenicity of the tumor increases, and a large number of bright dots soon covers most of the tumor volume. At that time, it is not unusual to hear a popping noise caused by bursting gas bubbles inside the tumor. Some echoes representing gas bubbles may be seen to "leak" into the adjacent veins. The hyperechogenicity of the tumor at the end of the session is usually considered a reliable indicator of an effective "burn." Unfortunately, it remains unclear to what portion of the thermal lesion the hyperechoic area on sonograms truly corresponds. In addition, the hyperechoic area is irregular in shape and rarely covers the entire tumor volume. In fact, the RFA-induced hyperechogenicity represents mostly gas microbubbles inside the tumor, not coagulated tissue. The hyperechogenicity of the treated volume decreases rapidly, and in the case of multisession RFA of large tumors, the first area treated has often reverted to normal echogenicity before the end of the procedure.

In hypervascular lesions, in particular in metastases from neuroendocrine tumors, extremely fast RFA action has been noted. In such lesions, roll-off occurs within a few minutes, and the lesion rapidly becomes markedly hyperechoic (Fig. 15.12). It is not rare to notice a combination of shadowing and reverberations distal to the lesion at the end of the procedure.

### Difficulties in US-Guided RFA of Large Lesions

For a successful ablation, the entire tumor volume must be subjected to cytotoxic temperatures. This is not difficult for round

**Figure 15.12.** Multiple liver metastases from a small bowel carcinoid tumor. In addition to a wedge resection of one lesion, 10 small lesions were ablated with US guidance. (A) Contrast-enhanced CT scan shows one (arrow) of several new liver metastases. (B) Pre-RFA sonogram shows the correct placement of the tip of the needle and of the deployed prongs through a small (0.6 cm), round, mildly echogenic solid mass (arrows).

*(continued)*

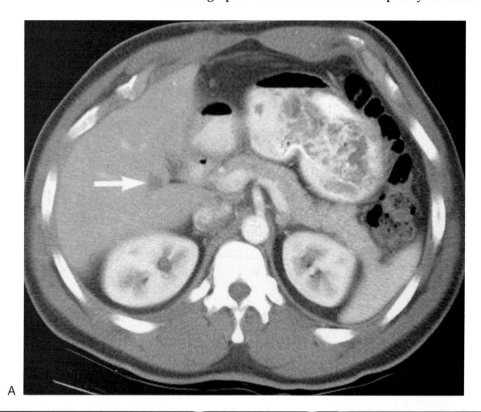

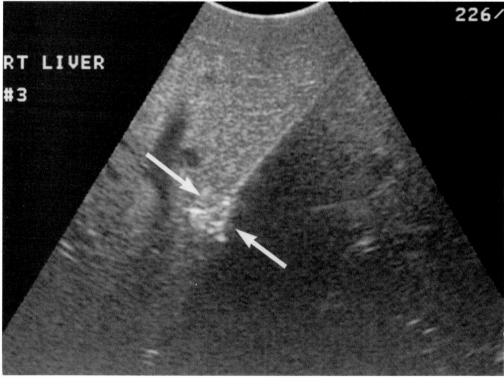

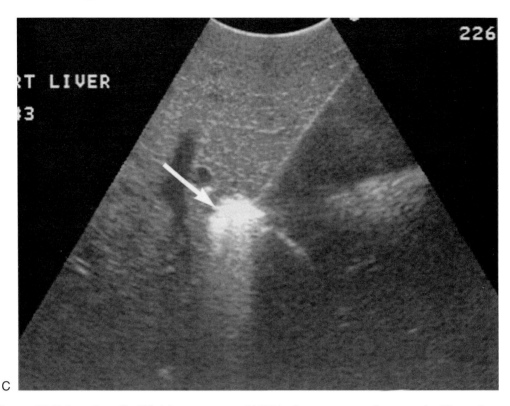

**Figure 15.12 (continued).** (C) After a very rapid RFA, the sonogram shows a significant increase in the echogenicity of the ablated area (arrow), with an unusual "snowstorm" appearance, a combination of reverberations and shadowing.

lesions less than 2.5 to 3.0 cm, because these are smaller than the thermal lesion created by the RFA device (assuming correct placement of the device through the lesion). The coverage in three dimensions of a larger volume with several small spherical elementary thermal lesions is much more complex to plan and difficult to achieve. Multiple sessions are needed to create overlapping grossly spherical thermal lesions that will ensure adequate ablation not only of the tumor but also of a sufficient (ideally 1 cm) surrounding rim of normal hepatic parenchyma. Unfortunately, the shape and size of the ablated volume vary significantly with a number of parameters, including the tissue inhomogeneity of the tumor, the amount and distribution of the tumor's internal vascularity, the presence of adjacent heat sinks, and the amount of vaporization or carbonization during the session. These parameters are not controllable, and the result is that the success of RFA of large masses is much less predictable than that of RFA of small masses, especially in light of the uncertainty of adequate coverage of a large tumor with multiple RFA lesions[7]

(Fig. 15.13). The ideal (and yet practical) technique to ablate large tumors (>2.5–3.0 cm) with multiple overlapping ablations using multiarray electrodes remains to be developed. In fact, a computer model of multisession ablation of large tumors has shown that the size of the composite RFA lesion created by overlapping a large number (up to 14) of elementary thermal ablation spheres remains surprisingly small relative to the large number of ablations performed.[24]

The deepest portion of a large tumor is treated first, starting with the most distal portion of the tumor. Once the session is finished, the prongs are retracted back into the cannula, the needle is pulled back 1.5 to 2.0 cm toward the proximal aspect of the tumor (pull-back technique), and the prongs are redeployed to create a second, overlapping spherical thermal lesion. Then the needle is completely withdrawn and reinserted parallel to the previous axis but at a distance of 2.0 to 2.5 cm from the first insertion site. Additional spheres of ablation are created to en-

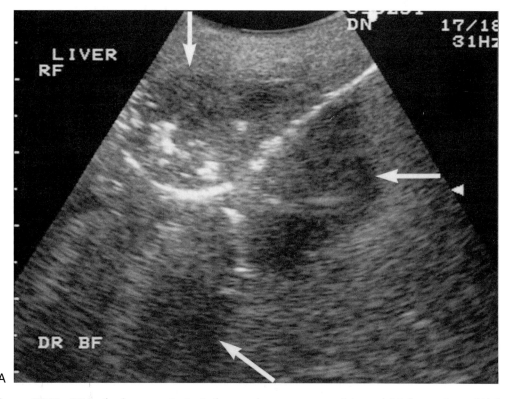

**Figure 15.13.** RFA of a large metastasis from colon cancer requiring multiple sessions. (A) Longitudinal sonogram obtained at the end of a session shows an echogenic area covering only part of the large tumor (arrows).

(*continued*)

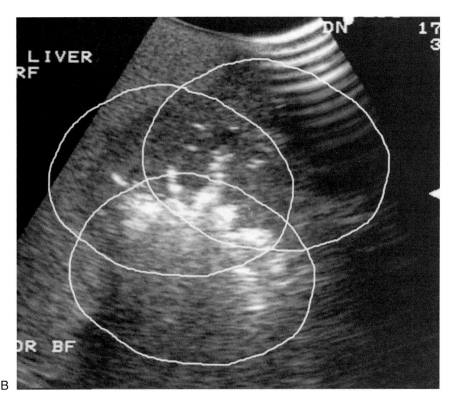

B

**Figure 15.13** (*continued*). (B) Transverse sonogram shows the echogenic recently ablated zone (deep white circle). The two superficial white circles represent areas remaining to be ablated. One year later, the patient developed a local recurrence that was treated with a second IOUS-guided RFA. Six months later, new small metastases developed with the patient being in otherwise good general condition.

compass the entire tumor volume, as needed (Fig. 15.13). We begin with the deepest aspect of the tumor because of the risk of obscuring the visibility of the deep portion of the tumor by the shadow that would result from RFA of the more superficial aspect of the tumor. This technique of tailored multisession ablation becomes even more challenging with tumors of irregular shape.

The multiple sessions that are needed for large tumors result in a lengthy procedure of up to 2 hours. However, the most significant obstacles to the use of RFA for large liver tumors remain the inability to clearly and reliably visualize the extent of the thermal lesion on real-time gray-scale US (in contrast to the easy visualization of ice-ball formation during cryotherapy) and the fact that the post-RFA US appearance of the tumor cannot guarantee that it has been completely ablated with a sufficient margin of normal liver parenchyma. Great hope has recently been placed on the use of US contrast agents at the end of the procedure to verify the absence of residual disease.[13]

Large lesions are likely to abut large veins (Fig. 15.9). In this case, complete ablation is difficult to achieve because of the heat-sink effect of these veins. It has been shown, however, that RFA can destroy tumors that are in contact with or even engulf a large vein and do so without damaging the wall of the vessel.[18]

Lesions located close to the hilum of the liver should not be treated with RFA because of the significant risk of bile duct injury and subsequent strictures.

## Follow-up of RFA Lesions and Detection of Local Recurrence

The follow-up of RFA lesions remains difficult. Subtle early recurrences are difficult to detect, and their treatment is problematic. Even with refined techniques such as contrast agents and harmonic imaging with pulse inversion, transabdominal US seems to have a very limited role in post-RFA follow-up, except perhaps for lesions located superficially in easy-to-scan areas of the liver. Contrast-enhanced CT and MRI are the standard imaging modalities used in the follow-up of RFA lesions. On CT, the ablated area appears hypodense and is not enhanced after injection of contrast medium. The area of necrosis seen on the early postablation CT scans should be larger than the original tumor. There is a close correlation between hypodense nonenhancing areas and pathologic evidence of coagulation necrosis.[25] In the first few days and weeks after treatment, a rim of enhancement surrounding the ablated area on CT and MRI represents peritumoral post-RFA inflammatory reaction.[17] Persistent hyperemia after this time, halo-like or nodular enhancement, and any gross enlargement of the ablated area are signs of recurrence.[26] An absence of such signs for 6 to 12 months indicates that treatment was successful.

Although local recurrence rates as low as 1.8% at 15 months have been reported,[18] recent reports indicate that higher rates of local recurrence are more likely. Solbiati et al[13] reported a 29.6% rate of local recurrence in a series of 172 metastases in 109 patients with a follow-up of 6 to 52 months. Although the recurrence rate was only 16.5% for lesions smaller than 3 cm, it reached 56.1% for lesions larger than 3 cm.

Repeat RFA of a recurrent lesion that appears as peripheral enhancing nodularity on CT or MRI is a challenge because the complete destruction of such a recurrence (which may be larger than suggested by the focal nodule seen on imaging) requires an even larger thermal lesion than the initial one (Fig. 15.14). In the case of repeat RFA for recurrence, the success rate has been reported at only 45.8%.[13]

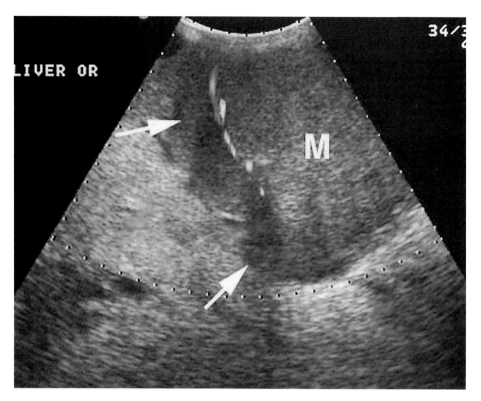

**Figure 15.14.** Repeat RFA for a local recurrence after RFA of a large metastasis from colon cancer 11 months previously. Intraoperative color Doppler sonogram shows the homogeneous necrotic mass (M) and a crescent-shaped markedly hypoechoic recurrence (arrows) with hypervascularity. Because of the high risk of additional occult recurrent nodules at the periphery of the lesion, this type of recurrence is particularly difficult to re-treat, as an even larger volume of ablation than the original one needs to be achieved.

## Conclusions

Because of its unique real-time capability, US has been recognized as the optimal imaging modality with which to guide the placement of the needle-electrode of the RFA device. The most accurate placement of the RFA device is achieved during laparotomy with sufficient exposure of the area of the liver to be treated. While US-guided RFA of small lesions (less than 2 cm) usually poses no technical difficulty as far as ensuring that the entire lesion has been heated to a sufficient temperature, there is still room for improvement of the RF devices and possibly of the US guidance technique in making 100% certain that the ablation of a large and irregular mass is complete. Considerable experience in both general and interventional (including intraoperative) US and a thorough understanding of the thermodynamics of RFA are prerequisites for a successful liver tumor RFA program, that is, one with a low recurrence rate.

## References

1. Sotsky TH, Ravikumar TS. Cryotherapy in the treatment of liver metastases from colorectal cancer. Semin Oncol 2002; 29:183–191.
2. Itamoto T, Katayama K, Fukuda S, et al. Percutaneous microwave coagulation therapy for primary or recurrent hepatocellular carcinoma: long-term results. Hepatogastroenterology 2001; 48:1401–1405.
3. LeVeen RF. Laser hyperthermia and radiofrequency ablation of hepatic lesions. Semin Intervent Radiol 1997; 14:313–324.
4. Numata K, Tanaka K, Kiba T, et al. Nonresectable hepatocellular carcinoma: improved percutaneous ethanol injection therapy guided by $CO_2$-enhanced sonography. Am J Roentgenol 2001; 177:789–798.
5. Dickson JA, Calderwood SK. Temperature range and selective sensitivity of tumors to hyperthermia: a critical review. Ann NY Acad Sci 1980; 335:180–205.
6. Goldberg SN. Radiofrequency tumor ablation: principles and techniques. Eur J Ultrasound 2001; 13:129–147.
7. Gazelle GS, Goldberg SN, Solbiati L, et al. Tumor ablation with radio-frequency energy. Radiology 2000; 217:633–646.
8. McGahan JP, Gu WZ, Brock JM, et al. Hepatic ablation using bipolar radiofrequency electrocautery. Acad Radiol 1996; 3:418–422.
9. McGahan JP, Dodd GD III. Radiofrequency ablation of the liver: current status. Am J Roentgenol 2001; 176:3–16.
10. Livraghi T, Goldberg SN, Monti F, et al. Saline-enhanced radiofrequency tissue ablation in the treatment of liver metastases. Radiology 1997; 202:205–210.
11. Solbiati L, Goldberg SN, Ierace T, et al. Hepatic metastases: percutaneous radio-frequency ablation with cooled-tip electrodes. Radiology 1997; 205:367–373.
12. Solbiati L, Goldberg SN, Ierace T, et al. Radio-frequency ablation of hepatic metastases: postprocedural assessment with a US microbubble contrast agent—early experience. Radiology 1999; 211:643–649.
13. Solbiati L, Ierace T, Tonolini M, et al. Radiofrequency thermal ablation of hepatic metastases. Eur J Ultrasound 2001; 13:149–158.
14. Rossi S, Buscarini E, Garbagnati F, et al. Percutaneous treatment of small hepatic tumors by an expandable RF needle electrode. Am J Roentgenol 1998; 170:1015–1022.
15. Lencioni R, Cioni D, Bartolozzi C. Percutaneous radiofrequency thermal ablation of liver malignancies: techniques, indications, imaging findings, and clinical results. Abdom Imaging 2001; 26:345–360.
16. Goldberg SN, Gazelle GS, Solbiati L, et al. Ablation of liver tumors using percutaneous RF therapy. Am J Roentgenol 1998; 170:1023–1028.
17. Rhim H, Dodd GD III. Radiofrequency thermal ablation of liver tumors. J Clin Ultrasound 1999; 27:221–229.
18. Curley SA, Izzo F, Delrio P, et al. Radiofrequency ablation of unresectable primary and metastatic hepatic malignancies: results in 123 patients. Ann Surg 1999; 230:1–8.
19. Scott DJ, Young WN, Watumull LM, et al. Accuracy and effectiveness of laparoscopic vs open hepatic radiofrequency ablation. Surg Endosc 2001; 15:135–140.

20. Siperstein A, Garland A, Engle K, et al. Laparoscopic radiofrequency ablation of primary and metastatic liver tumors. Technical considerations. Surg Endosc 2000; 14:400–405.

21. de Baere T, Bessoud B, Dromain C, et al. Percutaneous radiofrequency ablation of hepatic tumors during temporary venous occlusion. Am J Roentgenol 2002; 178:53–59.

22. Cervone A, Sardi A, Conaway GL. Intraoperative ultrasound (IOUS) is essential in the management of metastatic colorectal liver lesions. Am Surg 2000; 66:611–615.

23. Fornage BD. Sonographically guided needle biopsy of nonpalpable breast lesions. J Clin Ultrasound 1999; 27:385–398.

24. Dodd GD III, Frank MS, Aribandi M, et al. Radiofrequency thermal ablation: computer analysis of the size of the thermal injury created by overlapping ablations. Am J Roentgenol 2001; 177:777–782.

25. Goldberg SN, Gazelle GS, Compton CC, et al. Treatment of intrahepatic malignancy with radiofrequency ablation: radiologic-pathologic correlation. Cancer 2000; 88:2452–2463.

26. Chopra S, Dodd GD III, Chintapalli KN, et al. Tumor recurrence after radiofrequency thermal ablation of hepatic tumors: spectrum of findings on dual-phase contrast-enhanced CT. Am J Roentgenol 2001; 177:381–387.

# 16

# Radiographic Imaging Following Radiofrequency Ablation of Liver Tumors

Haesun Choi, Evelyne M. Loyer, and Chusilp Charnsangavej

Imaging has a crucial role in the follow-up of patients who have been treated with radiofrequency ablation (RFA) for hepatic neoplasms. Imaging is used to evaluate patients for residual or recurrent tumors and to diagnose rare complications secondary to treatment.

Computed tomography (CT) and magnetic resonance imaging (MRI) are the modalities of choice for post-RFA follow-ups. Both perform equally well, but because of greater availability, CT is more frequently used[1–5]; MRI is indicated if a patient is allergic to iodine, and is used as a problem-solving modality when, for example, a discrepancy exists between the clinical results and the CT findings or when a lesion is suspected on CT but is not definite. Ultrasonography is used to guide needle placement during the RFA procedure but has had a limited role in follow-up; however, recent studies have suggested that contrast-enhanced Doppler ultrasonography may be used to evaluate hypervascular tumors during and after ablation.[4,6,7]

## Imaging Findings

### Complete Ablation

Radiofrequency ablation induces an area of coagulative necrosis at the site of treatment. On nonenhanced CT, the necrosis is of low attenuation, but may contain areas of higher attenuation that will resolve at a variable rate during the following weeks or months.[8] Acutely, the lesion may contain gas, which will also resolve spontaneously.[1,3] The presence of gas always raises the possibility of an abscess. However, the decision about whether to perform a diagnostic aspiration should be based on the patient's symptoms, if any, since imaging findings are nonspecific.

The RFA defect is best evaluated following intravenous administration of a contrast agent.[1] The shape of the RFA defect varies,[2] but it is often round or ovoid. It sometimes has a more complex geometric shape depending on RFA needle placement or the proximity of large blood vessels. In comparison to pretreatment studies, the defect should be centered at the region of the tumor and should encompass the tumor in its entirety. To assure tumor-free margins, the defect, at early follow-up, should be larger than the tumor. Aside from size and location, the most important morphologic feature indicating complete ablation is the characteristic smooth margin of the defect. The interface between the liver and the lesion should be sharp, a consequence of an abrupt change in attenuation between the unenhanced necrosis and the adjacent liver parenchyma (Fig. 16.1). Any variation from this pattern should prompt a careful analysis to exclude residual tumor or recurrence.

These CT characteristics of the RFA defect have been reported by several groups and apply to MRI as well.[1,3,9–12] Specific to MRI are changes in signal intensity. On T2-weighted images, the ablated tumor is characterized by low signal intensity, while an untreated tumor produces high signal intensity.[9] At early follow-up, necrotic debris within the defect often produces heterogeneously high signal intensity and a hypointense rim on T2-weighted images (Fig. 16.2).

Enhancement on CT or MRI does not occur within the necrotic area but is sometimes present at the periphery of the RFA defect.[1–4,9,10] Peripheral enhancement is affected by the scanning technique and is more likely to occur in the arterial phase of enhancement.[4] When this happens, one needs to determine whether this enhancement is tumoral, particularly, but not only, when the treated tumor was hypervascular, or whether it is due to granulation tissue. Peripheral nontumoral enhancement due to granulation tissue varies in intensity and thickness. As a rule, nontu-

**Figure 16.1.** Complete ablation of hepatic metastasis from colon carcinoma. (A) CT scan obtained before radiofrequency ablation (RFA) shows a metastatic lesion in segment V (arrow). (B) CT scan obtained 1 month after RFA shows a low-attenuation defect (arrow) that is larger than the pretreatment lesion and has a smooth margin. (C,D) The defect (arrow) has decreased in size at 3 (C) and 9 (D) months of follow-up. © 2001 RadioGraphics. Reprinted with permission. See reference 1.

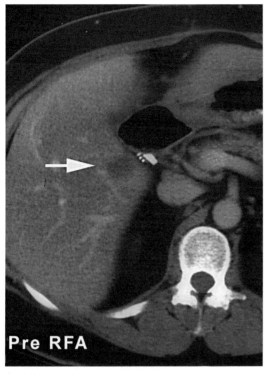

A

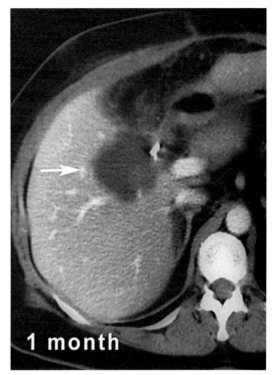

B

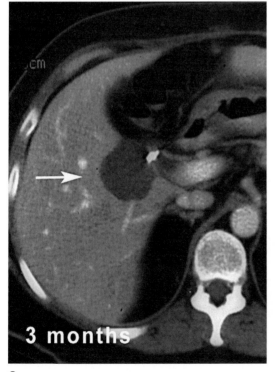

C

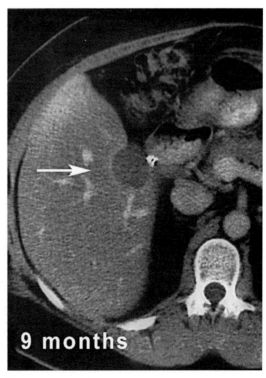

D

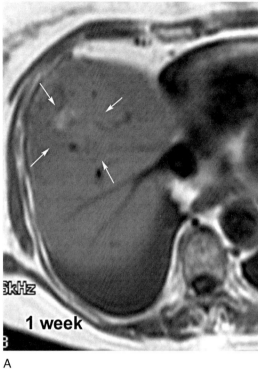

A

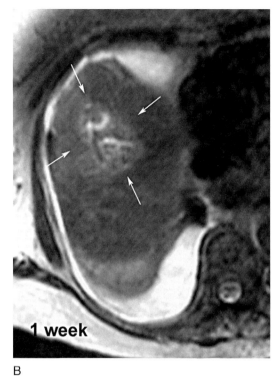

B

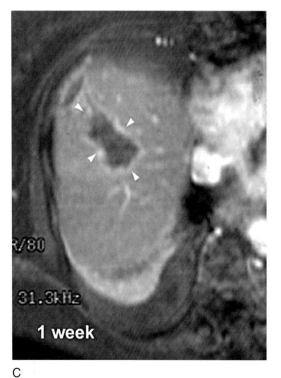

C

**Figure 16.2.** Complete ablation of hepatic metastasis from breast carcinoma. (A–C) One week after RFA, T1-weighted (A) and fat-saturated fast spin-echo T2-weighted image (B) of magnetic resonance imaging (MRI) show a heterogeneous defect (arrows) with internal hemorrhage; a rim enhancement (arrowheads) is seen on a contrast-enhanced T1-weighted image (C).
(*continued*)

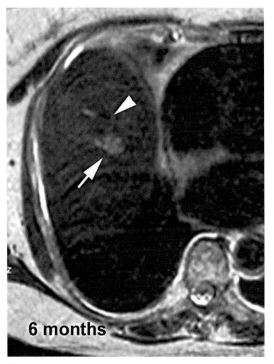

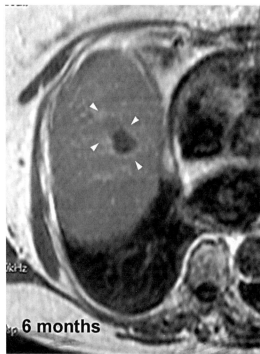

D

E

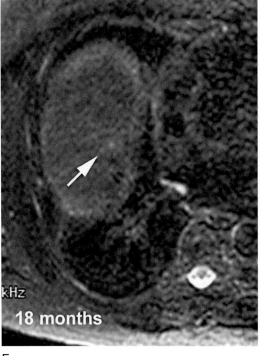

F

**Figure 16.2 (continued).** (D,E) Fat-saturated T2-weighted image (D) obtained at 6 months shows that the defect has decreased in size and become hypointense (arrowhead) anteriorly, with a small area of residual hyperintensity posteriorly (arrow). Significant resolution of the enhancing rim (arrowheads) is seen on a contrast-enhanced T1-weighted image (E). (F) The defect has further decreased in size and become less conspicuous (arrow) on a fat-saturated T2-weighted image obtained at 1.5 years. © 2001 RadioGraphics. Reprinted with permission. See reference 1.

moral enhancement is devoid of nodularity and forms a circumferential, or sometimes incomplete, homogeneous rim around the periphery of the treated tumor[6] (Fig. 16.3). In animal studies, histopathologic examination has shown a peripheral zone of congestion and sinusoidal hemorrhage immediately after ablation and a layer of granulation 5 weeks later.[13] Peripheral nontumoral enhancement may be more diffuse than tumoral enhancement and sometimes wedge-shaped owing to a compensatory increase

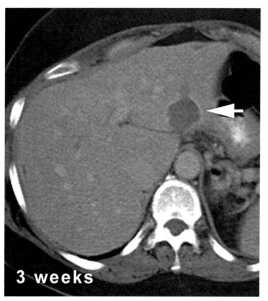

A

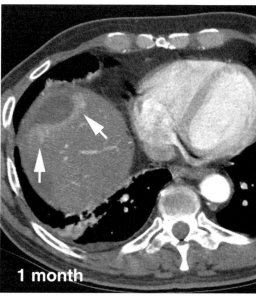

B

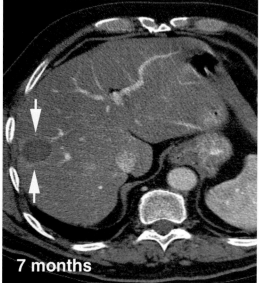

C

Figure 16.3. Benign peripheral enhancement. (A–C) CT scans obtained 3 weeks (A), 1 month (B), and 7 months (C) after RFA of hepatic metastases from colon carcinoma in three different patients. The rims are smooth, without nodularity (arrows). © 2001 RadioGraphics. Reprinted with permission. See reference 1.

in arterial flow in a territory where portal branches have been destroyed. Focal nodular enhancement at the margin of the defect is always very suspicious for recurrent or residual tumor.

An important criterion for complete ablation is the evolution over time of the size of the defect. While the evolution is unpredictable, when the ablation is complete, the size of the defect can only remain stable or decrease. Any enlargement is suspicious for tumor growth.[1–3]

### Incomplete Ablation and Local Recurrence

Incomplete ablation and local recurrence have similar appearances on CT and MRI. Only the clinical context differentiates them from each other.[14,15] For example, in patients with a recurrence findings from the post-RFA CT scan should have been compatible with complete ablation as defined above. Residual or recurrent tumor tissue may be obvious as a nodular area of low attenuation or enhancement that abuts or surrounds the defect or protrudes into the necrotic area (Fig. 16.4). Residual or recur-

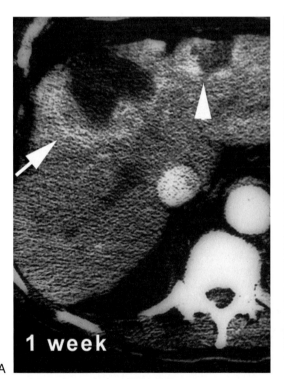
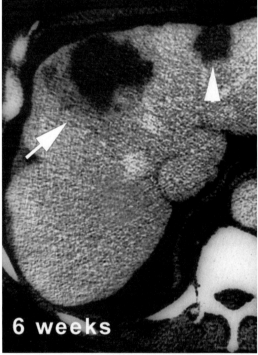

A                                                                                                                                    B

**Figure 16.4.** Incomplete ablation and local recurrence of hepatic metastasis from colon carcinoma. (A) CT scan obtained 1 week after RFA shows a postablation defect in segment III with an irregular enhancing rim (arrowhead). More diffuse, ill-defined enhancement (arrow) is seen around the defect in segments IV and VIII. These are indeterminate. (B) CT scan obtained at 6 weeks shows complete ablation in segment III (arrowhead) with resolution of the enhancing rim. In segments IV and VIII, recurrence or incomplete ablation (arrow) is seen as a low-attenuation margin along the border of the defect. © 2001 RadioGraphics. Reprinted with permission. See reference 1.

rent tumor also may be very subtle, indicated only by a distortion of the otherwise smooth interface between the RFA defect and the liver parenchyma. It may be a small nodule of only slightly higher attenuation protruding within the necrotic tissue (Fig. 16.5), or a faint zone of hypoattenuation that extends into

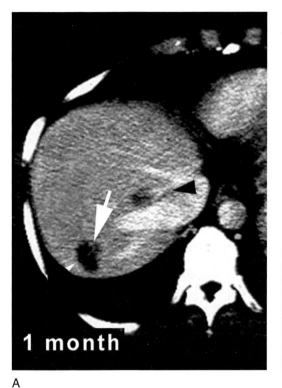

A

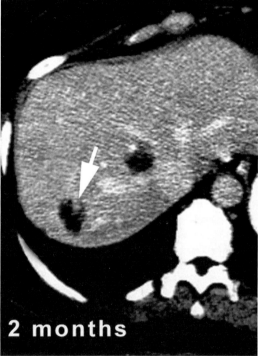

B

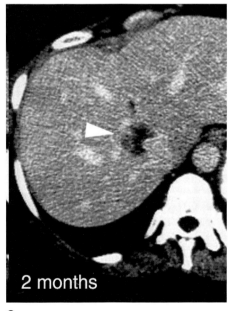

C

**Figure 16.5.** Incomplete ablation and local recurrence of hepatic metastasis from rectal carcinoma. (A) CT scan obtained 1 month after RFA shows incomplete ablation with a subtle soft tissue nodule (arrow) that protrudes into the ablation defect in segment VII. Ablation in segment VIII (arrowhead) was considered to be complete. (B,C) CT scan obtained at 2 months shows an enlarging residual tumor (arrow in B) in segment VII and local recurrence in segment VIII (arrowhead in C) at a slightly lower level. The ablation defect in segment VIII has become larger, and the contour is irregular. © 2001 RadioGraphics. Reprinted with permission. See reference 1.

the adjacent parenchyma.[1–3,8,16] Apparent enlargement of a defect is consistent with a recurrence[1,2] (Fig. 16.6). Chopra et al[2] have classified recurrences at the site of RFA into three morphologic patterns: nodular type, halo type, and gross enlargement.

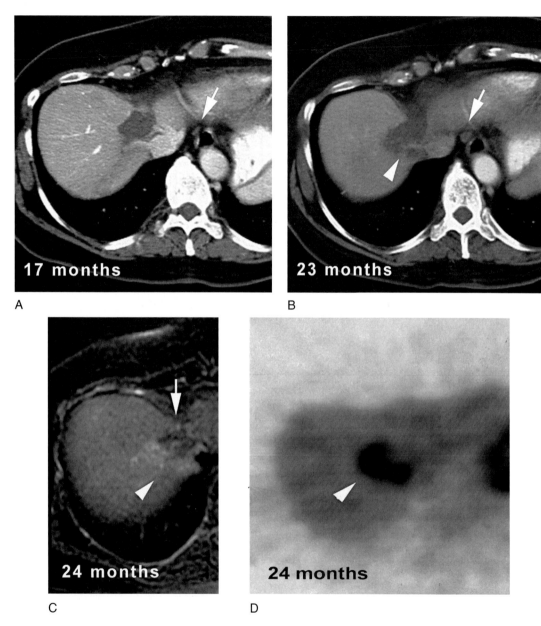

**Figure 16.6.** Local recurrence of hepatic metastasis from colon carcinoma. (A,B) CT scans obtained 17 (A) and 23 (B) months after RFA show an apparent increase in the size of the ablation defect in segment VIII. The area of low attenuation extends behind the right hepatic vein (arrowhead in B). The small lymph node (arrow) near the esophagus has enlarged. (C,D) Fat-saturated fast spin-echo T2-weighted MRI (C) and positron emission tomographic scan (D) obtained 24 months after ablation confirm the local recurrence (arrowhead) at the posterior aspect of the hypointense ablation defect (arrow in C). © 2001 RadioGraphics. Reprinted with permission. See reference 1.

The nodular and halo types are characterized, respectively, by a focal mass or a rim of tissue seen at the margin of the ablation.[8] The gross enlargement pattern is characterized by an increase in the overall tumor size.[2,9]

The contrast-enhancement pattern of recurrent tumors varies with the underlying pathology. The patterns of enhancement of hepatomas and hypervascular metastases from tumors such as neuroendocrine tumors, renal cell carcinomas, or breast carcinomas differ from those of most adenocarcinomas. Hypervascular tumors are typically hyperdense during the arterial phase of enhancement and become isodense or hypodense during later phases of enhancement (Fig. 16.7). In the study by Chopra et al,[2] all 10 local recurrences from hepatocelluar carcinomas were hyperattenuated during the arterial phase. In contrast, adenocarcinomas are relatively hypovascular tumors. A rim of enhancement at the periphery of residual or recurrent adenocarcinomas may appear similar to the peripheral enhancement observed at initial presentation.[3] The intensity and spatial distribution of enhancement of both tumor types vary over time.[17]

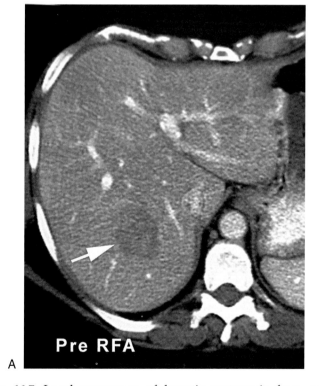

A

**Figure 16.7.** Local recurrence of hepatic metastasis from neuroendocrine tumor of the pancreas. (A) CT scan obtained before RFA shows a metastatic lesion (arrow) in segment VII.

(continued)

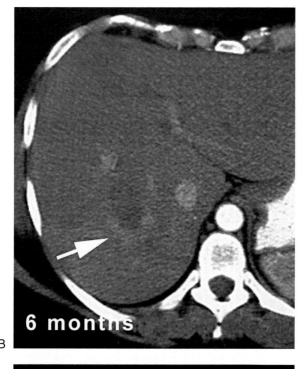

B

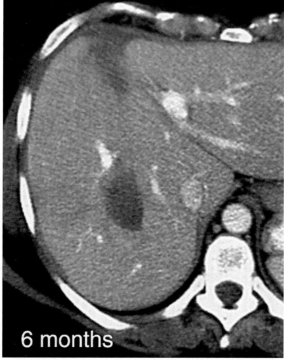

C

**Figure 16.7 (*continued*).** (B) Six months after RFA, a hypervascular tumor (arrow) is seen along the margin of the ablation defect in the arterial phase of triphasic CT. (C) This hypervascular recurrence is not appreciable in the portal phase. © 2001 RadioGraphics. Reprinted with permission. See reference 1.

From a practical standpoint, several elements besides the lack of nodularity help to differentiate peripheral reactive inflammation or abnormal perfusion from residual or recurrent tumor. At early follow-up, the enhancement should be clearly beyond the confines of the pretreatment tumor. With a multiphasic technique, hypervascular tumors tend to enhance early and briefly. These tumors often become hypodense relative to the surrounding parenchyma, while zones of perfusion abnormalities or area of fibrosis become isodense or hyperdense, respectively, over time.[3,11,17]

Another indication of recurrence could be an apparent increase in size or return of a zone of hyperemia,[2] assuming that no technical factors could account for this. In some cases, short-term follow-up or the use of other modalities such as MRI or positron emission tomography will be needed to make the diagnosis of residual or recurrent tumor. When appropriate, the radiographic findings should be correlated with tumor markers.

### Recurrences Outside the Ablation Site

Follow-up CT or MRI studies should also be scrutinized for new hepatic metastases and extrahepatic recurrences (Fig. 16.8). In a recent review of 304 patients treated with RFA for malignant hepatic tumors, new hepatic or extrahepatic metastases occurred in 47% of cases, compared with a local recurrence rate of only 9%.[14] In a smaller cohort, it was shown that, as could be expected from the patterns of spread of these tumors, recurrences were primarily intrahepatic in patients with ablated hepatocelluar carcinoma and both intra- and extrahepatic in patients with ablated hepatic metastases.[2]

## Technical Implications

The value of imaging studies after RFA is directly dependent on the quality of the technique. Some broad but important guidelines can be established. On CT or MRI, the liver should be assessed following intravenous administration of a contrast agent. Non–contrast-enhanced CT is helpful but not sensitive enough to detect subtle residual tumor or recurrence. With either modality, a dynamic technique allowing for the acquisition of images during the window of optimal hepatic parenchymal opacification is needed. This requires venous access with a large-bore needle (16 to 18 gauge). When optimal dynamic imaging is not possible, MRI using T2-weighted images can be more useful than CT.

Patients who have undergone RFA for hypervascular tumors, such as hepatocelluar carcinoma, need to be evaluated before and

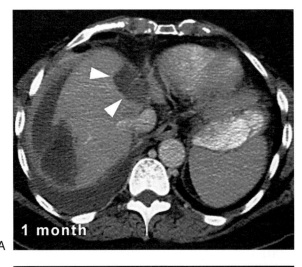

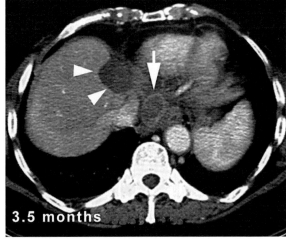

**Figure 16.8.** Recurrent disease with distant metastasis. CT scans obtained 1 (A) and 3.5 (B) months after RFA show complete ablation of a lesion (arrowheads) at the dome of the liver with no local recurrence. The postsurgical perihepatic fluid and pleural effusion resolved as well. However, at 3.5 months, nodal metastasis (arrow in B) is seen. © 2001 RadioGraphics. Reprinted with permission. See reference 1.

after intravenous administration of a contrast agent with a protocol that includes image acquisition during the arterial phase of enhancement. Small hypervascular tumor nodules could be overlooked if this phase is not performed. The RFA treatment induces morphologic changes that evolve over time.

The detection of subtle recurrent disease, superimposed on posttreatment changes, may be impossible without a comparison with a baseline evaluation. Depending on the investigators, a baseline evaluation is acquired within 1 to 3 months of the RFA procedure.[3,4,18,20] This difference in recommended timing of base-line evaluation could be likely related to differences in RFA tech-niques, protocols and types of clinical practice. With percuta-neous RFA, there is an option for immediate reablation if residual tumor is detected; with the surgical approach, the practical im-plications of immediate re-treatment are debatable.

Depending on the stage and known patterns of spread, the de-tection of extrahepatic recurrences may require additional stud-ies such as pelvic or chest CT. With colorectal carcinomas, for example, the pelvis should be evaluated for anastamotic, locore-gional or peritoneal recurrences while such a study would not be useful in the follow-up of the majority of hepatocelluar carcinomas.

## Conclusions

Enhanced CT and MRI are optimal imaging modalities in eval-uating the liver tumors following RFA.[10] Both techniques pro-vide reliable assessment of therapeutic results. With the benefit of T2-weighted images and superior tissue contrast, MRI can be particularly helpful in detecting recurrent tumor with a gross en-largement pattern and when CT findings are inconsistent with clinical pictures. Triphasic technique is essential when the treated tumor is hypervascular.

### References

1. Choi H, Loyer EM, DuBrow RA, et al. Radio-frequency ablation of liver tumors: assessment of therapeutic response and complications. RadioGraphics 2001; 21:S41–S54.
2. Chopra S, Dodd GD III, Chintapalli KN, et al. Tumor recurrence af-ter radiofrequency thermal ablation of hepatic tumors: spectrum of findings on dual-phase contrast-enhanced CT. AJR 2001; 1177:381–387.
3. Kim HK, Choi D, Lee WJ, et al. Hepatocellular carcinoma treated with percutaneous radio-frequency ablation: evaluation with fol-low-up multiphase helical CT. Radiology 2001; 221:447–454.
4. Rhim H, Goldberg N, Dodd GD III, et al. Essential techniques for successful radiofrequency thermal ablation of malignant tumors. RadioGraphics 2001; 21:S17–S19.
5. Sironi S, Livraghi T, Meloni F, et al. Small hepatocellular carcinoma treated with percutaneous RF ablation: MR imaging follow-up. AJR 1999; 173:1225–1229.
6. Cioni D, Lencioni R, Rossi S, et al. Radiofrequency thermal ablation of hepatocellular carcinoma: using contrast-enhanced harmonic power doppler sonography to assess treatment outcome. AJR 2001: 177:783–788.
7. Solbiati L, Goldberg SN, Ierace T, et al. Radiofrequency ablation of hepatic metastases: postprocedural assessment with a US mi-

crobubble contrast agent: early experience. Radiology 1999; 211:643–649.

8. Goldberg SN, Gazelle GS, Compton CC, et al. Treatment of intrahepatic malignancy with radiofrequency ablation: radiologic-pathologic correlation. Cancer 2000; 88:2452–2453.

9. Goldberg SN, Gazelle GS, Solbiati L, et al. Ablation of liver tumors using percutaneous RF therapy. AJR 1998; 170:1023–1028.

10. Livraghi T, Goldberg SN, Lazzaroni S, et al. Hepatocellular carcinoma: radiofrequency ablation of medium and large lesions. Radiology 2000;214:761–768.

11. Solbiati L, Goldberg SN, Ierace T, et al. Hepatic metastases: percutaneous radio-frequency ablation with cooled-tip electrodes. Radiology 1997; 205:367–373.

12. Solbiati L, Ierace T, Goldberg SN, et al. Percutaneous US-guided radio-frequency tissue ablation of liver metastases: treatment and follow-up in 16 patients. Radiology 1997; 202:195–203.

13. Kuszyk BS, Boitnott JK, Choti MA, et al. Local tumor recurrence following hepatic cryoablation: radiologic-histophathologic correlation in a rabbit model. Radiology 2000; 217:477–486.

14. Curley S, Izzo F, Delrio P, et al. Radiofrequency ablation of malignant liver tumor in 304 patients: recurrence complications (abstract). In: Program/Proceedings of the Annual Meeting of the American Society of Clinical Oncology, New Orleans, May 20–23, 2000.

15. De Beere T, Elias D, Dormain C, et al. Radiofrequency ablation of 100 hepatic metastases with a mean follow-up of more than 1 year. AJR 2000; 175:1619–1625.

16. McGahan JP, Dodd GD III. Radiofrequency ablation of the liver. AJR 2001; 176:3–16.

17. Loyer EM, Chin H, DuBrow RA, et al. Hepatocellular carcinoma and intrahepatic peripheral cholangiocarcinoma: enhancement patterns with quadruple phase helical CT—a comparative study. Radiology 1999; 212:866–875.

18. Solbiati L, Livraghi T, Goldberg SN, et al. Percutaneous radio-frequency ablation of hepatic metastases from colorectal cancer: long-term results in 117 patients. Radiology 2001; 221:159–166.

19. Lees WR, Gilliam AR. Complications of radiofrequency and laser ablation of liver metastases: incidence and management (abstract). Radiology 1999; 213(P):122.

20. Gazelle GS, Goldberg SN, Solbiati L, Livraghi T. Tumor ablation with radio-frequency energy. Radiology 2000; 217:663–646.

# 17

# Magnetic Resonance Imaging-Guided and -Monitored Radiofrequency Interstitial Thermal Cancer Ablation

Sherif Gamal Nour and Jonathan S. Lewin

Current trends in medical practice place increased emphasis on minimizing invasiveness while upgrading the efficacy of treatment and effectively utilizing medical resources in a cost-effective manner. Similarly, interventional radiology has emerged and evolved over the past quarter century so that a majority of its procedures are performed in the setting of cancer patient care. Under conventional fluoroscopic, ultrasound, or computed tomography (CT) guidance, interventions range from straightforward diagnostic procedures, such as biopsy and aspiration, to a more complicated array of palliative/therapeutic procedures, such as tumor embolization, biliary and hollow viscous stenting, percutaneous gastrostomy, celiac plexus and other nerve blocks, inferior vena cava filter application, and percutaneous image-guided brachytherapy.

As the art of oncologic therapy advances and extends the horizons for cancer management, parallel innovations in interventional radiology, particularly in interventional magnetic resonance imaging (MRI), have a tremendous potential to assume a central role in the continued progress of cancer therapy beyond the traditional surgery–radiotherapy–chemotherapy triad. There are numerous exciting topics in this field that are expected to enjoy substantial contributions from MRI. They include gene therapy,[1–3] and targeted drug delivery,[4,5] control of angiogenesis,[6] and the delivery of various forms of thermal energy such as radiofrequency, laser,[7] focused ultrasound,[8] microwave,[9] and cryotherapy[10] for tumor ablation.

Looking ahead at cancer patient care in the new millennium, this chapter highlights the current utility and future directions of interventional MRI in guiding and monitoring cancer ablation using radiofrequency energy.

## Radiofrequency Interstitial Thermal Therapy

Radiofrequency interstitial thermal ablation (RF-ITA) entails the deployment of radiofrequency (RF) current into the target tissue through an electrode connected to an RF generator. As the current flows from the source to the return (grounding pad) electrode, the ions in the tissues surrounding the monopolar source electrode begin to agitate, resulting in frictional (resistive) heating with consequent formation of an ovoid necrotic lesion surrounding the RF electrode tip. RF-ITA has been effectively and safely applied to treat a wide range of benign and malignant conditions. The vast majority of reports have described RF-ITA treatment of liver tumors.[11–13] However, other target organs and tissues have included the brain,[14] kidney,[15,16] prostate,[17,18] breast,[19] spleen,[20] lung,[21] and bone.[22]

Interstitial RF thermotherapy is an attractive treatment option for several reasons. This modality has a long history of use and, based on data from our site and others, complications resulting from radiofrequency ablation (RFA) are uncommon, with the coagulation effect of the heating process contributing to a very low incidence of hemorrhage in the central nervous system[23,24] and abdomen.[25,26] The equipment necessary to create RF lesions is typically readily accessible, as it is utilized by the neurosurgical community and is relatively inexpensive in comparison to laser light sources.

Reproducible tissue destruction has been observed in a variety of tissues. Furthermore, studies in both humans and animals have shown that thermal lesion shape and size can be controlled through electrode design as well as the duration and magnitude of the energy delivered.[23,24,27–29] Energy deposition is easy to control with RF ablation and allows gradual tissue heating.[23] The presence of a thermister in the electrode tip gives continuous temperature feedback, while impedance measurements provide another parameter related to tissue changes at the ablation site. These features are of particular importance when destroying tumors adjacent to neurovascular structures. Unlike radiation therapy but like other thermal ablative therapies, interstitial RF thermal ablation can be repeated multiple times without concern for the cumulative dose.

## Rationale for Image Guidance

As described above, RF therapy is not a new therapeutic modality, rather it has been used with great success by the neurosurgical community over the past three decades.[14] Placement of RF electrodes into pathologic tissue has typically been performed under direct visualization or stereotactic guidance based on preoperative CT data. Indications for this form of therapy have historically included cordotomy, pallidotomy, leukotomy, and thalamotomy for the treatment of intractable pain and involuntary movement disorders.[30–37] Radiofrequency catheter ablation has also been widely and successfully practiced during the past 15 years to treat cardiac arrhythmias.[38,39]

Although RF thermal treatment of localized malignancy has been practiced under direct surgical[12,40] and laparoscopic[41] visualization, much of the excitement over expanding the therapeutic uses of RF energy beyond the neurosurgical and cardiac fields has been engendered by the advancements in imaging technology. The ability to perform thermal treatment of cancer percutaneously under image guidance has changed RFA from an adjuvant surgical technique to a minimally invasive alternative to surgery that is more suited to the large sector of poor surgical candidates. The primary contribution of image guidance to needle-based thermal treatment is the safe and precise electrode delivery into targeted pathology. Not surprisingly, the ideal electrode trajectory during actual procedure execution is often significantly different from that suggested on the preprocedure imaging data due to the frequent shift of anatomic structures when using modified patient positions during treatment. Additionally, the guided approach provides updated information regarding the development of new pathologic conditions that may alter treatment decision making, such as the appearance of other tumor foci or the accumulation of ascites. Once the RF electrode is successfully delivered into the targeted tumor, image guidance adds to the efficacy of the procedure by optimizing the electrode position within the pathologic tissue and by showing the thickness of intact tissue between the targeted tumor and adjacent vital structures, such as the gallbladder, bowel loops, or renal pelvis, thereby enabling confident inclusion of an adequate "safety margin" to the ablated volume.

## MRI Guidance and Monitoring

As new imaging modalities have been developed and introduced into the diagnostic imaging armamentarium, their adoption for procedure guidance has inevitably occurred. With its incomparable attributes for diagnostic imaging, MRI has followed this pattern with burgeoning interest in the use of MRI techniques for interventional procedure guidance. The term *interventional MRI* was introduced into the medical terminology a few years ago to describe the use of this explicit imaging modality for rapid guidance or monitoring of minimally invasive diagnosis or therapy. To date, much of the effort in the development of MRI-guided therapy has concentrated on local treatment of cancer and cancer metastases using percutaneous MRI-guided thermal or chemical tumor ablation.

### Justification

In addition to the general benefits of image guidance for radiofrequency thermal ablation procedures, as discussed above, MRI guidance offers additional advantages (Table 17.1) that significantly enhance treatment safety and efficacy and that give MRI an edge over other imaging modalities for this use.

The use of interstitial RF thermotherapy under MRI guidance is based on the direct destruction of tissue through the application of RF energy. The methodology differs significantly from the empirical approach typically used in neurosurgical applications of RFA technology in which variations in lesion size and shape due to unanticipated thermal conduction during treatment cannot be predicted and are not usually recognized until follow-up imaging studies are performed. The major contribution of MRI to interstitial RF thermotherapy is its outstanding ability to mon-

**Table 17.1 Advantages of Magnetic Resonance Imaging (MRI) during the Guidance and Monitoring of Radiofrequency Interstitial Thermal Ablation (RF-ITA)**

| | |
|---|---|
| During the guidance of RF electrode into the target tumor | High soft tissue contrast<br>High spatial resolution<br>Multiplanar capabilities<br>High vascular conspicuity<br>Lack of ionizing radiation |
| During the monitoring of thermal tissue destruction | Ability to define treatment end point by providing immediate feedback about the extent of necrosis *during* ablation<br>Feasibility of temperature mapping |

itor the zone of thermal tissue destruction during the procedure and therefore to provide real-time guidance for deposition of the RF energy. Through MRI monitoring, thermal lesion size and configuration can be directly controlled by the operator and adjusted during the procedure to compensate for deviations from the preoperative predictions and to define the treatment end point without moving the patient from the interventional suite. This is an attribute of MRI imaging that cannot be reliably duplicated by any other currently utilized imaging modality. MRI is exceptionally well suited for this purpose because of the absence of ionizing radiation, excellent soft tissue discrimination, spatial resolution, multiplanar capabilities, and its sensitivity to temperature and blood flow.[42–44] This not only permits accurate tumor destruction, including the margins, but also extends the application of RFA to the safe destruction of tumor within the visceral organs and adjacent to vital neurovascular structures. Furthermore, MRI is not hampered by the difficulties caused by changes in tissue imaging characteristics brought about by RFA, as have been described by some authors using ultrasound guidance.[25]

### The Interventional MRI Suite

During the early years of MRI development, the relatively long imaging times and geometry of closed-bore superconducting cylindrical systems made MRI an unlikely guidance modality for radiologic procedures. Increasingly, many of these disadvantages have been overcome through system hardware and pulse sequence improvements that have allowed the development of rapid imaging on open systems.

The hardware and software developments that made interventional MRI and subsequently MRI-guided RF-ITA a reality are as follows:

### Hardware Developments

1. The development of "open" magnet imaging systems has facilitated the patient access necessary for performing the interventional procedures[45–50] (Fig. 17.1). Many different MRI system designs have been used to guide percutaneous procedures. Each of these systems has advantages and disadvantages with a constant trade-off among signal-to-noise ratio, access to the patient, usable field of view, and expense.
2. The construction of higher-quality, low-noise receiver chains has allowed lower field systems to provide relatively high signal-to-noise ratio images, thereby greatly improving image quality compared to earlier attempts at low-field MRI. These systems now provide sufficient image quality for the procedure guidance phases of minimally invasive procedures. Im-

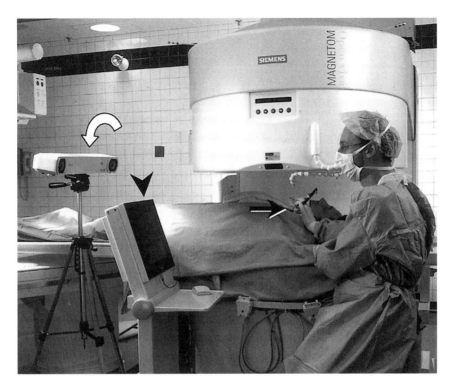

**Figure 17.1.** C-arm system for percutaneous intervention. The magnetic resonance imaging (MRI) suite setup for radiologic intervention has a video camera sensor array (curved arrow) that detects the location and orientation of a hand-held probe (black arrow). The system automatically acquires continuous MR images based on the probe position, and automatically updates display of four images on a shielded liquid-crystal display (LCD) monitor adjacent to the scanner (arrowhead). A computer mouse on the LCD console and foot pedals (not shown) allow the scanner to be operated by the radiologist throughout the procedure.

age acquisition times of 1 to 3 seconds or less per image provide the necessary temporal resolution.

3. The ability to operate the scanner and view images at the scanner side within the magnetic field was facilitated through the development of in-room, high-resolution, RF-shielded monitors[50–54] (Fig. 17.1). Combined with the patient access allowed by open imaging systems, this capability allows the entire procedure to be performed with the operator sitting next to the patient and with no need to remove the operator's hand from the interventional device at any time.

4. The development of frameless navigation devices (Fig. 17.1) utilizing an interface between an optically linked 3D digitizer and the measurement control software of the MR imager enables rapid and interactive MR images to be acquired in any arbitrary plane determined by a hand-held, sterilizable probe or other interventional device. This allows rapid planning and confirmation of complex trajectories for rigid instruments.

5. The development of needles and probes that are undeflected by the magnetic field creates little or no field distortions or image degradation.[46,55]

### Software Developments

The modification and development of rapid gradient-echo pulse sequences facilitated their use in interactive guidance during device placement. These sequences allow a wide range of tissue contrast in a time frame sufficient for device tracking even at low field strength and with the suboptimal coil position sometimes required to access a puncture site.[45,50,52,56–58]

Furthermore, the inherent inability of MRI to actively monitor a thermal lesion as it is created, due to imaging interference caused by the RF source, has been overcome. New software and hardware modifications have been developed that allow RF energy to be deposited during imaging (interrupted only during brief sampling periods), thereby maintaining tissue temperature while making interference-free real-time monitoring possible.[59]

### Clinical Experience and Technical Considerations

The primary focus at our institution has been the advancement of minimally invasive interstitial RF thermotherapy of tumors of the liver and retroperitoneum with electrode placement performed under direct MRI guidance within the MR imager. An MRI-guided RF-ITA procedure typically has three phases: guidance, confirmation, and ablation/monitoring. Our experience with 40 MRI-guided and -monitored RF-ITA procedures among 368 interventional MRI procedures is as follows:

### The Guidance Phase

Under conscious sedation, a custom-made MRI-compatible, 17-cm, 17-gauge shielded RF electrode with a 1- to 3-cm exposed tip (Radionics, Burlington, MA) is percutaneously placed into the liver or retroperitoneum and advanced into the targeted tumor under MRI fluoroscopic guidance, using short TR/short TE gradient-echo sequences (Fig. 17.2). This consists of a continuous imaging mode that allows automated sequential acquisition, reconstruction, and in-room display of multiple sets of three contiguous, parallel, 5-mm slices centered on the electrode position. Image sets in two orthogonal scan planes oriented along the shaft of the electrode are used during this continuous imaging mode to guide electrode insertion with respect to the three-dimensional geometry of the tumor. According to the radiologist's preference, the aforementioned optically linked frameless stereotaxy system [developed in collaboration with Radionics and Siemens Medical Systems (Erlangen, Germany)] can be used to interactively drive image acquisition (Fig. 17.1). A more detailed discussion regard-

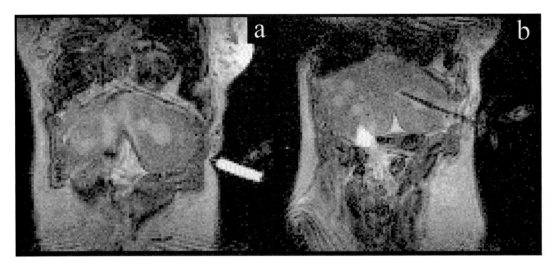

**Figure 17.2.** A 41-year-old woman with metastatic carcinoid tumor to the liver. Direct MR fluoroscopic guidance using coronal PSIF (a gradient reversed form of FISP; Fast Imaging with steady state precession) sequence (TR/TE 19.4/9.5; three acquisitions; 45-degree flip angle). (A) Typical initial localization of entry point using a saline-filled syringe. (B) The needle has been accurately introduced along the planned trajectory into the targeted tumor. The peculiar coronal orientation offered by MRI facilitates safe targeting of high hepatic lesions without risking the pleura, the near real-time MR fluoroscopic guidance allows a time-efficient redirection of needle tip during introduction, and the inherent high tissue contrast of MRI ensures precise localization of the target lesion. © 2000 Lippincott Williams & Wilkins. Reprinted with permission. See reference 45.

ing the fast imaging techniques used for electrode guidance and their temporal resolutions is discussed below (see General Safety Measures for Interventional MRI Suites).

### The Confirmation Phase

Once the RF electrode is delivered into the targeted tumor, the electrode position is confirmed using the higher spatial resolution turbo spin echo (TSE) scans (Fig. 17.3) prior to commencing the actual ablation session.

### The Ablation/Monitoring Phase

When the interventionalist is comfortable with the electrode position, the deployment of RF energy can be confidently instituted. In the early phase of our clinical series, when a nonperfused electrode was used, interstitial RF thermal ablation was performed at an electrode tip temperature of 90 ± 2°C. With this electrode design, lesion length is dependent on exposed tip length, while lesion diameter is limited to approximately 2 cm.[60] This limited ability to achieve a larger lesion diameter is thought to be due to charring at the electrode/tissue interface, which in turn impairs energy transfer. With the water-cooled (cool-tip) electrode concept, a pump is used to circulate chilled water inside the electrode to cool the tip temperature to 10° to 20°C, thereby pre-

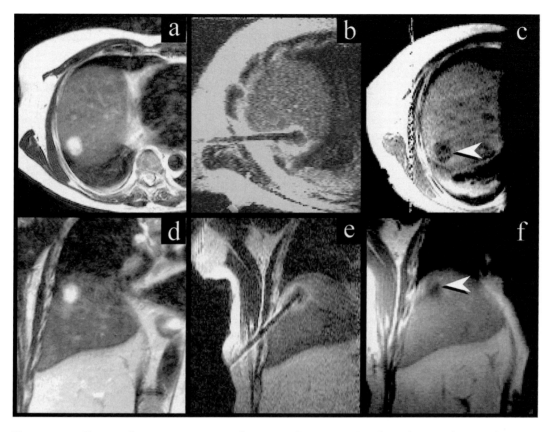

**Figure 17.3.** Hepatic dome metastasis. Turbo spin-echo T2-weighted axial (A) and coronal (D) images of the abdomen demonstrate hyperintense metastasis in the posterior dome of the right lobe of the liver. Turbo spin-echo T2-weighted oblique axial-sagittal (B) and coronal (E) images with similar parameters along the course of the MRI-compatible radiofrequency (RF) electrode confirm the electrode position within the tumor. The effects of radiofrequency interstitial thermal ablation (RF-ITA) are noted as marked hypointensity developed around the active distal 3 cm of the electrode, surrounded by a rim of hyperintensity reflecting edema and hyperemia. After RF-ITA, contrast-enhanced T1-weighted axial (C) and coronal (F) images demonstrate hypointensity corresponding to an avascular area of tumor necrosis. This approximates the volume of the originally identified tumor, along with a small margin of surrounding normal parenchyma. © 1998 John Wiley & Sons, Inc. Reprinted with permission. See reference 26.

venting charring at the interface and allowing energy to be transmitted farther from the source electrode. Lesions can be created with this electrode design that would have required multiple ablations with intervening electrode repositioning with a standard RF electrode. To maximize the area of resulting necrosis, we usually combine the use of the cool-tip electrode with pulsed application of RF energy where brief periods of current interruption are automatically triggered when tissue impedance rises beyond a preset threshold. Again, the intention is to prevent tissue charring and cavitation, which lead to the cessation of RF current deposition.

The ablation time usually ranges from 6 to 20 minutes at each electrode location prior to repositioning for larger tumors. However, the exact duration of an individual session is based on the MRI findings during that session to achieve maximal ablation tissue necrosis for the MRI-compatible electrode in use. Multiplanar STIR (Short Tau Inversion Recovery) and T2-weighted images are performed prior to the procedure. These sequences are repeated intermittently during the ablation session to monitor thermal lesion size and configuration. The size and shape of the developing thermal lesion is directly observed as an enlarging low-signal zone surrounded by high-signal tissue reaction on intermittently acquired TSE T2-weighted and/or TSE STIR MR images (Figs. 17.3 and 17.4).

At the conclusion of ablation sessions using cool-tip electrodes, a second application of RF energy at the same electrode position may be necessary, without cooling, when the desired margins are achieved, in order to destroy the area adjacent to the cooled electrode. A practical method to test the necessity for such additional RF application is to continue measuring the RF electrode tip temperature for 2 minutes after the RF power has been turned off. We re-ablate the center of the "doughnut" if its temperature falls below 60°C before the 2 minutes have elapsed.

Electrode repositioning into persistent foci of high-signal tumor, as detected on the T2 and STIR images, is performed in the scanner under continuous MRI guidance in an interactive manner similar to that used for initial electrode placement. The "guide–confirm–ablate/monitor" sequence of events is repeated until the induced thermal lesion is noted to encompass the entire tumor and a small cuff of normal adjacent tissue or when the developing thermal lesion approaches adjacent vital structures. The RF electrode is then withdrawn, and repeat images are obtained with the addition of gadopentetate dimeglumine-enhanced T1-weighted images to confirm the final zone of tissue destruction and to exclude complications (Figs. 17.3 and 17.4).

Temperature-sensitive MRI sequences have also been developed to enable accurate on-line monitoring of heat deposition.[61–63] The relationship of MRI signal intensity change to tissue temperature is a complex phenomenon, and precise MRI measurement of temperature is difficult. However, the phase transition from viable to necrotic tissue can also be imaged (Fig. 17.5) using changes in the tissue relaxation parameters, T1 and T2, that occur in the process of necrosis.[64,65] The accuracy of MRI findings in defining thermal lesion size has been repeatedly demonstrated using several different energy sources.[66–68]

After the ablation and postprocedure scanning, the patient is observed overnight before being discharged the following morning at our institution as part of a National Cancer Institute–reg-

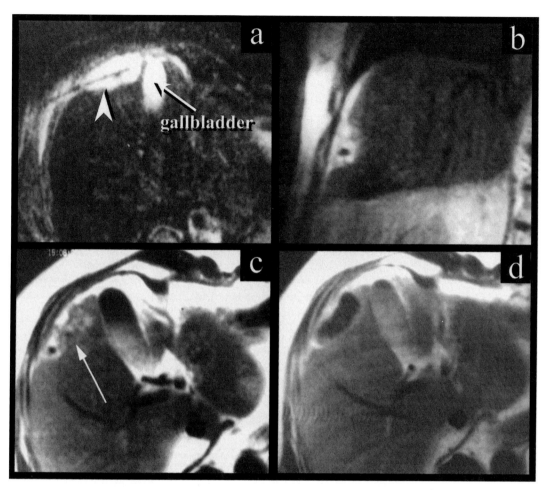

**Figure 17.4.** A 74-year-old patient with a large liver metastasis from a previously resected leiomyosarcoma of the stomach. (A) STIR axial image during the ablation procedure demonstrates a very bright 5 × 3 cm tumor mass bisected by the dark line of the titanium electrode within its center (arrowhead). The gallbladder is seen as another bright structure just medial to the tumor mass. (B) T2-weighted oblique image perpendicular to the titanium electrode demonstrates the electrode as a dark dot within the lower third of the lesion. Two longitudinal electrode passes through the lesion were performed, to ablate both the lower and upper halves of this large tumor. (C) Contrast-enhanced T1-weighted axial image obtained before ablation, at the same level as (A), demonstrates irregular enhancement in the region of the tumor (arrow). The gallbladder can be seen medial to the tumor, partially filled with contrast. (D) Immediately after the ablation session, a contrast-enhanced T1-weighted axial image at the same level as (C) demonstrates a markedly hypointense lesion completely replacing the enhancing mass, with a slight rim of marginal enhancement. This typical pattern of loss of vascularity with slight reactive marginal enhancement is seen in all patients and has demonstrated a very high correlation with pathologic evidence of tissue necrosis in animal models. This loss of vascularity can be seen on contrast-enhanced CT scan as well, and has been noted to persist for several months as the treated tumor is resorbed. © 1998 John Wiley & Sons, Inc. Reprinted with permission. See reference 26.

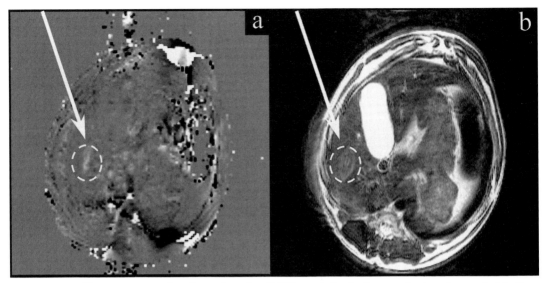

**Figure 17.5.** Phase maps and turbo spin-echo (TSE) magnitude image during thermal ablation. MRI parameters, including T1, T2, diffusion, and the resonant frequency of the protons, vary with temperature. In these images, the water proton resonant frequency method is used to generate images (A) that can be used quantitatively to measure temperature. Here, the image gray scale is proportional to temperature in the canine liver undergoing thermal ablation. While the conventional MRI (B) shows edema and coagulative necrosis at the site of the ablation, no direct assessment of temperature is possible. © 1999 John Wiley & Sons, Inc. Reprinted with permission. See reference 62.

istered phase II clinical trial. According to this thermal ablation protocol, we bring the patient back for follow-up clinical and MRI scanning at 2 weeks and then again at 3 months after ablation and at 3-month intervals thereafter. Follow-up MRI reveals essentially the same signal characteristics of the induced thermal lesion as noted on the intraprocedural and the immediate postablation scans (i.e., ovoid low-signal zone surrounded by high-signal tissue reaction on TSE T2-weighted and TSE STIR images with marginal enhancement on the postgadolinium T1-weighted scans). Gradual shrinkage of the central hypointense necrotic region and resolution of the reactive bright/enhancing rim surrounding the thermal lesion is noted on the sequential follow-up scans (Fig. 17.6).

## Safety Issues

Safe clinical application of MRI-guided RFA requires careful consideration of a number of measures related to both the interventional use of MRI and the medical application of RF energy.

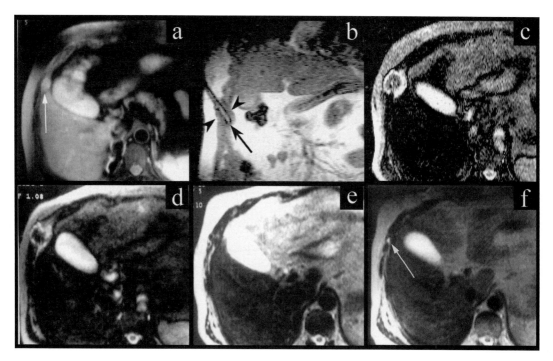

**Figure 17.6.** Images of a 49-year-old man with a metastatic renal cell carcinoma; status post–multiple previous resections. (A) Axial MRI at the level of the gallbladder and liver demonstrates a 2-cm mass projecting inward from the abdominal wall (arrow). This was the only remaining metastasis. (B) Coronal MRI (2-second acquisition time) during MRI-fluoroscopic guidance of a titanium electrode (arrow), which is placed through the long axis of the abdominal wall lesion (arrowheads). (C) Heavily T2-weighted MRI obtained at the completion of ablation demonstrates a low signal central zone, corresponding to tissue necrosis, surrounded by a ring of high signal representing tissue reaction. Ablation was continued until the central necrotic area encompassed the entire tumor as initially depicted, along with a small margin of a normal surrounding tissue. (D) Similar heavily T2-weighted axial image obtained 2 weeks after ablation still demonstrates the low signal central necrotic core. There has been slight extension of edema from thermal injury along the muscle groups of the abdominal wall, appearing as bright fingers extending anteriorly and posteriorly from the central thermal lesion. (E) T2-weighted axial image obtained 3 months after ablation demonstrates a marked reduction in size of both the edema and central low signal core. (F) T2-weighted axial image obtained 6 months after treatment demonstrates complete resolution of treated mass, with only a punctate area of scarring at the position of the electrode tip (arrow). CT scan at this time was completely normal, without abnormal enhancement or residual mass. © 1998 John Wiley & Sons, Inc. Reprinted with permission. See reference 26.

## General Safety Measures for Interventional MRI Suites

While interventional radiologists performing MRI-guided RFA will essentially be using the basic skills they develop during their earlier experience with the more conventional ultrasound- and CT-guided interventions, they must always be aware of the major basic difference, that is, the magnetic field. Although risks are less prominent on the low- and medium-field (0.2–0.5 T) strength magnets typically used for MRI-guided RFA, hazardous consequences can result when ferromagnetic instruments become attracted and accelerated in the fringe field of the scanner and can cause serious or even fatal injuries. As a rule, no ferromagnetic materials should be brought within the 5-gauss line of any scanner. Scalpels, needles, RF electrodes, and anesthesia equipment should be made of MRI-compatible materials. Physiologic monitors need to be either nonferromagnetic or kept outside the fringe field of the magnet. Electric burns can result from direct electromagnetic induction in a conductive loop, induction in a resonant conducting loop, or electric field resonant coupling with a wire (the antenna effect).[69–71] The last mechanism is more relevant when performing interventions with catheters and guidewires rather than with rigid needles and electrodes. Generally, the risk of electric burns may be minimized by limiting conductive loops, wire–patient contact, and cable lengths. Finally, acoustic noise during interventions on open low- and medium-field scanners does not normally reach the occupational exposure limit (15 minutes per day at 115 dB), and ear protection is therefore generally not needed during routine MRI-guided RFA, in contrast to other high-field MRI-guided interventions.

### Specific Safety Measures for Percutaneous MRI-Guided Needle Procedures

In addition to the general measures discussed above, knowledge of several operator-dependent parameters and of the effects of their modification during procedure planning and execution is central to the conduction of safe, efficient tumor ablation using MRI guidance. These parameters are best addressed under the two broad categories of those pertinent to visualization of the tumor and those pertinent to visualization of the RF electrode.

#### Adequate Visualization of the Target Pathology and Surrounding Anatomy

Because speed is critical in pulse sequences designed primarily for the guidance phase of RF electrode placement, the resultant images will not have the quality expected from a purely diagnostic sequence. However, they should provide sufficient anatomy/pathology contrast along with good vascular conspicuity for safe device navigation toward the target tumor. Different near–real-time pulse sequences are available that allow multiple tissue contrasts to be obtained depending on the implemented pulse sequence parameters.[57,58,72] The most commonly used sequences for the guidance phase of MRI-guided RF-ITA are FISP (fast imaging with steady-state precession) (0.3–1 image/sec, keyhole 3/sec), true FISP (1 image/sec, keyhole 3/sec), and PSIF (a gradient reversed form of FISP) (4–5 seconds/image). Adequate visualization of anatomy and pathology varies in different applications and requires selection of the appropriate pulse sequence and tissue contrast mechanism. We often dedicate a separate planning session prior to the ablation session for selection of the optimal sequence to best depict the anatomy/pathology contrast and the ideal RF electrode trajectory and treatment position for each patient.

*Adequate Visualization of the Ablation Device*
Unlike guidance using x-ray–based techniques, such as fluoroscopy and CT, there are a number of user-defined imaging parameters and electrode trajectory decisions that can markedly alter ablation device visibility and therefore affect the accuracy and safety of MRI-guided RF-ITA.[73]

*Pulse Sequence-Dependent Factors*

1. Sequence design (SE, TSE, GRE): The most important pulse sequence issue with regard to needle visibility is the sensitivity of the sequence to magnetic susceptibility effects.[73] The commonly used rapid gradient echo (GRE) sequences (FISP, true FISP, and PSIF) are associated with more prominent susceptibility artifacts from needles and electrodes than with the relatively slower spin-echo (SE) or turbo spin-echo (TSE) sequences. Therefore, to reduce artifactual needle widening, the use of TSE imaging for position confirmation or primary guidance, should be strongly considered when needle/electrode placement within 5 mm of major neurovascular structures is contemplated rather than relying on the more rapid GRE sequences for guidance of the entire procedure.[50,52]
2. Field strength: The higher the MR field strength, the larger the apparent width of the needles and electrodes used (Fig. 17.7). On the low-field (0.2 T) system we utilize for MRI-guided RFA procedures, the apparent needle/electrode width under GRE image guidance ranges from approximately 4 mm for smaller gauges to 9 mm for larger gauges.[73] Although this degree of artifactual widening is acceptable for larger lesions in areas of low neurovascular density, such as the abdomen and extremities, it is clearly unacceptable for lesions located in complex anatomic regions or adjacent to major vessels. The degree of artifactual widening can be reduced by approximately a factor of two by using a TSE pulse sequence or higher sampling bandwidth.[73]
3. Pulse sequence sampling bandwidth: The higher the sampling bandwidth, the less apparent the needle/electrode widening.[73]
4. Frequency encoding direction: When frequency encoding is perpendicular to the needle, it results in artifactual widening. When parallel to the needle, it results in less obvious artifact at the tip and hub of the needle. Depending on needle com-

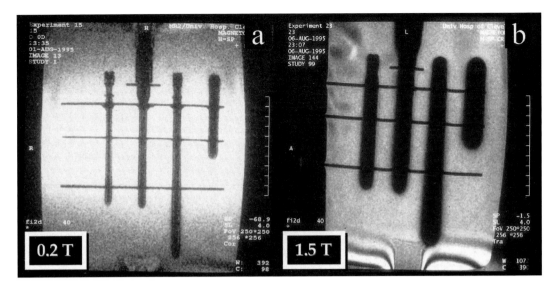

**Figure 17.7.** Effect of magnetic field strength on needle visualization. MRI of the same set of various needles taken at 0.2 T (A) and 1.5 T (B). Both sets were imaged with a fast gradient echo sequence commonly used to guide interventions [fast imaging with steady-state free precession (FISP)] with the shafts of needles perpendicular to the static magnetic field. Note the marked artifactual widening of the needles caused by the higher magnetic field strength (B). © 1996 The American Roentgen Society. Reprinted with permission. See reference 73.

position and orientation, swapping the frequency and phase-encoding axes relative to the needle shaft can reduce or increase the apparent needle width by a factor of 0.33 to 2.5 for TSE sequences[73] (Fig. 17.8). This effect can be used to decrease the apparent needle width when the needle artifact obscures adjacent anatomic structures by setting the frequency-encoding axis of the image parallel to the needle shaft.[50,52] In the presence of even mild respiratory motion, the needle tip for thinner, e.g., 22-gauge, needles can be difficult to visualize with certainty in tissue. Therefore, in our experience this effect is usually more useful to more confidently identify the needle tip location on TSE images by maximizing the needle artifact through frequency-encoding the image in a direction perpendicular to the needle shaft.

*Needle-Dependent Factors*

1. Needle composition: The optimal material for needle fabrication varies with MRI system field strength. Relatively less expensive materials, such as high-nickel, high-chromium stainless steel, may be adequate at 0.2 T but may give rise to unacceptable artifact at 1.5 T.[73,74] Conversely, small-caliber needles constructed from low-artifact materials such as tita-

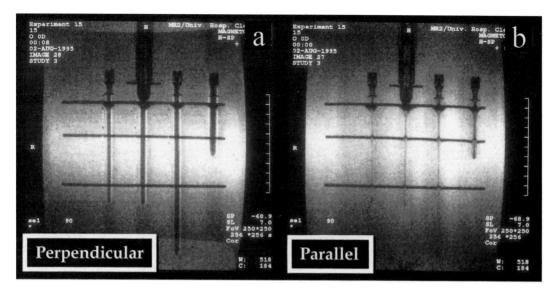

**Figure 17.8.** Effect of frequency-encoding direction on needle visualization. Spin-echo MRI of the same set of needles as in Fig. 17.7 obtained with the frequency encoding direction perpendicular to needle shafts (A) and parallel to needle shafts (B). Sequence used in (A) resulted in more artifactual needle widening than in (B), yet rendered the needle tip more visible. © 1996 The American Roentgen Society. Reprinted with permission. See reference 73.

nium may be difficult to identify in certain clinical settings at low field.

2. Needle orientation relative to the main magnetic field ($B_0$): The apparent needle diameter diminishes markedly from a decrease in artifact as the needle shaft approaches the axis of the static magnetic field[73–75] (Fig. 17.9). Artifacts resulting from field distortion arise most significantly where the field enters and exits objects of differing magnetic susceptibility, such as the needle and surrounding tissue.

When the needle is parallel to the field, distortion of the field (and therefore image artifact) occurs mostly at the tip and hub and to a lesser extent along the shaft. The field is increased within the needle shaft. However, because there are no protons to image within the needle, no image distortion occurs. The field is also distorted slightly adjacent to the shaft. At low fields, the distortion adjacent to the shaft is much less than the effect of the applied imaging gradients, and therefore little mismapping occurs, with the artifact along the shaft related primarily to mild signal loss caused by decreased $T2^*$. When the needle is perpendicular to the main magnetic field, the field enters and exits throughout the length of the shaft. Local field distortion and therefore more prominent artifact, can thus be observed along the entire needle.

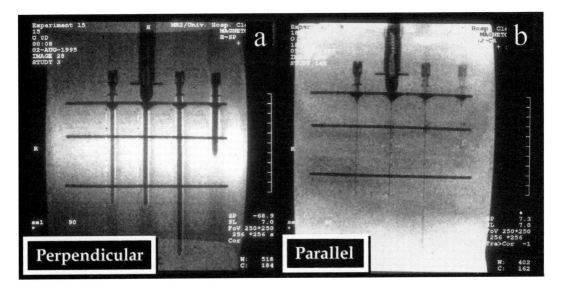

**Figure 17.9.** Effect of needle orientation relative to the main magnetic field ($B_0$) and its visualization. Spin-echo MRI of the same set of needles as in Figs. 17.7 and 17.8 obtained with needle shafts perpendicular (A) and parallel (B) to static magnetic field at 0.2 T. Note the marked reduction in artifactual needle widening when needles are parallel to static magnetic field. This effect can render smaller needles invisible during interventions. © 1996 The American Roentgen Society. Reprinted with permission. See reference 73.

Although the apparent needle width decreases as it is positioned parallel to the static magnetic field (vertically for most biplanar magnets and along the long axis of cylindrical or "double-doughnut" systems), artifact at the device tip blooms and obscures the true tip position. Steep needle trajectories may be more familiar or may appear advantageous in some anatomic locations but may be prohibited due to poor needle conspicuity and loss of tip position information.

### Safety Issues for the Use of Radiofrequency Energy

#### Adequate System Grounding

The deposition of high currents during RFA procedures can result in serious burns at the grounding pad site.[76] This is due to the fact that when RF current passes through its complete electric circuit, an equal amount of current is deposited at the return electrodes (grounding pads) as at the source electrode. Therefore, the amount of heat deposited at the grounding pads is actually equivalent to that used for "cooking the tumor" at the source electrode. Heating is maximal at the edges of the pads, particularly the leading edges facing the RF electrode.[77] To avoid serious burns at the grounding pad site, multiple large-surface-area foil pads should be placed on well-prepared skin and oriented

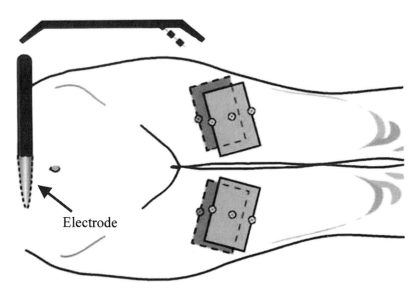

**Figure 17.10.** Proper placement of grounding pads for RF ablation. Schematic drawing depicts the placement of the grounding pads (gray rectangles) in relation to the RF electrode. To minimize grounding pad burn, multiple pads should be placed horizontally, with their long axis facing the electrode. This facilitates a more even distribution of heat dissipation minimizing untoward heating along the grounding pad surface. © 2001 Elsevier. Reprinted with permission. See reference 77.

with the longest surface edge facing the RF electrode[76] (Fig. 17.10).

### Adequate RF Current Deposition

The optimal outcome of an RFA session is creating a thermal lesion that covers the whole targeted tumor plus a rim of safety margin comparable to the 0.5- to 1-cm rim generally targeted during surgery. While undertreatment is an unacceptable outcome, overablation is also not free from risks. Injury of vital structures adjacent to the target tumor can complicate the treatment, and organs such as the gallbladder and biliary radicles as well as bowel loops are particularly sensitive to thermal injury.[77] Careful planning and image guidance, particularly with MRI in which the induced thermal lesion can be observed as it forms in near–real-time, are important in order to avoid such complications. In addition to the concern about collateral damage, it is also important when planning extensive ablations to consider whether sufficient organ function can be preserved and to be aware that large-volume tissue necrosis is associated with a higher incidence of infection and postablation syndrome. Keltner et al[78] reported a case of prolonged RF liver ablation for metastatic carcinoid tumor complicated by hemolysis, rhabdomyolysis, and transient acute renal failure.

## Financial Considerations

During the early period of interventional MRI, there was a debate over the cost-effectiveness of using such technology to guide procedures already being performed under the guidance of other more conventional, less expensive, and widely available imaging modalities. Compared to current ultrasound- and CT-guided procedures, MRI-guided interventions are slightly more expensive. (At our institution, the charges for an MRI-guided procedure are currently approximately 10% to 15% more than for a similar procedure performed under CT guidance.) Therefore, it is warranted, when the procedure is carried out for a diagnostic purpose, to use the most cost-effective choice of either ultrasound or CT unless there is a specific need for the higher soft tissue contrast or vascular conspicuity offered by MRI.

However, when thermal therapy is the issue, the unparalleled ability of MRI to detect residual untreated tumor foci during the ablation session outweighs the extra cost associated with the use of this technology. In fact, in many practices where thermal therapy is performed under ultrasound or CT guidance, the patient is ultimately transferred to the MRI scanner following ablation to confirm the extent of necrosis; this makes the cost of a conventionally guided procedure even higher.

Although the current availability of interventional MRI suites is limited to the academic setting, a growing number of radiology practices are expected to develop interventional MRI capability in the future. Open MRI systems are the fastest growing sector of the U.S. MRI market, and an increasing number of radiology practices have access to open units. Several vendors offer interventional accessories for less than $160,000, making the cost of performing percutaneous MRI-guided procedures relatively low for those sites with preexisting open MRI scanners.

Compared to the surgical approach, the use of MRI for RF-ITA procedure guidance is associated with tremendous cost reduction, from a decrease in the cost of the procedure itself relative to surgery to the equal or greater savings realized by avoiding both intensive care unit usage as well as routine hospitalization. This is in addition to the patient benefits resulting from the reduction in morbidity, mortality, postprocedure discomfort, and required recovery time when open surgical procedures can be avoided.[79]

## Current Research and Future Directions

The developed clinical expertise in image-guided RFA of tumors and the acknowledgment of the obvious advantages MRI offers in this setting (Table 17.1), have sparked researchers` interest to further investigate the full potential of this new technique of RFA. In this section, we broadly outline the current status of MRI-guided RFA in terms of recent and ongoing research efforts that are likely to have pertinent effects on this developing technique.

The feasibility and safety of RF-ITA on various body organs solely under MRI guidance have been investigated in animal models. Several reports have shown that the applicability of this technique extends beyond the results already achieved in the current clinically recognized applications. Encouraging results from pancreatic,[80] long bone,[81] vertebral,[82] and other organ ablations promise the expanding future of cancer treatment by taking advantage of the minimally invasive nature of RFA along with the superb value of MRI for guiding and monitoring therapy.

Developing the RF technology necessary to create larger thermal lesions with the least number of RF electrode insertions is another popular research topic that attempts to address an important existing limitation in the more widespread use of RF energy for tumor ablation. Overcoming this limitation is essential to reduce such risks as tumor seeding, bleeding, and infection. It is also important in order to reduce the procedure time and thus improve patient compliance, particularly when managing large tumors. Techniques already investigated include the use of multiple-probe RF electrode arrays[83] or internally cooled (cool tip) RF electrodes that prevent charring at the electrode/tissue interface, thereby allowing a higher maximum energy to be deposited into the tissue.[84,85] Cool-tip RF electrodes are already commercially available and are widely used in clinical practice. Other investigators have proposed the creation of larger thermal lesions through the reduction of the blood supply to an organ in order to reduce perfusion-mediated tissue cooling, that is, the "heat sink,"[86] or through direct intraparenchymal injection of hypertonic saline either as a bolus before or as continuous infusion during ablation to create a high local ion concentration in the tissue being treated.[87–89]

Parallel to these investigations, there has been ongoing research to justify the future utility of MRI in light of the developing technology of RF thermal treatment. It has been reported that MRI accurately guides and monitors the effect of reduced tissue perfusion on the induced thermal lesion size in both rabbit livers[90] and pig kidneys.[91] Previous work in our laboratory has also already demonstrated the feasibility of interactive MRI monitoring of intraparenchymally injected hypertonic saline in ex-vivo tissues[92]; we are currently investigating this finding in vivo and testing whether the alteration of local tissue biology by injection of hypertonic NaCl solution might affect the proven capability of MRI[26] to monitor a thermal lesion as it develops.

Another interesting subject related to our investigation of the validity of MRI as an excellent real-time predictor of tumor necrosis is the three-dimensional registration of thermal lesions as they appear on MRI compared to the real cellular damage seen histologically. Results have shown that the central hypointense region seen on T1, T2, and STIR images reliably corresponds to the area of actual cell death.[93] Further survival animal experiments are ongoing to address whether the cellular elements within the bright/enhancing rim marginating the thermal lesion also progress to complete necrosis.

Finally, the practice of RFA under MRI guidance is backed, as mentioned earlier, by extensive complementary MRI physics research primarily focusing on MRI pulse sequence development[72] and device tracking optimization. Interactive MRI scan plane definition for rigid interventional devices, such as RF electrodes, without the need for stereotactic cameras, is now possible using wireless, tuned fiducial markers mounted to the device[94] or by using real-time keyhole imaging that enables the interventionalist to orient the imaging slice position, slice orientation, and the axes' rotation within the slice and to view the newly oriented images as they are reconstructed with an ample temporal resolution of 4 images/sec.[95]

It is hoped that the integrated efforts of researchers working in these interrelated fields will converge in a state-of-the-art practice of the already established paradigms of MRI-guided and -monitored radiofrequency interstitial thermal tumor ablation. The implication of this will serve the ultimate goal of achieving a higher standard of care for cancer patients.

### Acknowledgments
The authors would like to acknowledge the members of the Interventional MR Imaging Research Program at the University Hospitals of Cleveland and Case Western Reserve University for their ongoing commitment to the development of interventional MRI techniques. We would like also to thank Bonnie Hami, M.A., for her invaluable editorial assistance.

### References

1. Allport JR, Weissleder R. In vivo imaging of gene and cell therapies. Exp Hematol 2001; 29(11):1237–1246.
2. Yang X, Atalar E, Li D, et al. Magnetic resonance imaging permits in vivo monitoring of catheter-based vascular gene delivery. Circulation 2001; 104(14):1588–1590.
3. Floeth FW, Aulich A, Langen KJ, Burger KJ, Bock WJ, Weber F. MR imaging and single-photon emission CT findings after gene therapy for human glioblastoma. AJNR 2001; 22(8):1517–1527.

 4. Guerquin-Kern JL, Volk A, Chenu E, et al. Direct in vivo observation of 5-fluorouracil release from a prodrug in human tumors heterotransplanted in nude mice: a magnetic resonance study. NMR Biomed 2000; 13(5):306–310.
 5. Calvo BF, Semelka RC. Beyond anatomy: MR imaging as a molecular diagnostic tool. Surg Oncol Clin North Am 1999; 8(1):171–183.
 6. Fuss M, Wenz F, Essig M, et al. Tumor angiogenesis of low-grade astrocytomas measured by dynamic susceptibility contrast-enhanced MRI (DSC-MRI) is predictive of local tumor control after radiation therapy. Int J Radiat Oncol Biol Phys 2001; 51(2):478–482.
 7. Eichler K, Mack MG, Straub R, et al. Oligonodular hepatocellular carcinoma (HCC): MR-controlled laser-induced thermotherapy. Radiologe 2001; 41(10):915–922.
 8. Huber PE, Jenne JW, Rastert R, et al. A new noninvasive approach in breast cancer therapy using magnetic resonance imaging-guided focused ultrasound surgery. Cancer Res 2001; 61(23):8441–8447.
 9. Chen JC, Moriarty JA, et al. Prostate cancer: MR imaging and thermometry during microwave thermal ablation—initial experience. Radiology 2000; 214(1):290–297.
10. Mala T, Edwin B, Samset E, et al. Magnetic-resonance-guided percutaneous cryoablation of hepatic tumours. Eur J Surg 2001; 167(8):610–617.
11. Pawlik TM, Tanabe KK. Radiofrequency ablation for primary and metastatic liver tumors. Cancer Treat Res 2001; 109:247–267.
12. Nicoli N, Casaril A, Marchiori L, Mangiante G, Hasheminia AR. Treatment of recurrent hepatocellular carcinoma by radiofrequency thermal ablation. J Hepatobiliary Pancreat Surg 2001; 8(5):417–421.
13. Buscarini L, Buscarini E, Di Stasi M, Vallisa D, Quaretti P, Rocca A. Percutaneous radiofrequency ablation of small hepatocellular carcinoma: long-term results. Eur Radiol 2001; 11(6):914–921.
14. Anzai Y, Lufkin R, DeSalles A, Hamilton DR, Farahani K, Black KL. Preliminary experience with MR-guided thermal ablation of brain tumors. AJNR 1995; 16(1):39–48; discussion 49–52.
15. Lewin JS, Connell CF, Duerk JL, Nour SG, Resnick MI, Haaga JR. A phase II clinical trial of interactive MR-guided interstitial radiofrequency thermal ablation of primary kidney tumors: preliminary results. Chicago: Proceedings of the Radiological Society of North America (RSNA) 87th Scientific Meeting, 2001:261.
16. Pavlovich CP, Walther MM, Choyke PL, et al. Percutaneous radio frequency ablation of small renal tumors: initial results. J Urol 2002; 167(1):10–15.
17. Syed AH, Stewart LH, Hargreave TB. Day-case local anaesthetic radiofrequency thermal ablation of benign prostatic hyperplasia: a four-year follow-up. Scand J Urol Nephrol 2000; 34(5):309–312.
18. Zlotta AR, Djavan B, Matos C, et al. Percutaneous transperineal radiofrequency ablation of prostate tumour: safety, feasibility and pathological effects on human prostate cancer. Br J Urol 1998; 81(2):265–275.
19. Izzo F, Thomas R, Delrio P, et al. Radiofrequency ablation in patients with primary breast carcinoma: a pilot study in 26 patients. Cancer 2001; 92(8):2036–2044.

20. Wood BJ, Bates S. Radiofrequency thermal ablation of a splenic metastasis. J Vasc Intervent Radiol 2001; 12(2):261–263.
21. Dupuy DE, Zagoria RJ, Akerley W, Mayo-Smith WW, Kavanagh PV, Safran H. Percutaneous radiofrequency ablation of malignancies in the lung. AJR 2000; 174(1):57–59.
22. Rosenthal DI, Hornicek FJ, Wolfe MW, Jennings LC, Gebhardt MC, Mankin HJ. Percutaneous radiofrequency coagulation of osteoid osteoma compared with operative treatment. J Bone Joint Surg 1998; 80(6):815–821.
23. Zervas NT, Kuwayama A. Pathological characteristics of experimental thermal lesions. Comparison of induction heating and radiofrequency electrocoagulation. J Neurosurg 1972; 37(4):418–422.
24. Farahani K, Mischel PS, Black KL, De Salles AA, Anzai Y, Lufkin RB. Hyperacute thermal lesions: MR imaging evaluation of development in the brain. Radiology 1995; 196(2):517–520.
25. Rossi S, Di Stasi M, Buscarini E, et al. Percutaneous RF interstitial thermal ablation in the treatment of hepatic cancer. AJR 1996; 167(3):759–768.
26. Lewin JS, Connell CF, Duerk JL, et al. Interactive MRI-guided radiofrequency interstitial thermal ablation of abdominal tumors: clinical trial for evaluation of safety and feasibility. J Magn Reson Imaging 1998; 8(1):40–47.
27. Aronow S. The use of radio-frequency power in making lesions in the brain. J Neurosurg 1960; 17:431 438.
28. Zervas NT. Eccentric radio-frequency lesions. Confin Neurol 1965; 26(3):143–145.
29. Chung YC, Duerk JL, Lewin JS. Generation and observation of radio frequency thermal lesion ablation for interventional magnetic resonance imaging. Invest Radiol 1997; 32(8):466–474.
30. Sweet WH, Mark VH, Hamlin H. Radiofrequency lesions in the central nervous system of man and cat: including case reports of eight bulbar pain-tract interruptions. J Neurosurg 1960; 17:213–225.
31. Tew JM, Keller JT. The treatment of trigeminal neuralgia by percutaneous radiofrequency technique. In: Keener EB, ed. Clinical Neurosurgery. Baltimore: Williams & Wilkins, 1977: 557–578.
32. Siegfried J. 500 percutaneous thermocoagulations of the gasserian ganglion for trigeminal pain. Surg Neurol 1977; 8(2):126–131.
33. Hitchcock ER, Teixeira MJ. A comparison of results from center-median and basal thalamotomies for pain. Surg Neurol 1981; 15(5):341–351.
34. Broggi G, Franzini A, Giorgi C, et al. Radiofrequency percutaneous trigeminal rhizotomy. Considerations in 1000 consecutive cases of essential trigeminal neuralgia. J Neurosurg Sci 1985; 29:165.
35. Laitinen LV, Bergenheim AT, Hariz MI. Leksell's posteroventral pallidotomy in the treatment of Parkinson's disease. J Neurosurg 1992; 76(1):53–61.
36. Rosomoff HL, Brown CJ, Sheptak P. Percutaneous radiofrequency cervical cordotomy: technique. J Neurosurg 1965; 23(6):639–644.
37. Nashold BS Jr, Ostdahl RH. Dorsal root entry zone lesions for pain relief. J Neurosurg 1979; 51(1):59–69.

38. Huang SK. Radio-frequency catheter ablation of cardiac arrhythmias: appraisal of an evolving therapeutic modality. Am Heart J 1989; 118(6):1317–1323.

39. Soejima K, Suzuki M, Maisel WH, et al. Catheter ablation in patients with multiple and unstable ventricular tachycardias after myocardial infarction: short ablation lines guided by reentry circuit isthmuses and sinus rhythm mapping. Circulation 2001; 104(6):664–669.

40. Elias D, Debaere T, Muttillo I, Cavalcanti A, Coyle C, Roche A. Intraoperative use of radiofrequency treatment allows an increase in the rate of curative liver resection. J Surg Oncol 1998; 67(3):190–191.

41. Yohannes P, Pinto P, Rotariu P, Smith AD, Lee BR. Retroperitoneoscopic radiofrequency ablation of a solid renal mass. J Endourol 2001; 15(8):845–849.

42. Schenck JF, Jolesz FA, Roemer PB, et al. Superconducting open-configuration MR imaging system for image-guided therapy. Radiology 1995; 195(3):805–814.

43. Cline HE, Schenck JF, Watkins RD, Hynynen K, Jolesz FA. Magnetic resonance-guided thermal surgery. Magn Reson Med 1993; 30(1):98–106.

44. Cline HE, Hynynen K, Watkins RD, et al. Focused US system for MR imaging-guided tumor ablation. Radiology 1995; 194(3):731–737.

45. Lewin JS, Nour SG, Duerk JL. Magnetic resonance image-guided biopsy and aspiration. Top Magn Reson Imaging 2000; 11(3):173–183.

46. Lufkin R, Teresi L, Hanafee W. New needle for MR-guided aspiration cytology of the head and neck. AJR 1987; 149(2):380–382.

47. Lufkin R, Duckwiler G, Spickler E, Teresi L, Chang M, Onik G. MR body stereotaxis: an aid for MR-guided biopsies. J Comput Assist Tomogr 1988; 12(6):1088–1089.

48. Kaufman L, Arakawa M, Hale J, et al. Accessible magnetic resonance imaging. Magn Reson Q 1989; 5(4):283–297.

49. Gronemeyer DH, Kaufman L, Rothschild P, Seibel RM. New possibilities and aspects of low-field magnetic resonance tomography. Radiol Diagn (Berl) 1989; 30(4):519–527.

50. Lewin JS. Interventional MR imaging: concepts, systems, and applications in neuroradiology. AJNR 1999; 20(5):735–748.

51. Gehl HB, Frahm C, Schimmelpenning H, Weiss HD. A technic of MRT-guided abdominal drainage with an open low-field magnet. Its feasibility and the initial results. Rofo Fortschr Geb Rontgenstr Neuen Bildgeb Verfahr 1996; 165(1):70–73.

52. Lewin JS, Petersilge CA, Hatem SF, et al. Interactive MR imaging-guided biopsy and aspiration with a modified clinical C-arm system. AJR 1998; 170(6):1593–1601.

53. Silverman SG, Collick BD, Figueira MR, et al. Interactive MR-guided biopsy in an open-configuration MR imaging system. Radiology 1995; 197(1):175–181.

54. Lee MH, Lufkin RB, Borges A, et al. MR-guided procedures using contemporaneous imaging frameless stereotaxis in an open-configuration system. J Comput Assist Tomogr 1998; 22(6):998–1005.

55. Lufkin R, Teresi L, Chiu L, Hanafee W. A technique for MR-guided needle placement. AJR 1988; 151(1):193–196.

56. Mahfouz AE, Rahmouni A, Zylbersztejn C, Mathieu D. MR-guided biopsy using ultrafast T1- and T2-weighted reordered turbo fast low-angle shot sequences: feasibility and preliminary clinical applications. AJR 1996; 167(1):167–169.

57. Duerk JL, Lewin JS, Wendt M, Petersilge C. Remember true FISP? A high SNR, near 1-second imaging method for T2-like contrast in interventional MRI at .2 T. J Magn Reson Imaging 1998; 8(1):203–208.

58. Chung YC, Merkle EM, Lewin JS, Shonk JR, Duerk JL. Fast T(2)-weighted imaging by PSIF at 0.2 T for interventional MRI. Magn Reson Med 1999; 42(2):335–344.

59. Zhang Q, Chung YC, Lewin JS, Duerk JL. A method for simultaneous RF ablation and MRI. J Magn Reson Imaging 1998; 8(1):110–114.

60. McGahan JP, Schneider P, Brock JM, et al. Treatment of liver tumors by percutaneous radiofrequency electrocautery. Semin Intervent Radiol 1993; 10:143–149.

61. Vogl TJ, Muller PK, Hammerstingl R, et al. Malignant liver tumors treated with MR imaging-guided laser-induced thermotherapy: technique and prospective results. Radiology 1995; 196(1):257–265.

62. Chung YC, Duerk JL, Shankaranarayanan A, Hampke M, Merkle EM, Lewin JS. Temperature measurement using echo-shifted FLASH at low field for interventional MRI. J Magn Reson Imaging 1999; 9(1):138 145.

63. Botnar RM, Steiner P, Dubno B, Erhart P, von Schulthess GK, Debatin JF. Temperature quantification using the proton frequency shift technique: in vitro and in vivo validation in an open 0.5 tesla interventional MR scanner during RF ablation. J Magn Reson Imaging 2001; 13(3):437–444.

64. Matsumoto R, Oshio K, Jolesz FA. Monitoring of laser and freezing-induced ablation in the liver with T1-weighted MR imaging. J Magn Reson Imaging 1992; 2(5):555–562.

65. Bleier AR, Jolesz FA, Cohen MS, et al. Real-time magnetic resonance imaging of laser heat deposition in tissue. Magn Reson Med. 1991; 21(1):132–137.

66. Anzai Y, Lufkin RB, Hirschowitz S, Farahani K, Castro DJ. MR imaging-histopathologic correlation of thermal injuries induced with interstitial Nd:YAG laser irradiation in the chronic model. J Magn Reson Imaging 1992; 2(6):671–678.

67. Matsumoto R, Selig AM, Colucci VM, Jolesz FA. MR monitoring during cryotherapy in the liver: predictability of histologic outcome. J Magn Reson Imaging 1993; 3(5):770–776.

68. Tracz RA, Wyman DR, Little PB, et al. Comparison of magnetic resonance images and the histopathological findings of lesions induced by interstitial laser photocoagulation in the brain. Lasers Surg Med 1993; 13(1):45–54.

69. Dempsey MF, Condon B, Hadley DM. Investigation of the factors responsible for burns during MRI. J Magn Reson Imaging 2001; 13(4):627–631.

70. Dempsey MF, Condon B. Thermal injuries associated with MRI. Clin Radiol 2001; 56(6):457–465.

71. Nitz WR, Oppelt A, Renz W, Manke C, Lenhart M, Link J. On the heating of linear conductive structures as guide wires and catheters in interventional MRI. J Magn Reson Imaging 2001; 13(1):105–114.

72. Duerk JL, Butts K, Hwang KP, Lewin JS. Pulse sequences for interventional magnetic resonance imaging. Top Magn Reson Imaging 2000; 11(3):147–162.

73. Lewin JS, Duerk JL, Jain VR, Petersilge CA, Chao CP, Haaga JR. Needle localization in MR-guided biopsy and aspiration: effects of field strength, sequence design, and magnetic field orientation. AJR 1996; 166(6):1337–1345.

74. Frahm C, Gehl HB, Melchert UH, Weiss HD. Visualization of magnetic resonance-compatible needles at 1.5 and 0.2 Tesla. Cardiovasc Intervent Radiol 1996; 19(5):335–340.

75. Mueller PR, Stark DD, Simeone JF. MR-guided aspiration biopsy: needle design and clinical trials. Radiology 1986; 161(3):605–609.

76. Goldberg SN, Solbiati L, Halpern EF, Gazelle GS. Variables affecting proper system grounding for radiofrequency ablation in an animal model. J Vasc Intervent Radiol 2000; 11(8):1069–1075.

77. Goldberg SN. Radiofrequency tumor ablation: principles and techniques. Eur J Ultrasound 2001; 13(2):129–147.

78. Keltner JR, Donegan E, Hynson JM, Shapiro WA. Acute renal failure after radiofrequency liver ablation of metastatic carcinoid tumor. Anesth Analg 2001; 93(3):587–589.

79. Lewin JS. MR guides intervention and keeps costs down. Diagn Imaging (San Franc). 1998; suppl open MRI:MR22–24.

80. Merkle EM, Haaga JR, Duerk JL, Jacobs GH, Brambs HJ, Lewin JS. MR imaging-guided radio-frequency thermal ablation in the pancreas in a porcine model with a modified clinical C-arm system. Radiology 1999; 213(2):461–467.

81. Aschoff AJ, Merkle EM, Emancipator SN, Petersilge CA, Duerk JL, Lewin JS. Femur: MR imaging-guided radio-frequency ablation in a porcine model-feasibility study. Radiology 2002; 225(2):471–478.

82. Nour SG, Aschoff AJ, Mitchell IC, Emancipator SN, Duerk JL, Lewin JS. MR-guided radiofrequency (RF) thermal ablation of the lumbar vertebrae in a porcine model. Radiology 2002; 224(2):452–462.

83. Goldberg SN, Gazelle GS, Dawson SL, Rittman WJ, Mueller PR, Rosenthal DI. Tissue ablation with radiofrequency using multiprobe arrays. Acad Radiol 1995; 2(8):670–674.

84. Goldberg SN, Gazelle GS, Solbiati L, Rittman WJ, Mueller PR. Radiofrequency tissue ablation: increased lesion diameter with a perfusion electrode. Acad Radiol 1996; 3(8):636–644.

85. Lorentzen T. A cooled needle electrode for radiofrequency tissue ablation: thermodynamic aspects of improved performance compared with conventional needle design. Acad Radiol 1996; 3(7):556–563.

86. Goldberg SN, Hahn PF, Tanabe KK, et al. Percutaneous radiofrequency tissue ablation: does perfusion-mediated tissue cooling limit coagulation necrosis? J Vasc Intervent Radiol 1998; 9(1 pt 1):101–111.

87. Livraghi T, Goldberg SN, Monti F, et al. Saline-enhanced radiofrequency tissue ablation in the treatment of liver metastases. Radiology 1997; 202(1):205–210.

88. Goldberg SN, Ahmed M, Gazelle GS, et al. Radio-frequency thermal ablation with NaCl solution injection: effect of electrical conductivity on tissue heating and coagulation—phantom and porcine liver study. Radiology 2001; 219(1):157–165.
89. Miao Y, Ni Y, Mulier S, et al. Ex vivo experiment on radiofrequency liver ablation with saline infusion through a screw-tip cannulated electrode. J Surg Res 1997; 71(1):19–24.
90. Aschoff AJ, Merkle EM, Wong V, et al. How does alteration of hepatic blood flow affect liver perfusion and radiofrequency-induced thermal lesion size in rabbit liver? J Magn Reson Imaging 2001; 13(1):57–63.
91. Aschoff AJ, Sulman A, Martinez M, et al. Perfusion-modulated MR imaging-guided radiofrequency ablation of the kidney in a porcine model. AJR 2001; 177(1):151–158.
92. Nour SG, Lewin JS, Duerk JL. Saline injection in ex-vivo liver: monitoring with fast gradient echo sequences at 0.2T. Glasgow, Scotland: Proceedings of the International Society for Magnetic Resonance in Medicine (ISMRM) 9th Scientific Meeting, 2001.
93. Breen MS, Lancaster TL, Lazebnik RL, et al. Three dimensional correlation of MR images to muscle tissue response for interventional MRI thermal ablation. In: Proceedings of SPIE Medical Imaging 2001: visualization, display, and image-guided procedures, vol 4319. Bellingham, WA: SPIE, 2001: 211–220.
94. Flask C, Elgort D, Wong E, et al. A method for fast 3D tracking using tuned fiducial markers and a limited projection reconstruction FISP (LPR-FISP) sequence. J Magn Reson Imaging 2001; 14(5):617–627.
95. Hwang K-P, Hillenbrand C, Shankaranarayanan A, et al. Interactive scan plane adjustment for real-time keyhole imaging. Proceedings of the ISMRM workshop on minimum MR data acquisition methods, October 2001, pp. 106–108.

# Index